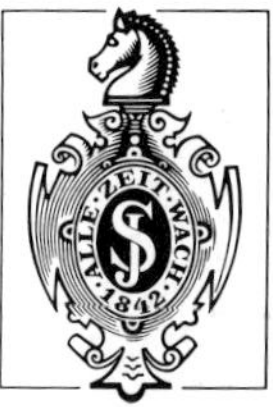

Y. Higashi   A. Mizushima   H. Matsumoto

Introduction to Abdominal Ultrasonography

With Forewords by
M.L. Skolnick and W.J. Russel

With 471 Figures in 950 Separate Illustrations

Springer-Verlag
Berlin Heidelberg New York
London Paris Tokyo
Hong Kong Barcelona
Budapest

Yoshitaka Higashi, MD
Department of Radiology
Fukuoka University
7-45-1 Nanakuma, Jonan-Ku
Fukuoka 814, Japan

Akira Mizushima, MD
Department of Radiology
Kyushu University
3-1-1 Maidashi, Higashi-Ku
Fukuoka 812, Japan

Hirotsugu Matsumoto, MD
Department of Surgery
Chubu Hospital
208-3 Aza Miyazato, Gushikawa-city
Okinawa 904-22, Japan

ISBN 3-540-51889-4 Springer-Verlag Berlin Heidelberg New York
ISBN 0-387-51889-4 Springer-Verlag New York Berlin Heidelberg

Library of Congress Cataloging-in-Publication Data
Higashi, Yoshitaka, [Fukubu ekō nyūmon. English] Introduction to abdominal ultrasonography / Y. Higashi,
A. Mizushima, H. Matsumoto. p. cm. Rev. and expanded translation of: Fukubu ekō nyūmon.
ISBN 3-540-51889-4 (alk. paper). –
ISBN 0-387-51889-4 (alk. paper)
1. Abdomen–Ultrasonic imaging. I. Mizushima, A. (Akira), 1955– . II. Matsumoto, H. (Hirotsugu), 1949– .
III. Title. [DNLM: 1. Abdomen–pathology. 2. Ultrasonography. WI 900 H634f] RC944.H5413 1991
617.5′507543–dc20 DNLM/DLC for Library of Congress 90-10459 CIP

The use of general descriptive names, registered names, trademarks, etc. in this publication, does not imply, even in
the absence of a specific statement, that such names are exempt from the relevant protective laws and regulations and
therefore free for general use.

Product Liability: The publisher can give no guarantee for information about drug dosage and application thereof
contained in this book. In every individual case the respective user must check its accuracy by consulting other
pharmaceutical literature.

Typesetting, printing and binding: Triltsch, Würzburg
21/3145-543210 – Printed on acid-free paper

Foreword

Ultrasound is unlike any other cross-sectional imaging modality. In CT and MRI, serial cross-sectional images are obtained in predetermined planes by a technologist and the images are then interpreted by a physician. The ultrasound study is an interactive procedure tailored to evaluating the patient's specific clinical problem. The person performing the examination is essentially interpreting the study as it is being done. One should appreciate that the study is more than just an examination of the requested regional anatomy. Depending upon the initial ultrasound findings and the patient's history, one may wish to image adjacent or even more remote regions to clarify or expand upon initial imaging findings.

The images produced by an ultrasound scanner display a small cross-sectional region of anatomy in real time. To appreciate the total anatomy of the region, the operator must scan through a volume of tissue, while mentally integrating images of the multiple small fields of view. A limited number of still images are recorded only to document specific normal or abnormal structures (assuming that the entire study is not videotaped for subsequent review). What the operator fails to image, or images but fails to record is lost forever. Thus, the diagnostic quality of the ultrasound examination is very dependent upon the skill of the examiner.

The demands upon the examiner are great, and greater than in any other cross-sectional imaging study. One must have an intimate knowledge of the regional anatomy so as to choose the optimal plane to display specific normal or pathologic anatomy. One must also appreciate the physics of ultrasound and its effects upon image formation so as to recognize the anatomic distortions that can occur from improper instrument settings or unavoidable artifacts of scanning.

The essence of teaching is effective communication of information from teacher to student. Drs. Higashi, Mizushima, and Matsumoto use graphics, well labeled images, and concise text to clearly convey to the reader a basic understanding of ultrasound physics, of normal anatomy in the upper abdomen, and of a variety of pathologic conditions as displayed by ultrasound, and as correlated with gross anatomy. The responsibility of the sonographer is very great; he or she must therefore be well trained. This book provides an effective beginning.

Pittsburgh, March 1991   M. Leon Skolnick, MD

Foreword

It has been my pleasure to work with Yoshitaka Higashi and Akira Mizushima for nearly a decade. Higashi's true artistry in composing ultrasonograms is vivid and stimulating to observe. The commentaries he provides examining patients serve to guide students and medical specialists alike through normal and abnormal anatomical structures. Higashi has contributed heavily to educating medical students and resident physicians, and to helping compile the examinations of the Japanese Board of Radiology. For years, he has been an active consultant to manufacturers, striving to improve ultrasonographic apparatus.

Publication of this text brings to mind many improvements I have witnessed in Japanese radiology – toward its achieving the status of a true medical specialty. During these years I have had the privilege of assisting a large number of Japanese doctors preparing for training in one of the outstanding US radiology residency and fellowship programs. All of them have enviable "track records" and are now teachers and leaders in the development of diagnostic radiology in Japan. Currently, six of this group are professors, five being the chairman of the radiology departments at reputable Japanese universities.

Among the effective means strengthening the bonds between American and Japanese radiologists are the examinations of the Japanese Board of Radiology, which began in 1970; the increasing exchange of information among radiologists participating in Japanese and American radiological meetings during the past two decades; and the more recent efforts of the Japanese Radiological Society and the Association of American University Radiologists.

With increasing frequency, Japanese radiologists are publishing their scientific reports in English in American and European journals. Their publications, which hitherto often appeared only in Japanese, are now being widely read in English.

In the past, the preponderance in the overall flow of ideas and achievements in diagnostic radiology favored American radiology. As a consequence of the above developments, this flow can hopefully achieve a better balance. I sincerely hope that this authoritative text on ultrasonography will be an additional milestone in promoting increased dialogue between Japanese and American colleagues in radiology.

Mercer Island, Washington, March 1991   Walter J. Russel, MD, DMSc, FACR

Preface

This textbook is intended for medical students, residents in diagnostic radiology, and ultrasonologists who have just begun detailed studies in ultrasound diagnosis. One of the book's distinguishing features are the clear schematic drawings designed to facilitate the reader's understanding of ultrasonographic images. These illustrations are the work of Yuichi Kuramoto, M.D., whose expertise in ultrasound diagnosis is strongly reflected in their quality.

Unlike other imaging modalities, such as computed tomography, angiography, upper gastrointestinal series, and magnetic resonance imaging, the moving images observable during ultrasound examination provide much more information then those frozen on films or photographs. Thus, three-dimensional anatomy is much more easily understood during the examination than afterwards. However, textbooks in which only static images can be included, are very limited. To compensate for this, three-dimensional presentations of anatomy, such as the ultrasonographically imaged tubular structures in the liver, are supplemented with numerous multicolored schemata.

In the United States and other Western countries, there are many well-trained, experienced ultrasound technicians; consequently, some radiologists make their diagnosis only on the basis of "frozen" images which technicians have recorded on film. However, we believe that radiologists' active participation in scanning and in recording the images enhances the quality and diagnostic accuracy. For this reason, the scanning techniques are carefully discussed from the standpoint of both the technician and the radiologist-in-training.

The clinical discussions are brief and clear. Vivid ultrasonographic images were carefully selected so as to clearly convey the characteristic features of each disease entity.

This is a revised and expanded English version of a very popular textbook which was originally published in Japanese by the Shujunsha Co., LTD in June 1986.

Fukuoka and Okinawa, February 1991

Y. Higashi, MD
A. Mizushima, MD
H. Matsumoto, MD

Acknowledgements

We gratefully acknowledge the assistance of Drs. Takafumi Koganemaru, Tsunako Sata, Michiyo Oku, Ritsuko Fujimitsu, Kazuaki Kido, and Kyoko Hayashida of the Department of Radiology, and Drs. Keiko Matsumoto, Seiko Kumagai, Shusuke Nii, Yasuko Ichioka, Kazuhiro Fujimitsu, Hideaki Tanaka, Yoshiyuki Nishioka, and Tomoe Urabe of the Department of Health Care of Fukuoka University School of Medicine, without whose help this book could not have been completed.
We also thank Dr. Yuichi Kuramoto of the Department of Health Care of Fukuoka University for his high quality illustrations, Dr. David Paushter of the Cleveland Clinic Foundation for providing the examples of renal transplantation, and Dr. Ellen Abeln of the Cleveland Clinic Foundation for her advice and assistance in preparing the English manuscript.
Special thanks goes to Dr. Walter J. Russell of the Radiation Effects Research Foundation, who has continually encouraged us to publish this book in English.

Fukuoka and Okinawa, February 1991

Y. Higashi, MD
A. Mizushima, MD
H. Matsumoto, MD

Contents

1 Principles of Ultrasound

What Is Ultrasound?

The normal range of sound that human beings can perceive is 20–20 000 Hz. A sound wave with a frequency higher than 20 000 Hz is called ultrasound. The ultrasound used in abdominal imaging has a frequency of 3.5 or 5 MHz (1 MHz $= 10^6$ Hz). Ultrasound of such high frequency is barely transmitted in air but is transmitted well in solid or fluid materials (Fig. 1.1). In the human body, ultrasound is transmitted well in the abdominal organs and soft tissues but is not transmitted in air-containing organs such as the lungs or the gastrointestinal tract. Since bones do not transmit ultrasound, organs surrounded by bones cannot be examined.

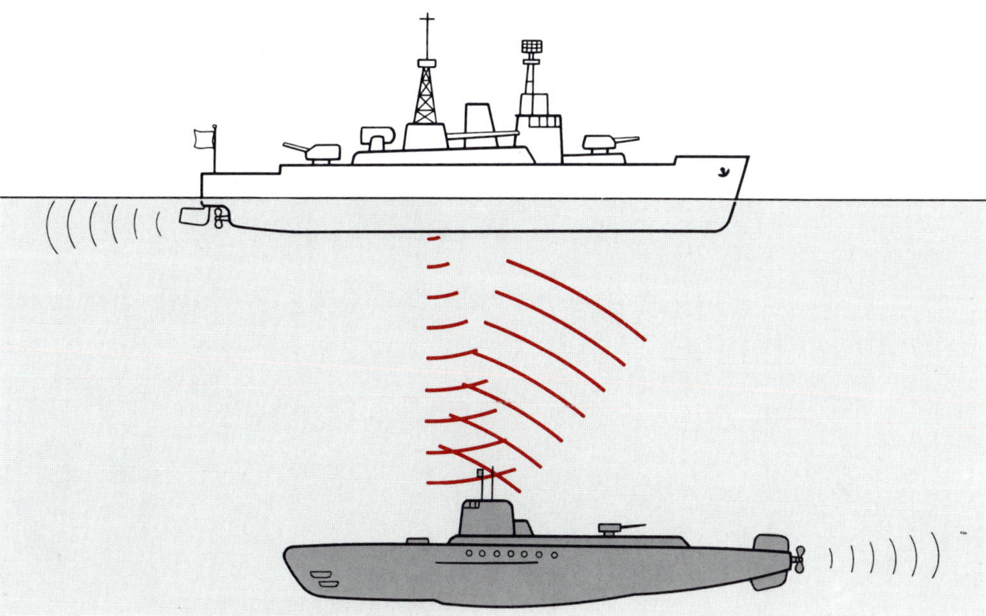

Fig. 1.1. Sonar, an application of ultrasound

Production of Ultrasound

Figure 1.2 illustrates what happens when electrical current is applied to each side of a piece of quartz coated with silver. The quartz expands or contracts from its original thickness, depending on the polarity of the current applied. This phenomenon is called the piezoelectric effect, and a substance with this property is called a piezoelectric element. Ultrasonographic transducers are made of ceramic materials, commonly lead zirconate titanate. Newer piezoelectric elements are also being developed.

When alternating current is applied to each surface of the piezoelectric element, ultrasound is produced, vibrating at a stable frequency determined by the thickness of the element (also called the resonant frequency). When the piezoelectric element is physically compressed by externally applied ultrasound, it produces a current. Hence, the piezoelectric element serves a dual function as both transmitter and receiver.

The part of the ultrasonographic equipment which transmits and receives ultrasound on the skin surface of the patient is called the transducer head. The piezoelectric element is located near the surface of the transducer head and is coated with a water-tight, insulated cover.

In the transducer head of a contact compound scanner, there is only one round crystal element of 10–20 mm in diameter, whereas the linear electronic scanner is composed of multiple thin rectangular crystals lined up side by side (Fig. 1.3).

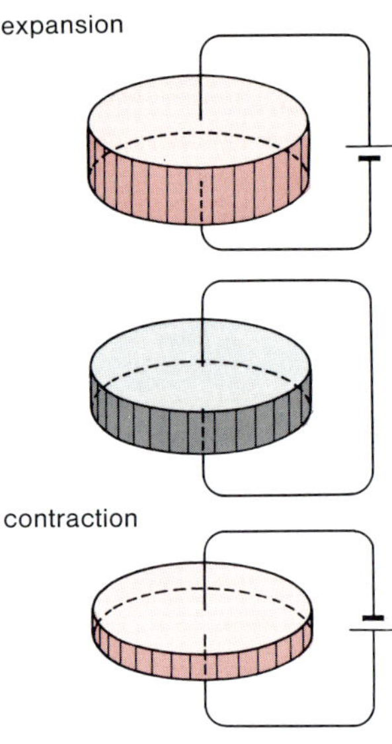

Fig. 1.2. *Piezoelectric effect.* A piezoelectric element changes its thickness when an electric current is applied

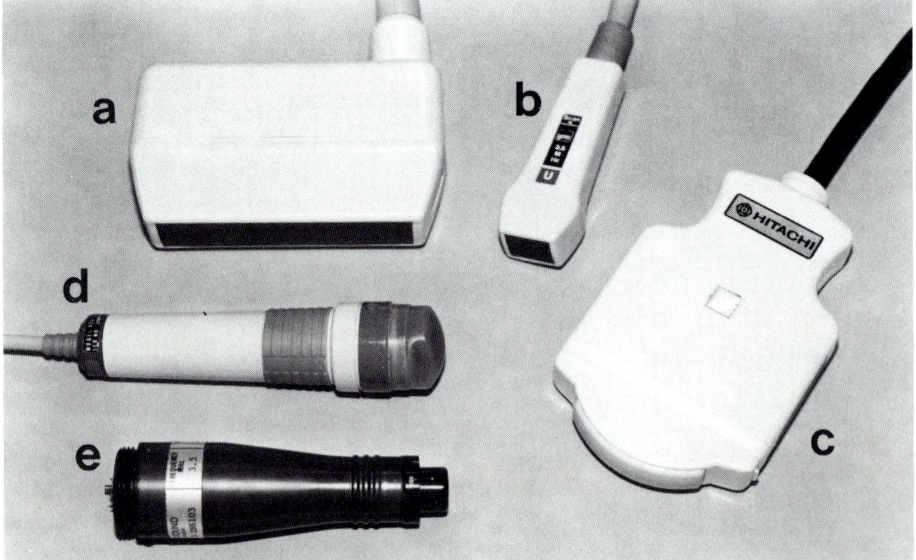

Fig. 1.3. *Various types of transducer heads:* a, linear electronic (linear array); b, electronic sector (phased array); c, convex electronic (curved linear array); d, mechanical sector; e, contact compound

Properties of Ultrasound

Transmission of Ultrasound

The velocity of ultrasound in most soft tissues is close to 1540 m/s. As it is transmitted, the intensity of the ultrasound beam is decreased by absorption, reflection, and scatter. Tissue absorption increases with the increasing frequency of the ultrasound beam. Ultrasound is transmitted well in fluids such as urine, bile, blood, ascites, pleural infusion, or cyst contents, with little loss in intensity.

Reflection, Refraction, and Scatter

When the ultrasound beam passes from a tissue of one acoustic impedance to a tissue of different acoustic impedance, a portion of the beam is reflected. Reflection requires a smooth surface which is larger than the wave length of the beam. When the beam encounters an interface that is irregular or smaller than the ultrasound beam, the beam is scattered in all directions. Only the portion of the scattered beam which comes back to the probe contributes to the ultrasonographic image. The contour of the tissue or organ being scanned is determined by reflection, whereas the inner echo pattern is primarily determined by scatter.

Refraction is the bending of the ultrasound beam when it crosses the interface of tissues of different acoustic impedance at an oblique angle.

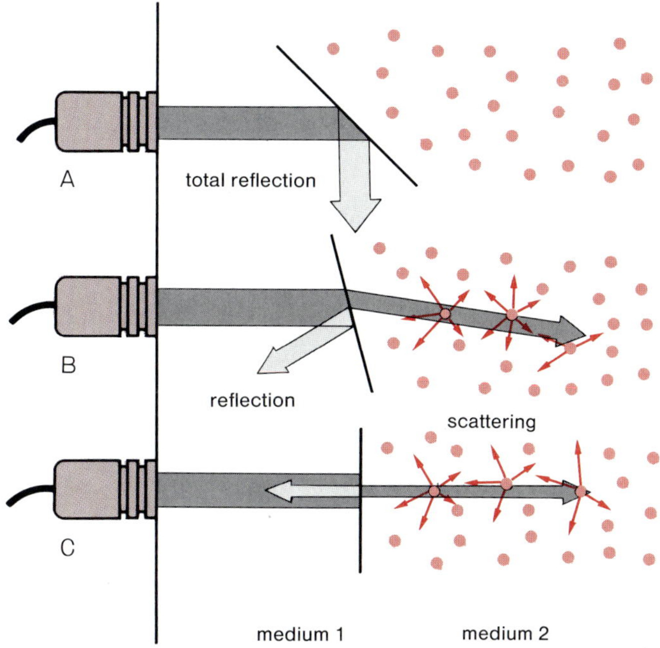

Fig. 1.4 A–C. *Reflection, scatter, and refraction of ultrasound.* **A** When the angle of incidence is larger than a certain critical angle, the entire beam is reflected. **B** A portion of ultrasound beam is reflected, and the remainder is refracted and continues on. The transmitted beam is partially scattered. **C** When the beam is perpendicular to the interface, most of the reflected beam comes back to the transducer, yielding a strong signal

Focus

A transducer with a flat face produces an ultrasound beam of the same width as the diameter of the face. The beam then diverges in the far field after traveling a certain distance. Using a transducer with a concave face, the ultrasound beam is focused in its focal zone and diverges beyond the focal zone (Fig. 1.5). A second way to focus a transducer is to place an acoustic lens in front of the piezoelectric crystal. The distance from the transducer face to the focal zone is called the focal length.

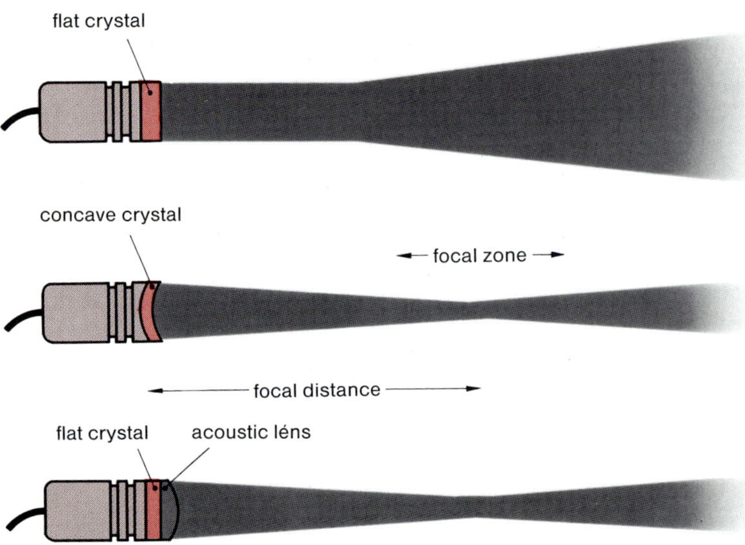

Fig. 1.5. *Focusing the ultrasound beam.* A concave face on the transducer or an acoustic lens can be used to focus sound. An acoustic lens is used in linear scanners

Resolution

Resolution refers to the ability to separate two small objects which are placed close together (Fig. 1.6). There are two types of ultrasound resolution:

1. Axial resolution is the ability to separate two objects along the path of the beam. Principles of physics state that axial resolution will be half the pulse length. However, there are several waves in a single pulse, and, therefore, in practice axial resolution is approximately 1 mm at the typically used frequency of 3.5 MHz.
2. Lateral resolution is the ability to separate two objects in a plane perpendicular to the beam. The narrower the ultrasound beam is, the better the lateral resolution becomes. Lateral resolution is best at a distance equal to the focal length.

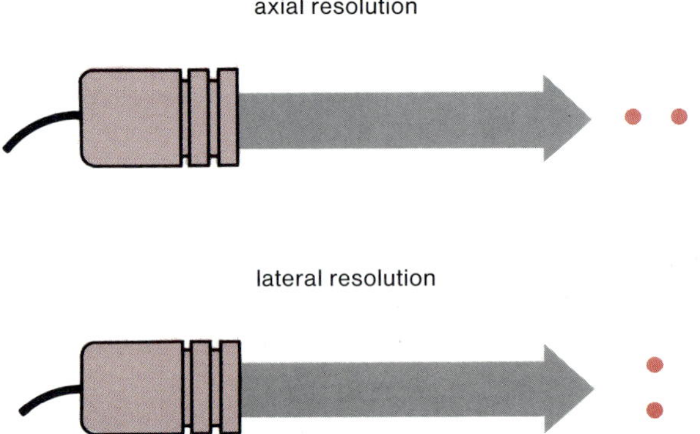

Fig. 1.6. *Resolution.* Resolution is the minimal distance at which two closely spaced reflectors can be distinguished as separate

Production of Ultrasonographic Images

The mechanics of a fish detector device can be used to illustrate the production of ultrasonographic images (Fig. 1.7). The ultrasound beam transmitted from the fishing boat at location *a* is reflected from the sea bed and returns to the detector. On the monitor, a spot of light indicates the depth of the sea. This depth is calculated as the product of half the transmit time and the velocity (ultrasound velocity in water is approximately 1500 m/s). If there is a school of fish in the path, ultrasound will be reflected from it, and therefore the presence and depth of the fish can be determined as well.

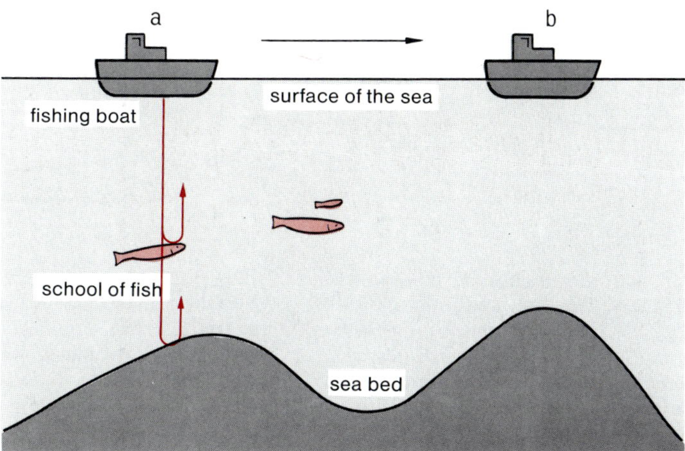

Fig. 1.7. *Mechanics of a fish detector.* The ultrasound beam emitted from the boat at point *a* provides depth information from immediately below point *a*. Continuous detection of the reflected beam as the boat moves toward point *b* delineates the topography of the sea bed and locates the school of fish

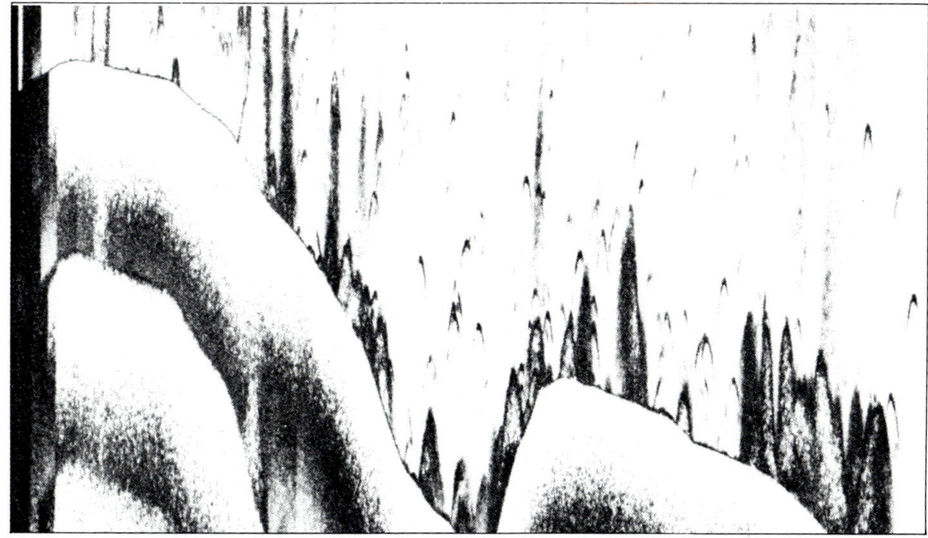

Fig. 1.8. *An image on a fish detector screen.* The sea bed appears to have two layers due to reverberation artifact. The shallower structure is the actual sea bed. Multiple small echoes in the water represent schools of fish

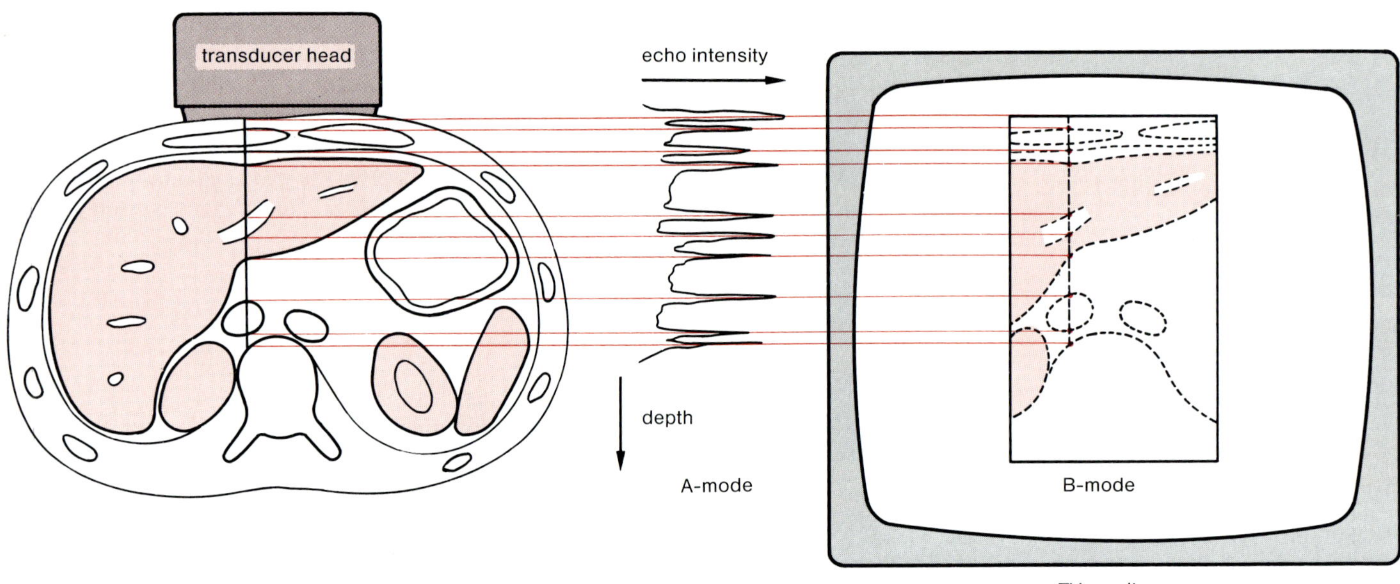

Fig. 1.9. *A-mode and B-mode*. In A-mode (amplitude mode), echo intensity is proportional to spike height. The distance (time) is usually on the *x*-axis, although on this figure it is on the *y*-axis for illustrative purposes. In B-mode (brightness mode), echo intensity is displayed as brightness on the monitor. A B-mode display obtained from a single static transducer cannot reproduce a slice of tissue, just as a stationary fishing boat cannot visualize the topography of the sea bed (Fig. 1.7). When the transducer is moved, the plane of the body traversed by the ultrasound beam is reproduced on the monitor. The transducer head of a linear electronic scanner has 60–130 thin rectangular crystals lined up side by side. The crystals are turned on sequentially, yielding the same results as moving the transducer manually

If the fishing boat remains stationary at location *a*, information is obtained from the school of fish immediately below it and from the sea bed. When the fishing boat moves, information produced by the reflected ultrasound beam can be recorded on a moving roll of paper similar to an electrocardiogram. Consequently, the topography of the sea bed and the schools of fish can be recorded on paper as two-dimensional images.

Instead of moving the fishing boat, if multiple fish detectors were positioned on the surface of the sea and each detector were turned on in sequential order, the same information could be obtained as though the boat were moving at high speed on the surface.

Diagnostic ultrasonographic equipment applies the same principles as the fish detector, but with higher accuracy. When a short pulse of ultrasound is emitted on the patient's skin surface, the beam is reflected at interfaces of different tissues. The transducer detects this reflected beam and records its intensity and transit time. This is called A-mode scanning in which the *x*-axis represents depth (calculated from the time for the beam to return), and the spike height in the *y*-axis is proportional to the echo intensity. The A-mode is seldom used for diagnostic purposes; instead, the B-mode, which displays intensity as degrees of brightness on the monitor is usually used.

Pulse-Echo Method

Ultrasonographic equipment utilizes the pulse-echo method. The transducer vibrates in the transmit mode only 0.1% of the time and receives the returning echoes the rest of the time. Currently, only the reflected ultrasound is used for medical imaging. The use of transmitted ultrasound has been attempted, but has met with little success.

What Is Real Time?

If the information from the examination is displayed on the monitor without significant delay, it is called real time. Fluoroscopic examinations (for example, cardiac catheterization or an upper gastrointestinal examination) produce real-time images, whereas CT scans, which require 3–5 s for scanning and several additional seconds to a few minutes to reconstruct the image, are not real-time images. In order to obtain real-time images ultrasonographically, linear electronic, electronic sector, convex electronic, or mechanical sector scanners must be used.

Ultrasonographic Equipment

Initially, most abdominal imaging was done with contact compound scanners. More recently, mechanical sector and linear electronic systems have been used for this purpose.

Contact Compound Scanner

The transducer head of a contact compound scanner is moved manually to image a cross-section of the patient. The position and the direction of the transducer are calculated by the angles of the three joints of the arm to which the transducer is attached. In this way, the shape of the body surface and the internal structures are accurately visualized in a large visual field. The disadvantages of the contact compound scanner are that it suffers from motion artifact because of relatively long (3–10-s) scanning times for each section, that skill is required to obtain good smooth images, that only static images can be obtained, and that the equipment is expensive.

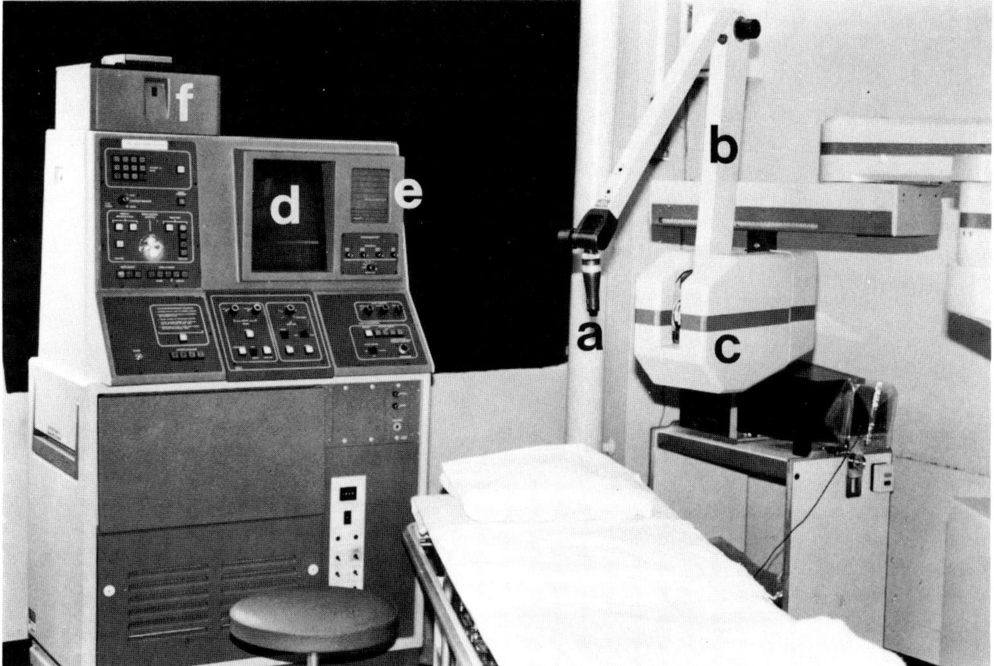

Fig. 1.10. *Contact compound scanner. a,* Probe; *b,* arm; *c,* scanner head; *d,* TV monitor; *e,* monitor for TGC adjustment; *f,* Polaroid camera

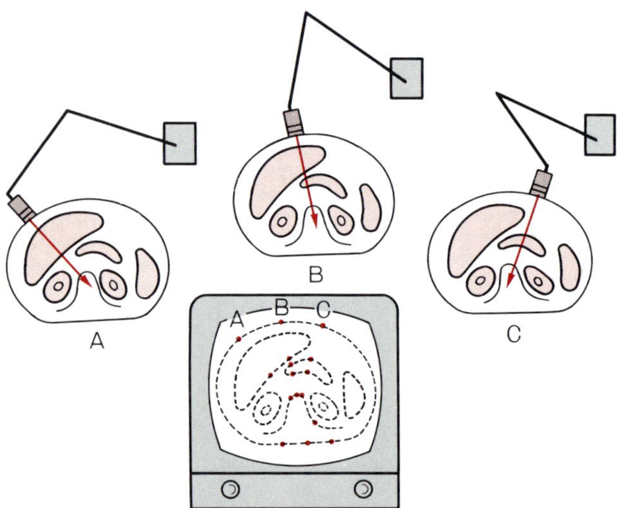

Fig. 1.11 A–C. *Principle of a contact compound scanner*. As the tip of the transducer is moved, images of the body surface and the internal structures are reconstructed by a scan converter

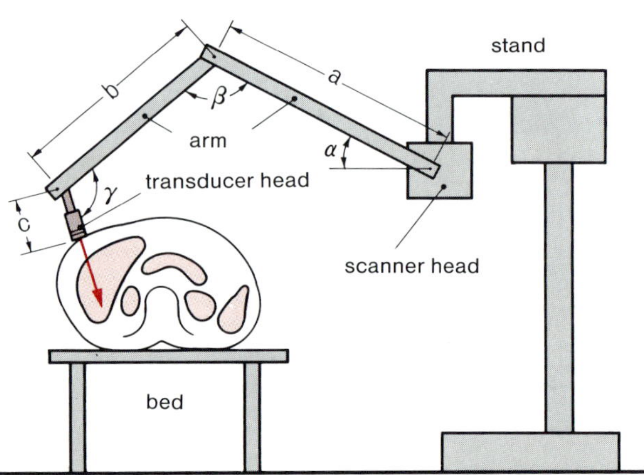

Fig. 1.12. *Scanner arm*. The position and the direction of the transducer in relation to the scanner head can be calculated by the angles of the three joints (α, β, γ) because the length of the arms (a and b), and the length of the transducer (c) are constant

A

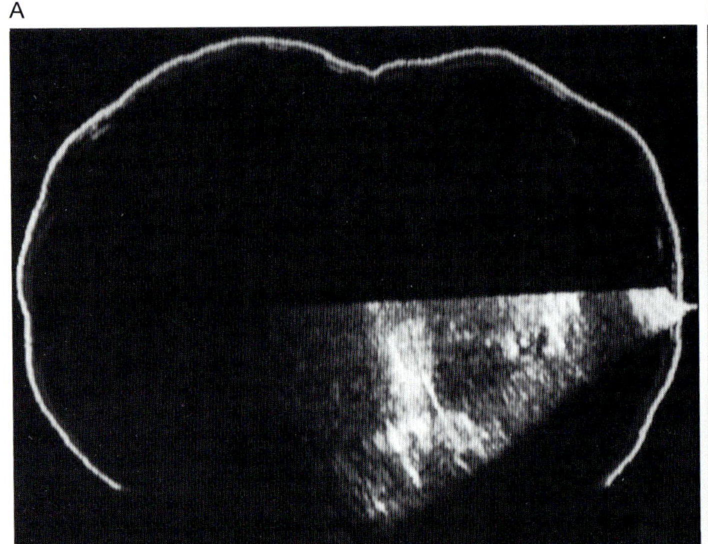

B

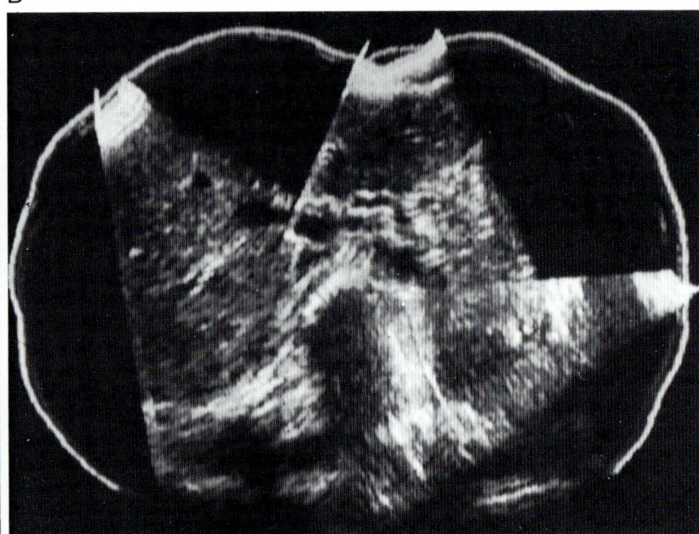

Fig. 1.13 A, B. *Contact compound scanning*. Each step of obtaining the image is shown separately. To facilitate understanding, the skin surface is drawn first. Actual scanning is continuous without any "gap" as is shown here. Partial images obtained during each scan are synthesized by a memory circuit of the scan converter to produce one section of the body

Linear Electronic Scanner

Linear electronic scanners are also known as linear array scanners. The inner structure of a linear electronic transducer head is shown in Fig. 1.14. The transducer face is 5–12 cm in length (most often 8 cm), and there are 60–130 thin rectangular crystals. In order to produce a focused beam, seven or eight crystals are used as a group. By varying the time at which individual crystals are fired, with the more central crystals delayed relative to the outer ones, the ultrasound beam from this group focuses to form

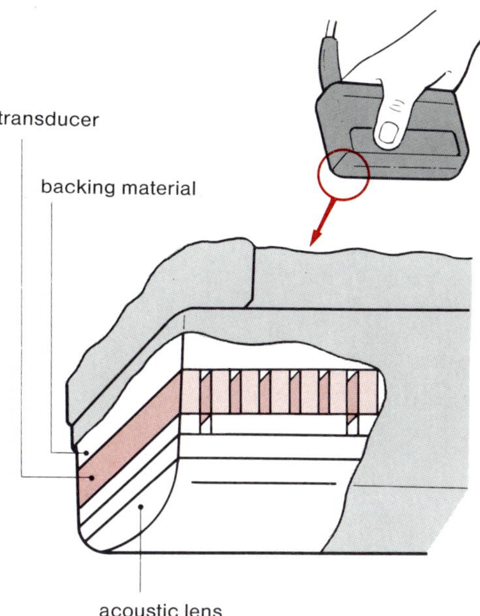

Fig. 1.14. *Transducer head of a linear electronic scanner.* There are many small rectangular crystals in the transducer

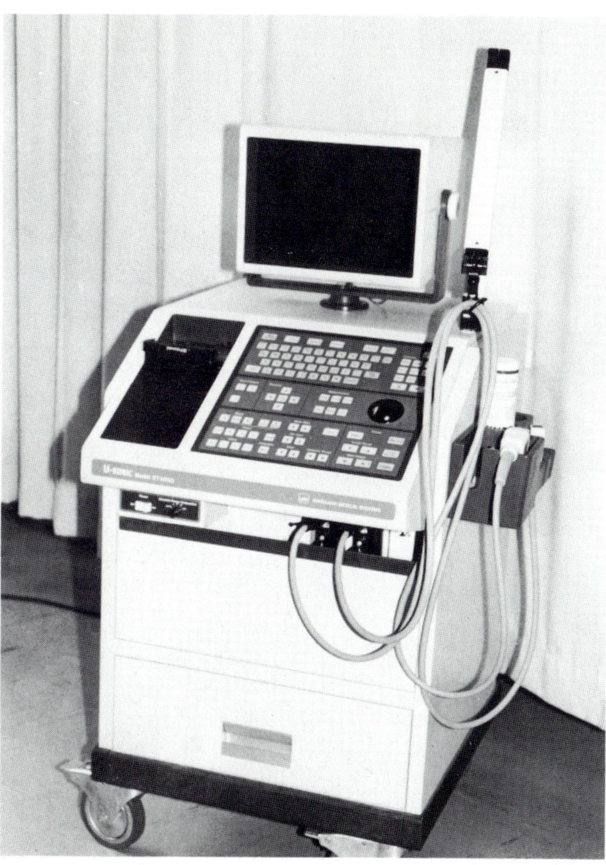

Fig. 1.15. *Linear electronic scanner.* This scanner also has a sector electronic scanner

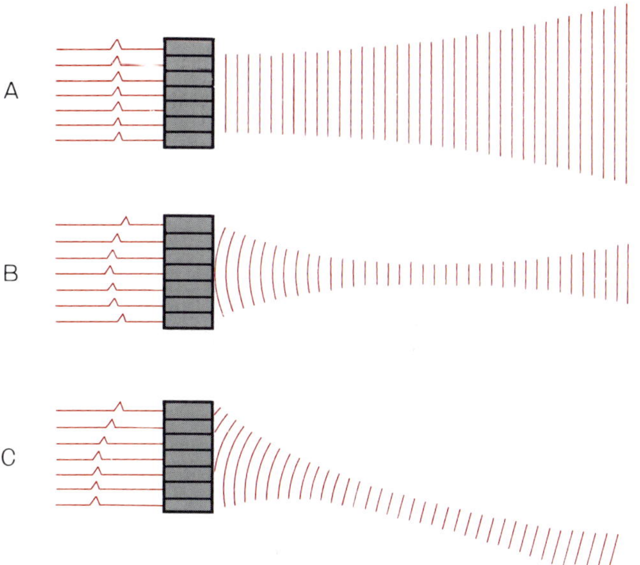

Fig. 1.16A–C. *Principles of electronic focusing.* When all seven elements in a group are fired simultaneously, there is no focusing effect (**A**). When a slight delay in timing is applied to the central elements, the beam is focused (**B**). The beam can also be emitted obliquely by altering the timing (**C**)

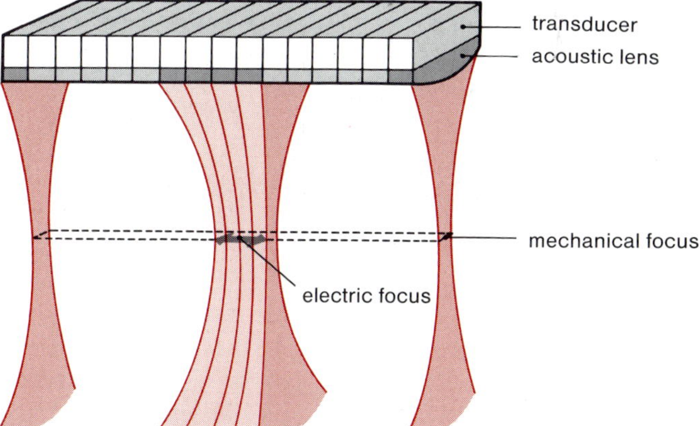

Fig. 1.17. *Focusing of linear electronic transducers.* Electronic focusing occurs in the longitudinal direction of the transducer, whereas mechanical focusing occurs in the direction of the short axis by using an acoustic lens

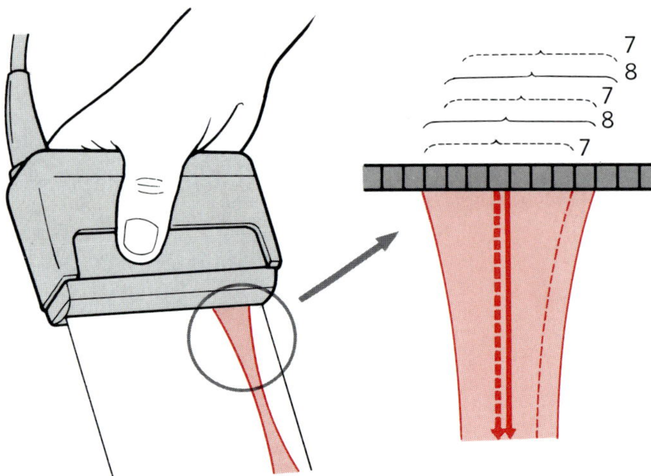

Fig. 1.18. *Scanning technique of a linear electronic transducer head.* When seven crystals are vibrated, the central axis of the ultrasound beam is aligned with the fourth crystal (*dashed line*). When eight crystals are used as a group, the axis of the beam passes between the fourth and fifth crystals (*solid line*). By progressing down the transducer and changing the groupings of the vibrating crystals one by one and alternating the numbers of crystals in a group (seven or eight), the number of distinct ultrasound beams which can be produced by a transducer head will be about twice the number of crystals within that head

a narrow beam. By changing the timing when the elements are fired, the focal distance or beam direction can be changed. This technique is called electronic focusing. By changing the number of elements in a group, 120–260 beams of ultrasound can be produced by a single transducer head (Fig. 1.18).

All the transducers complete one firing series in about 1/30 s. Thirty images are displayed on the monitor each second, enabling one to observe motion in the body. For this reason, using a linear electronic scanner is referred to as real-time scanning.

A special technique is not required to operate a linear electronic scanner as electronic functions are performed automatically. The disadvantages of the linear electronic scanner include a relatively small visual field compared to the contact compound scanner and consequent difficulty in identifying the orientation.

Electronic Sector Scanner

An electronic sector scanner, also known as a phased array scanner, employs the same principles as a linear electronic scanner, but the transducer surface is smaller. By altering the timing when each individual crystal is fired, both electronic focusing and the direction of the beam are controlled.

An electronic sector scanner is more expensive than a linear electronic scanner because of more complicated electrical circuitry to produce accurate timing and because each piezoelectric crystal is approximately half the size of the crystals in a linear scanner and are therefore more difficult to manufacture.

The electronic sector scanner was originally developed for echocardiography. However, it is suitable for intercostal examinations of the liver as it has a smaller blind spot at the dome of the liver when compared to the linear scanner (Fig. 1.21). An electronic sector scanner is also indispensible for examination of the pelvis.

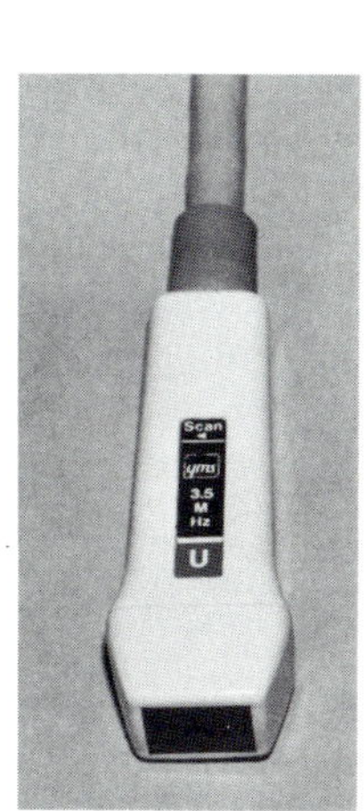

Fig. 1.19. Electronic sector scanner

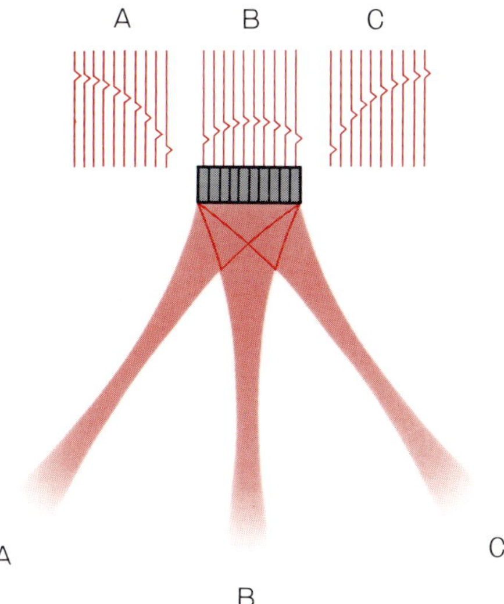

Fig. 1.20. *Beam pattern of electronic sector scanner*

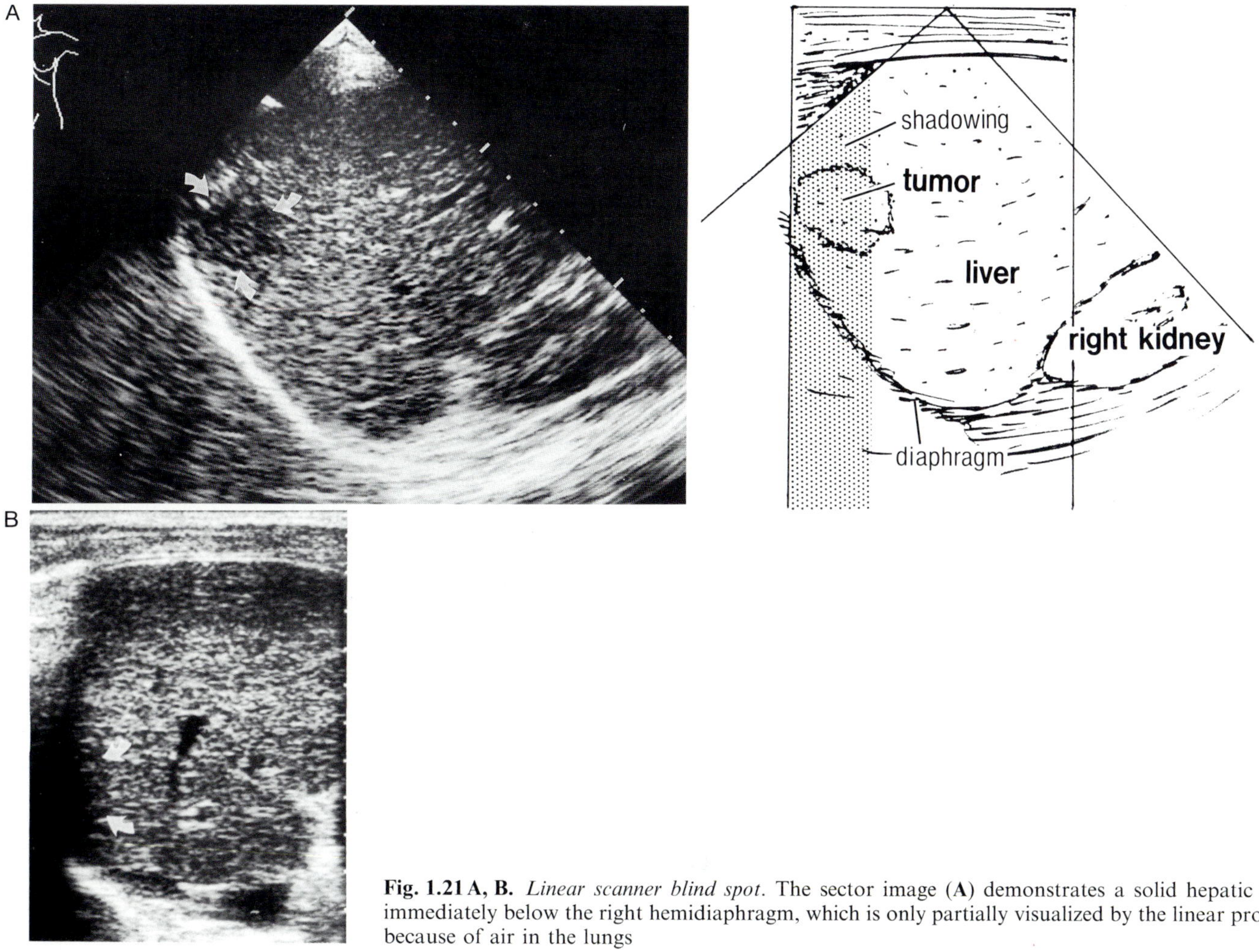

Fig. 1.21 A, B. *Linear scanner blind spot.* The sector image (**A**) demonstrates a solid hepatic tumor immediately below the right hemidiaphragm, which is only partially visualized by the linear probe (**B**) because of air in the lungs

Convex Electronic Scanner

The convex electronic sanner, also known as a curved linear scanner, is similar to the linear electronic scanner, except that the surface is convex. It differs from the scanner of an electronic sector system in that the ultrasound beam is always perpendicular to the surface of the transducer head. Since the electronic circuitry of the linear electronic system can be used to control a convex electronic transducer, it is not as expensive as the electronic sector system. Its visual field is similar to that of the electronic sector scanner. Superficial structures are better imaged (i.e., better near field discrimination) than with an electronic sector scanner, since the convex electronic transducer face is longer. However, when the skin surface is convex, the probe will not be in full contact with the skin. In addition, intercostal scanning cannot be performed perpendicular to the ribs (this is possible with a sector scanner). The angle of the beam spread is usually 60°, but recently some of the convex electronic scanners (called microconvex systems) can produce beam spreads close to 100°, but resolution in the far field is suboptimal.

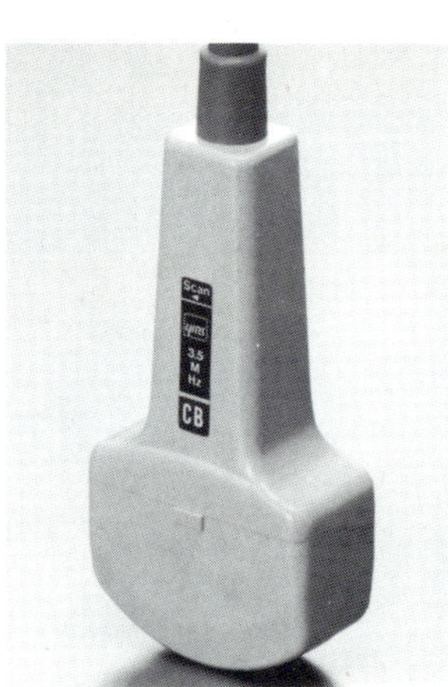

Fig. 1.22. Convex electronic scanner

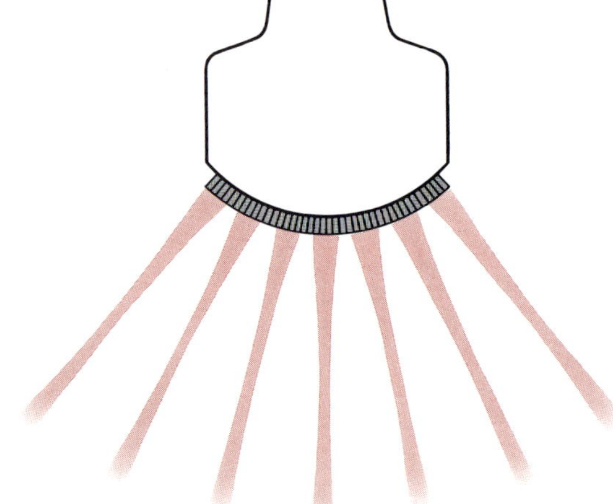

Fig. 1.23. *Ultrasound beam pattern of the convex electronic scanner*

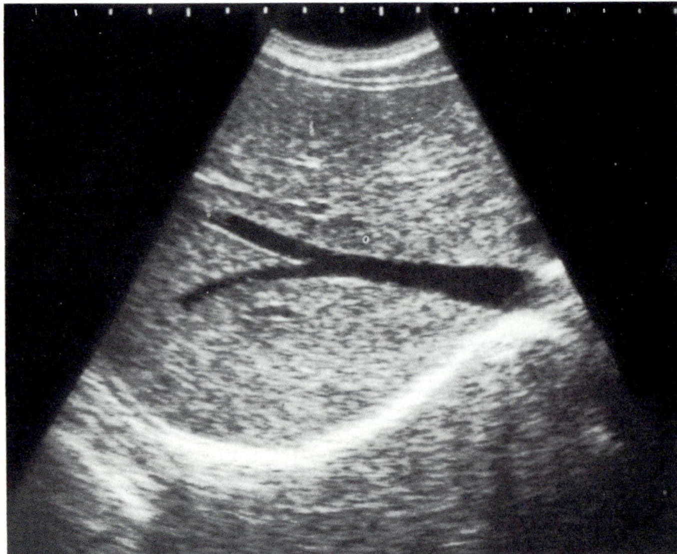

Fig. 1.24. *An image produced by a convex electronic scanner (right hepatic vein)*

Mechanical Sector Scanner

In order to obtain a fan-shaped real-time image, three or four transducers are mounted on a wheel that is rotated, or a single transducer rocks back and forth within transducer head. These types of mechanical sector scanners are less expensive than electronic sector scanners; however, in contrast to electronic sector scanners, the focal zone is fixed and vibration of the probe can be felt by the operator.

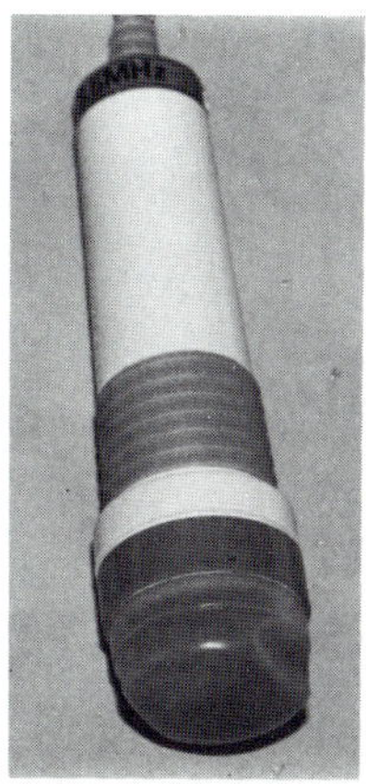

Fig. 1.25. *Mechanical sector scanner*

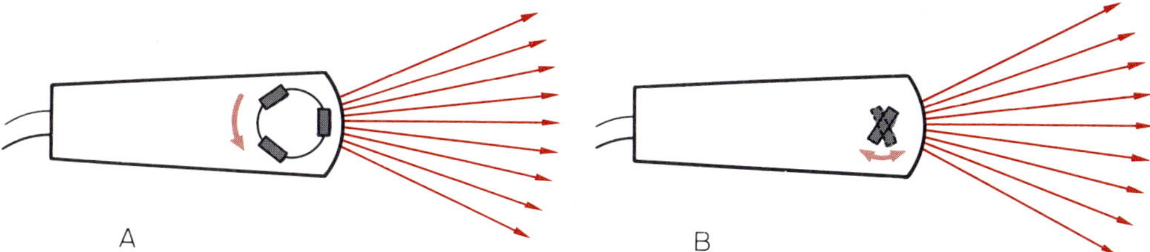

Fig. 1.26 A, B. *Scanning methods of mechanical sector scanners.* **A)** Rolling wheel type; **B)** oscillating type

Water Bath Method

When scanning superficial organs such as the breast or thyroid gland, a water-filled bag should be interposed between the transducer head and the skin surface. There are three reasons for using a water bag:

1. To bring the tissue to be examined into the focal zone. Standard transducers have a focal length of 6 cm. Using a water bag of 4 cm thickness, the superficial tissues 1–2 cm from the skin surface will be brought into the focal zone.
2. To make scanning easier. On a skin surface which is irregular, manual scanning can be difficult. The water bag also eliminates motion artifacts and the deformity of an organ which may occur by direct contact of the transducer head on the skin.
3. To eliminate reverberation artifact (see p. 22) in the field of interest. By creating a space between the probe and the skin surface, reverberation echoes in the tissues of interest can be eliminated.

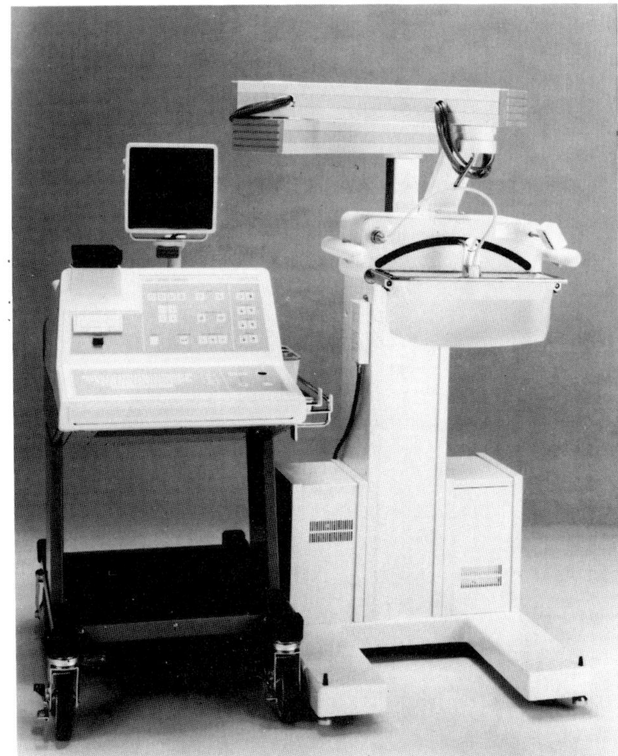

Fig. 1.27. *Equipment for the water bath method*

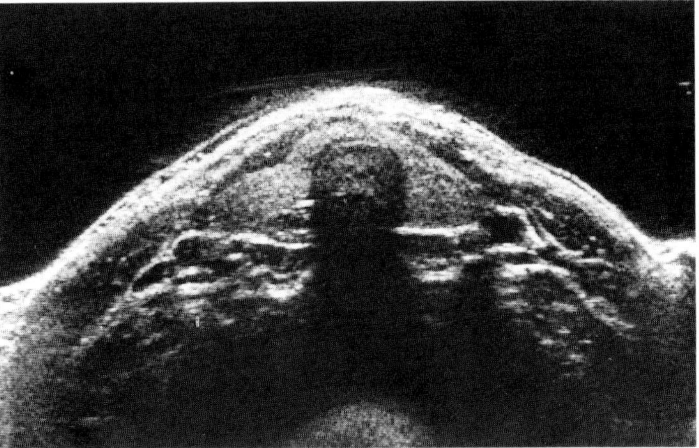

Fig. 1.28. *An image of a normal thyroid* (obtained with the equipment shown in Fig. 1.27)

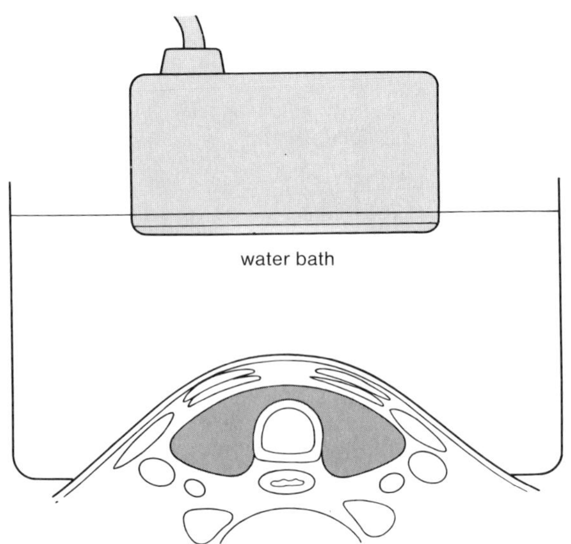

Fig. 1.29. *Water bath method using a linear electronic scanner*

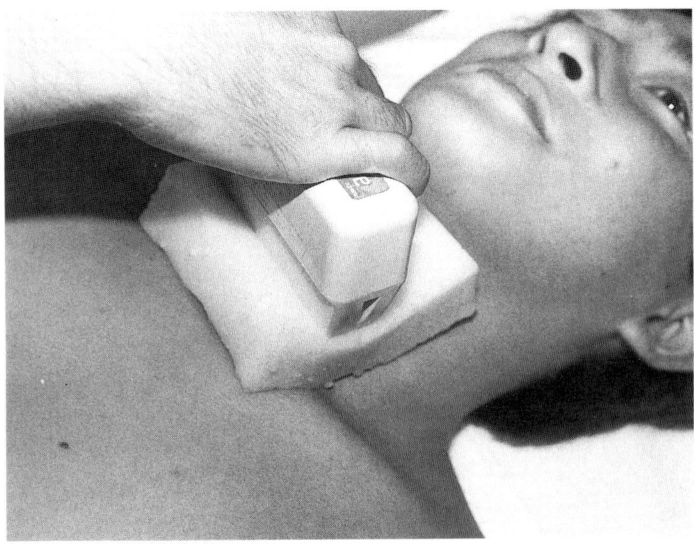

Fig. 1.30. *Use of polymer gel*

There is ultrasonographic equipment which is specially designed for the water bath method with a built-in water bag and a single transducer head which is used to scan automatically, with its tip in the water (Fig. 1.27). Using a water bag or a synthesized polymer gel material, linear electronic scanners can be used for superficial organs to yield real-time images (Fig. 1.29, 1.30).

Specialized Types of Transducers

1. Radial transducer head for the prostate gland: the ultrasound beam is transmitted radially from a rotating probe.
2. Endoscopic scanner: a small real-time transducer is attached to the tip of the endoscope for examination of the mediastinum or abdomen from inside the esophagus or stomach.
3. Octoson scanner: there are eight large transducers in a water tank. The patient is examined by lying prone on a plastic membrane which is on the top of a water tank.

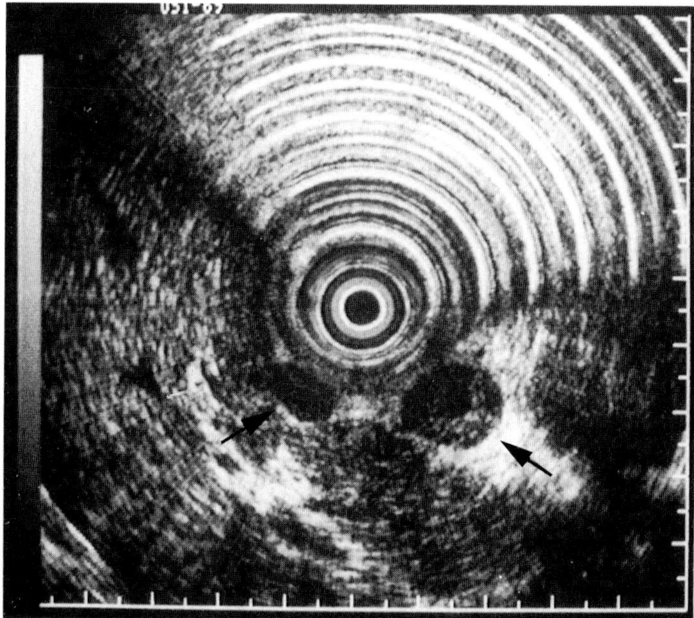

Fig. 1.31. *Endoscopic ultrasonography:* mediastinal lymph node enlargement (*arrows*). This image was obtained with a transducer in the esophagus, which is in the center of this picture

Adjusting the Scanner

Gain

The echo signal returning from the body is converted into an electronic signal by the transducer. This electronic signal has to be amplified to produce images on the monitor. The amplification of the electronic signal is called "gain" and it regulates the strengths of the echoes from all depths. The gain must be optimally set for good visualization as in Fig. 1.32 A.

Time Gain Compensation

The signal returning from the deep tissues (far field) of a patient is attenuated and much weaker than the signal returning from tissues close to the transducer. Simply increasing the gain cannot resolve this problem as the superficial echoes become too strong. In order to compensate for signal loss from the far field, adjustment of the sensitivity at each depth is necessary, and this is called time gain compensation (TGC) or sensitivity time control (STC). TGC is set so that a solid organ, such as the liver, will have uniform brightness at all depths.

Dynamic Range

The dynamic range is the range of echo levels from the highest to the lowest amplitudes that can be displayed on the monitor. Using a wide dynamic range, the image will appear soft, but small differences in echo levels cannot be detected. When the dynamic range is narrow, the differences in echo levels in a certain range will be exaggerated on the monitor.

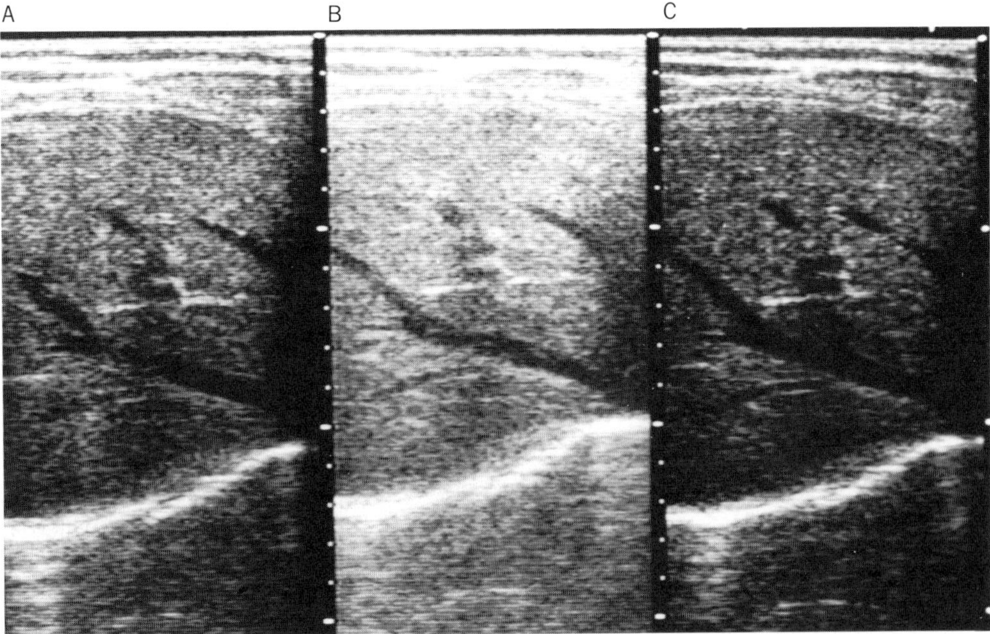

Fig. 1.32 A–C. *Gain settings.* **A** Optimal gain setting; **B** gain too high; **C** gain too low

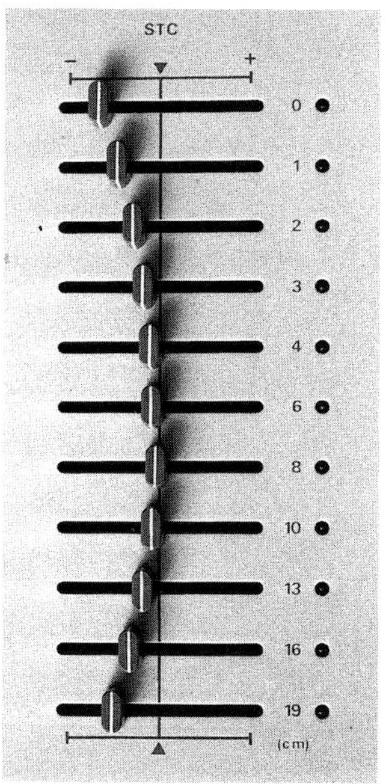

Fig. 1.33. *TGC controls*

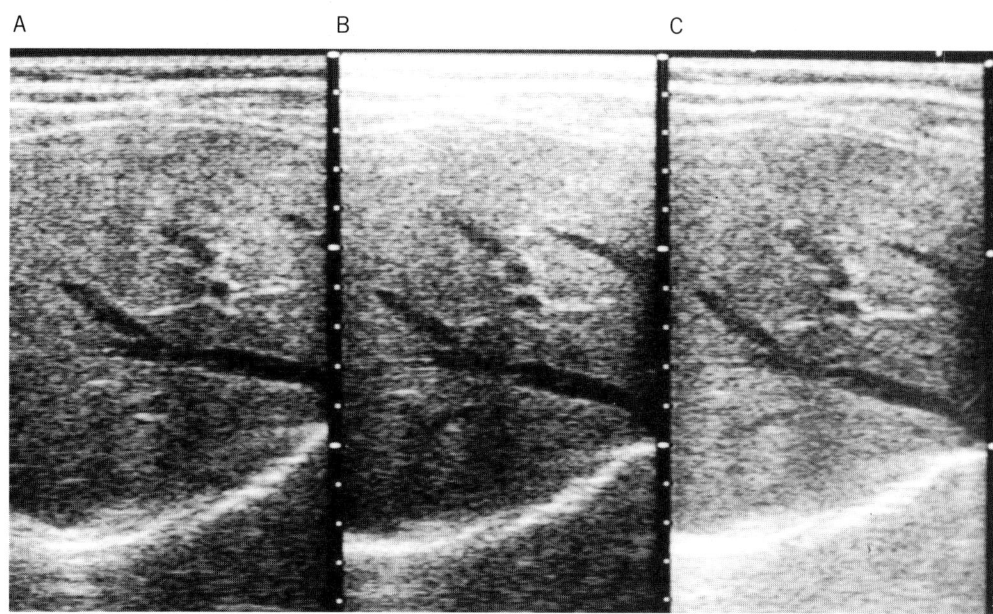

Fig. 1.34 A–C. *TGC adjustments*. **A** Optimal TGC; **B** near gain is too high; **C** far gain is too high

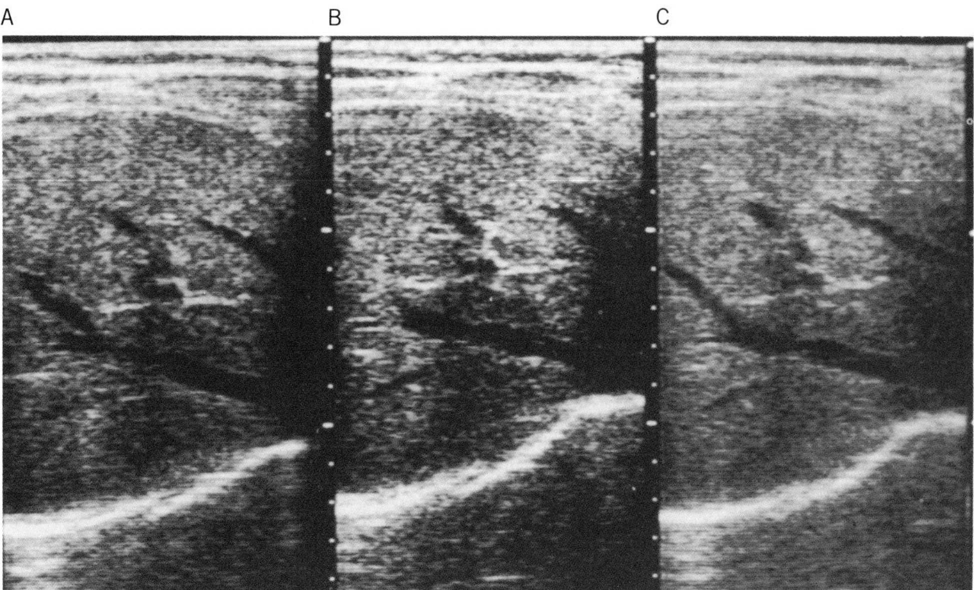

Fig. 1.35 A–C. *Dynamic range adjustments*. **A** Optimal dynamic range; **B** narrow dynamic range; **C** wide dynamic range

Techniques

Compression

Gently compressing the abdomen with the transducer head during subcostal scanning may help in visualizing the dome or anterior segment of the right lobe of the liver. This may also displace intestinal gas and improve visualization of the pancreas.

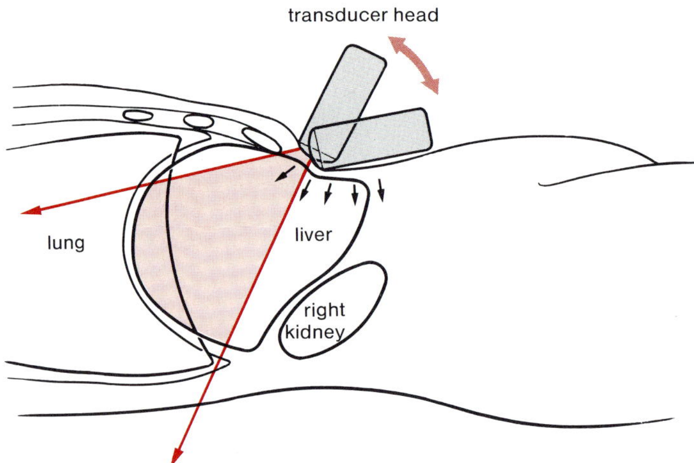

Fig. 1.36. *Visualization of the dome of the liver.* The transducer head should be pressed subcostally and tilted so that the beam is directed cephalad

Changing the Plane

Two planes, perpendicular to each other, should be obtained for every area of interest. This will help in the identification of the organ being examined and in the recognition of artifacts. For example, if a structure is round on two sections which are perpendicular to each other, then it must be spherical.

Fanning Movement of the Probe

By moving the probe in fan-shaped fashion, the shape of a structure can be determined. If it is a tubular structure, the direction of its long axis can be ascertained.

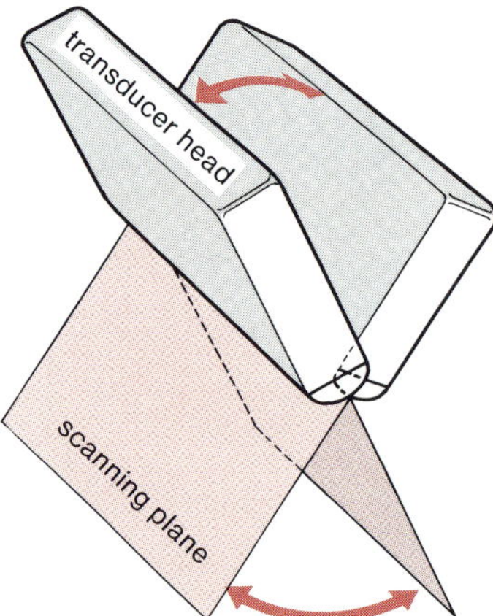

Fig. 1.37. *Fan-shaped movement of the transducer head.* The surface of the transducer head is fixed on the skin, and the opposite end of the transducer head is rocked in a fan-shaped fashion

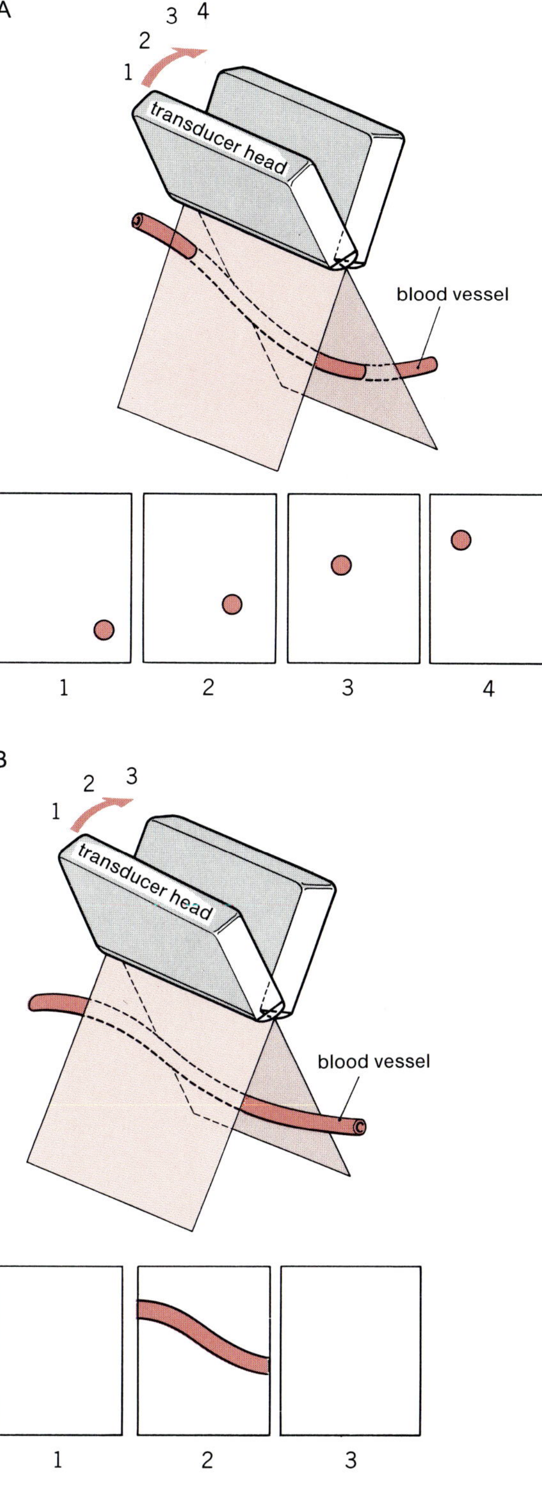

Fig. 1.38 A, B. *Fan-shaped movement of the transducer head and a vessel.* **A** When the probe is rocked in a fan-shaped fashion and crosses the longitudinal axis of a vessel, the cross-section of the vessel will slowly move on the monitor. **B** The vessel will be visualized as a linear structure when it is in the plane of the beam during fan-shaped movement of the transducer head

Artifacts

Knowing the nature and cause of artifacts is important for accurate diagnosis. Four common ultrasonographic artifacts are explained here.

Side Lobe Artifact

An ultrasound beam includes a single strong main lobe along the central axis and several weaker side lobes slightly off axis from the main lobe. Similarly to the main lobe, the side lobes are also reflected by interfaces in the body and are converted to an electrical signal. Since the ultrasonographic equipment cannot distinguish the signal

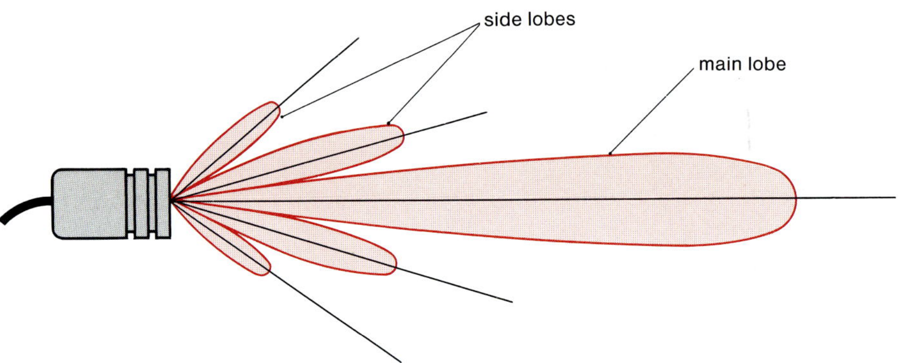

Fig. 1.39. *Shape of the ultrasound beam.* There is a strong main lobe along the central axis. Several weaker beams (side lobes) are present slightly off axis. In this figure, a transducer with only one crystal is shown, but similar pattern is seen with linear electronic scanners which have more than one crystal

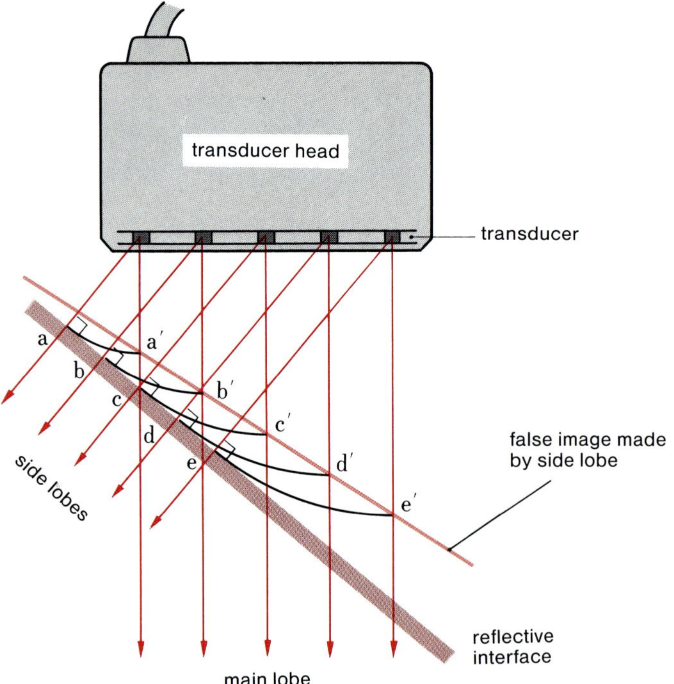

Fig. 1.40. *Generation of side lobe artifact.* The false images due to side lobes are produced because the echoes resulting from the side lobes are indistinguishable from the echoes resulting from the main lobe of the beam. When there are reflective interfaces perpendicular to the axis of a side lobe (*a, b, c, d, e*), they will be projected at the same distance from the transducer but on the axis of the main lobe (*a'*, *b'*, *c'*, *d'*, *e'*) and consequently falsely produce a structure *a'−e'*

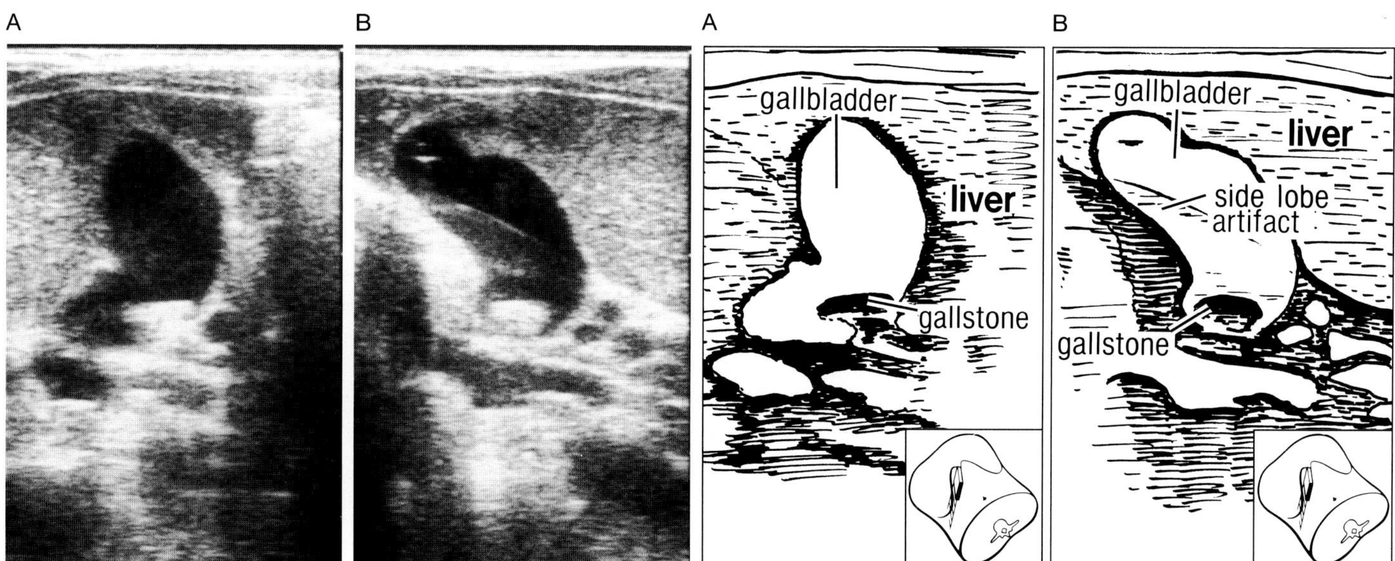

Fig. 1.41 A, B. *Side lobe artifact in the gallbladder due to intestinal gas.* Image **A** demonstrates a gallstone within the lumen of the gallbladder, which is otherwise normal. By altering the angle of the transducer head slightly (**B**), an oblique line appears within the lumen; this is a side lobe artifact due to intestinal gas adjacent to the gallbladder. Bile suldge may produce a similar appearance, but the echoes from sludge will not disappear by changing the angle of the transducer head

from the side lobes from the main lobe signal, the side lobe signal (which originates from a direction different from the main axis) is interpreted as if it originated from the main lobe. The signal from the side lobes is usually low in amplitude and therefore does not cause problems on properly designed and adjusted units. However, when there is a highly reflective interface in the direction of a side lobe or when the signal from the main lobe is weak due to an absence of reflectors along the main axis, false images created by the side lobes will become prominent.

Side lobe artifacts are commonly encountered during examination of the gallbladder. While the main lobe passes through the lumen of the gallbladder, the side lobes can be reflected by intestinal gas near the fundus of the gallbladder. This strong echo signal from the side lobes may be projected into the lumen of the gallbladder (Fig. 1.41).

Reverberation Artifact

When there are two or more highly reflective interfaces perpendicular to the ultrasound beam, complicated sequences of reflection can occur. For example, in Fig. 1.42 where there are two planes of reflection (*a*, *b*), sound does not simply reflect off each plane as in *A*, but will also produce more complicated reflection patterns between each plane and the surface of the probe (*B–E*). This phenomenon is called reverberation.

As previously stated, the time for the beam to make a round trip is used to calculate depth. Owing to these additional reflections prior to reception of the echo, a false image is created deeper than the actual depth of the reflector.

Reverberation echoes are frequently produced by the fascia of the abdominal muscles or by the peritoneum, producing multiple thin linear false echoes immediately below the abdominal wall. Consequently, small lesions in the superficial portions of the liver or in the fundus of the gallbladder may be obscured, and a hepatic cyst near the surface of the liver will not appear anechoic.

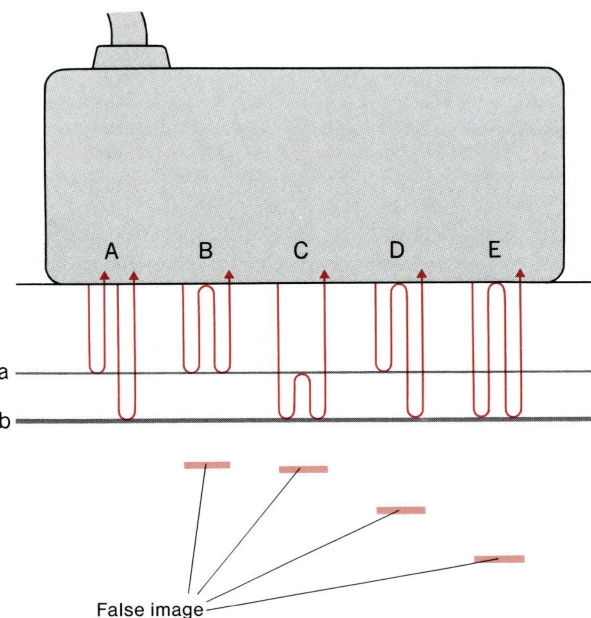

Fig. 1.42. *Reverberation artifact.* When there is more than one highly reflective interface parallel to the skin surface, the ultrasound beam will be reflected in several different ways. False images will be displayed on the monitor, deeper than the true image, because of the longer travel time of the reverberation echo returning back to the transducer

Causes of Unsharp Ultrasonographic Images

Several different factors cause unsharp images: an improperly focused beam, motion at the time of freezing the image, refraction of the ultrasound beam, differences in velocity of ultrasound in different tissues in the body (image reconstruction is based upon the assumption that sound travels at a velocity of 1540 m/s), and the fact that one ultrasound pulse usually includes two or three wave lengths rather than just one.

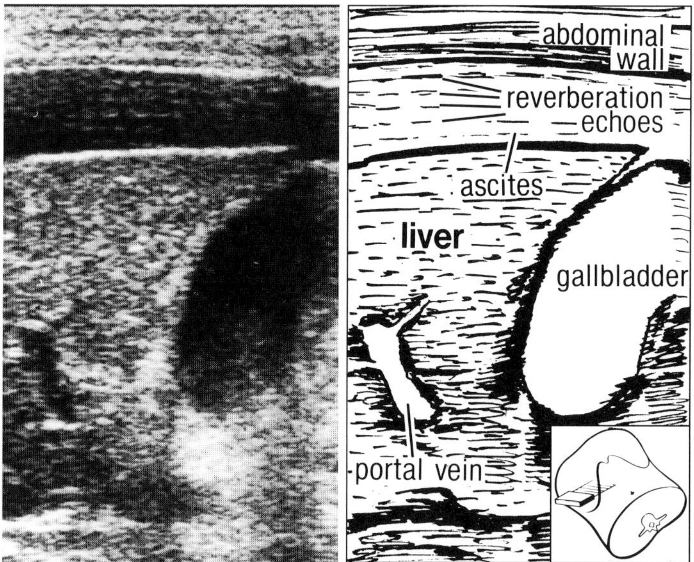

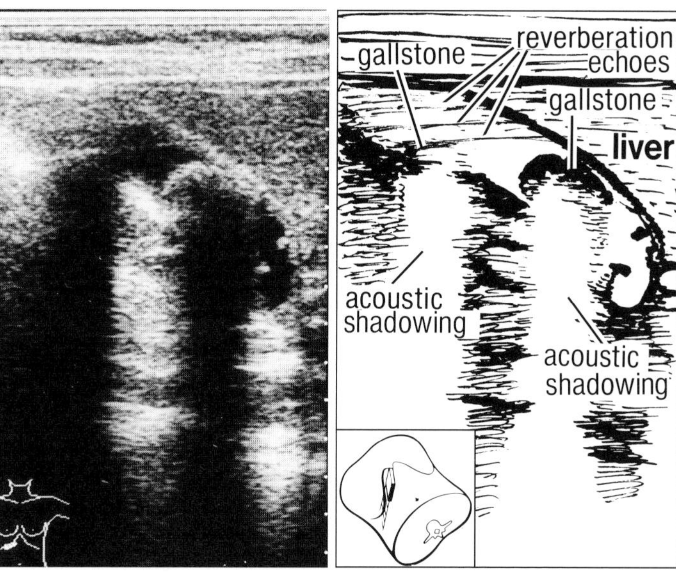

Fig. 1.43. *Reverberation artifact caused by the abdominal wall.* Reverberation echoes caused by the multiple reflecting planes in the abdominal wall are projected into the ascites. When there is no ascites, this artifact will be projected into the superficial portion of the liver, obscuring lesions in this location

Fig. 1.44. *A gallstone obscured by reverberation artifact.* Reverberation artifact produced by the abdominal wall is projected into the area of the gallbladder fundus, obscuring a stone. Only the acoustic shadowing caused by the stone is visualized

Snowflake-Like Echo Caused by Gas
Reverberation echoes may be ladder-shaped, as in Fig. 1.45, but more often they have a snowflake-like appearance. Small punctate echoes are densely packed in the superficial portion of the tissues, becoming progressively coarser with increasing depth, and finally disappearing at a certain depth.

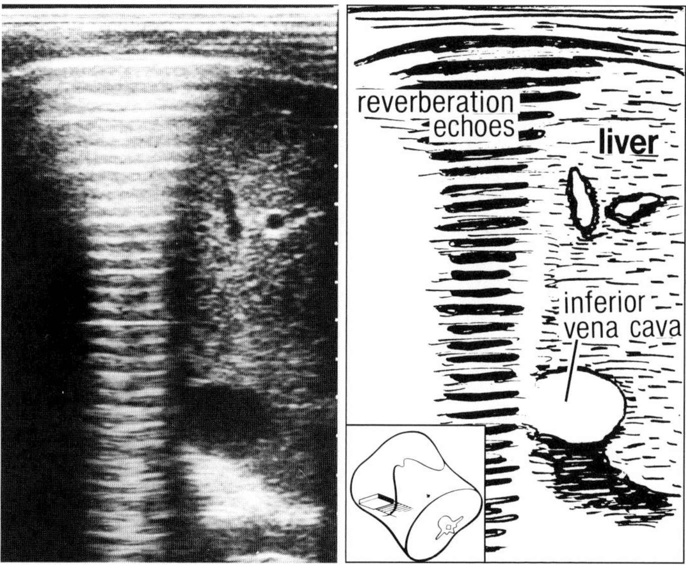

Fig. 1.45. *Ladder-shaped reverberation artifact caused by air in the lung*

Mirror Effect

At times, the ultrasound beam passes through the liver and is reflected by the diaphragm. If this beam is then reflected by a structure in the liver and then once more reflected by the diaphagm before returning to the transducer, these echoes will be displayed on the same axis as the original ultrasound beam, creating a false image on the monitor. For example, in Fig. 1.46 an intrahepatic structure (*A*) is projected superior to the diaphragm. This artifact is called the mirror effect. An echo pattern similar to the liver is uncommonly projected above the diaphragm into the lung due to the mirror effect.

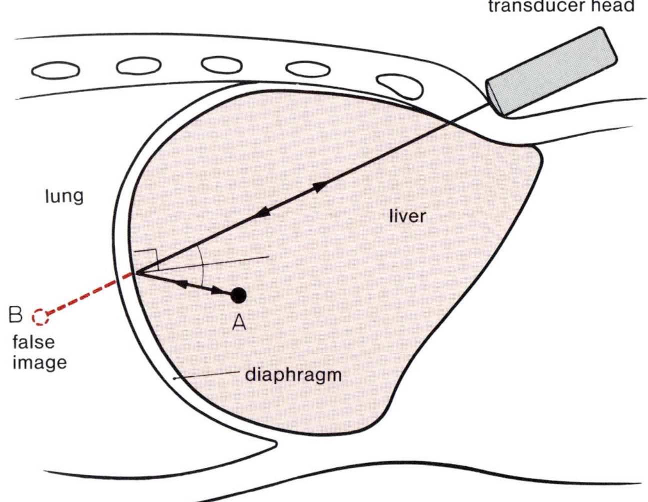

Fig. 1.46. *Principles of the mirror effect* (see text)

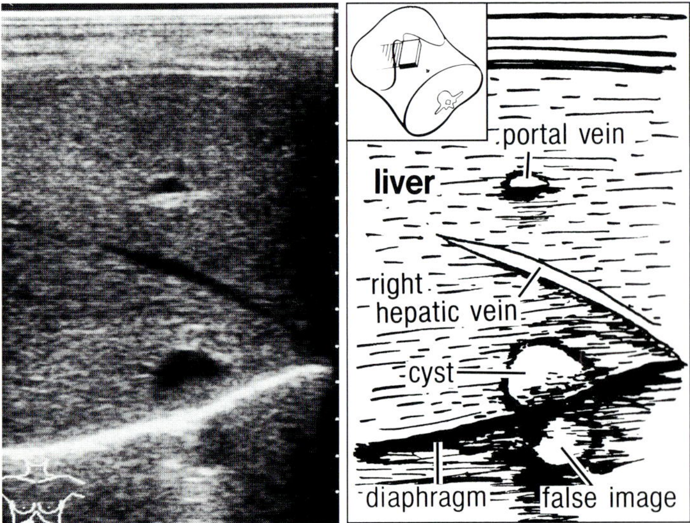

Fig. 1.47. *Mirror image of a hepatic cyst*

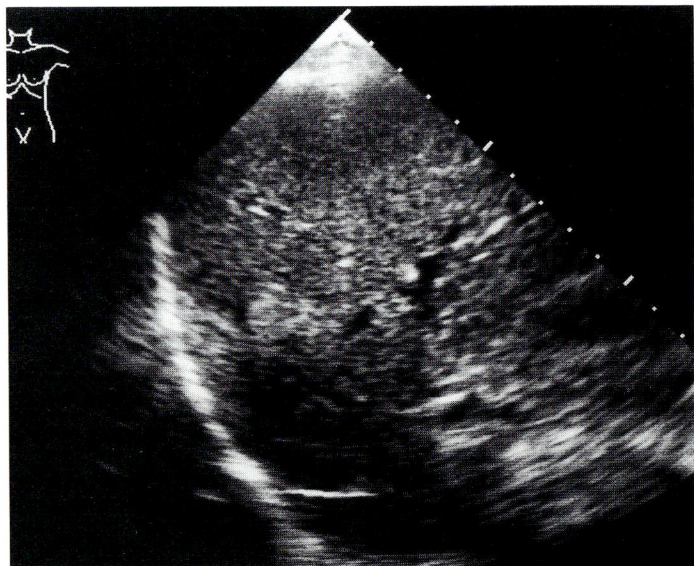

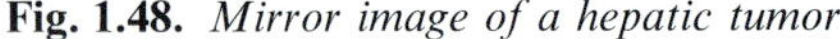

Fig. 1.48. *Mirror image of a hepatic tumor*

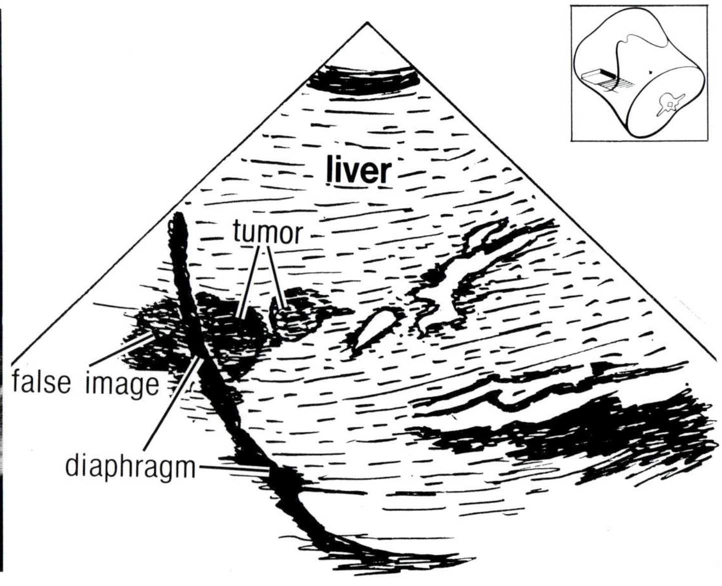

Lens Effect

Transverse scanning in the upper abdomen sometimes exhibits side-by-side duplication of midline structures. This is due to medial refraction of the ultrasound beam when it passes the border of the rectus abdominis muscle and fat. By altering the direction of the transducer, this effect may disappear.

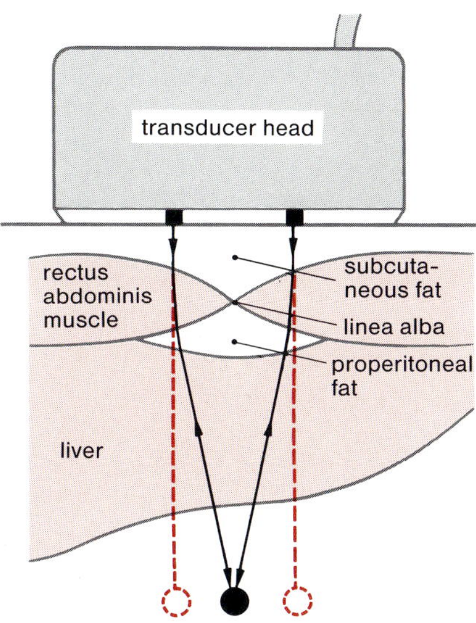

Fig. 1.49. *Principle of the lens effect.* Two ultrasound beams from different crystals refracted by the rectus muscles are reflected by the same structure (e.g., vessel) and return to each transducer. These reflected signals are displayed immediately below each transducer (*red circles*). Because of poor penetration through the linea alba in the midline, the true image (*black circle*) is seldom visualized

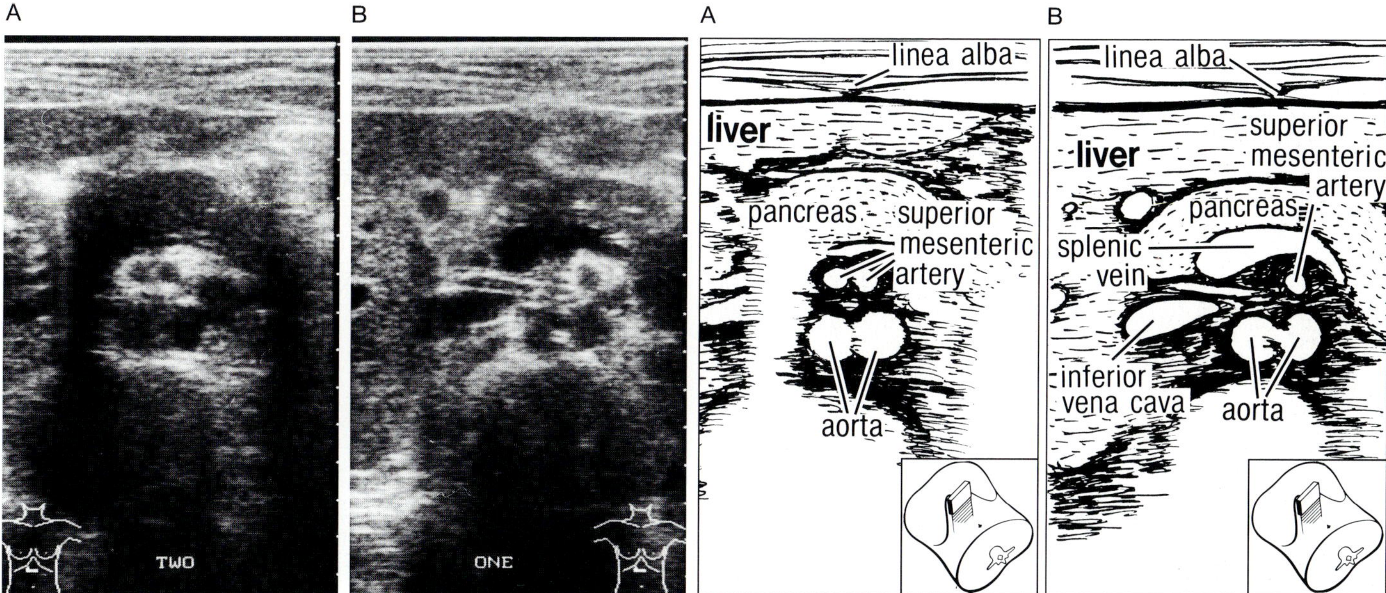

Fig. 1.50 A, B. *Lens effect seen on images of the superior mesenteric artery and abdominal aorta.* Image **A** demonstrates an apparent duplication of the superior mesenteric artery and abdominal aorta. Image **B** was obtained with a slight change in the direction of the beam, demonstrating a single superior mesenteric artery and a duplicated aorta

2 Scanning Techniques and Anatomy

Scanning Methods

To scan means to acquire information by moving the transducer head on the skin surface of the patient. With real-time equipment, simply placing the transducer head on the abdominal wall is called scanning as the transducer head performs this function electronically. In this section, various scanning methods are explained with illustrations.

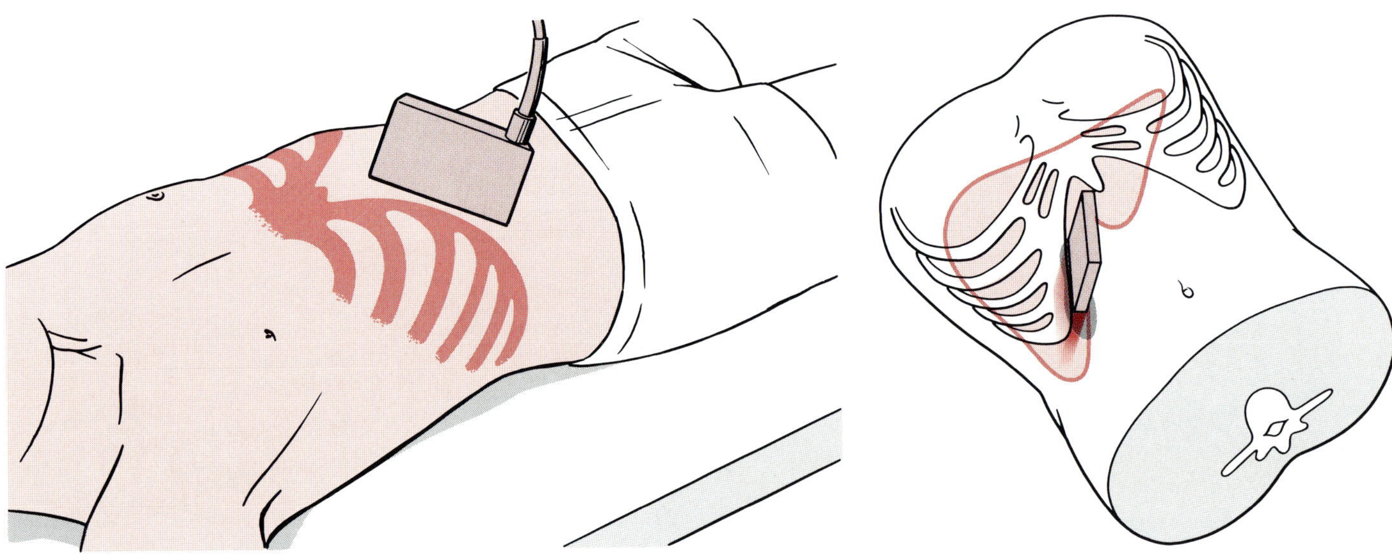

Subcostal Scanning

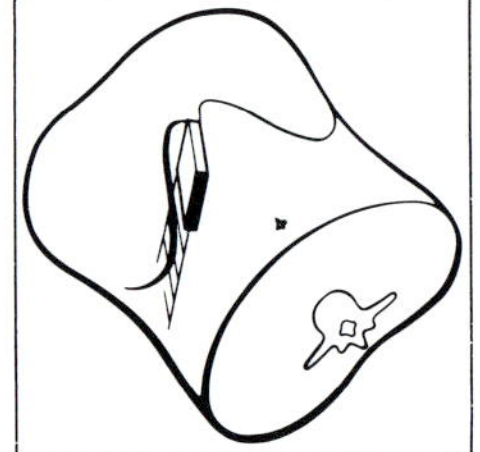

Fig. 2.1. The transducer head is placed along the right subcostal margin. The lower portions of the right lobe of the liver, the gallbladder, and the right kidney are visualized. By tilting the tip of the transducer head toward the head on deep inspiration, the upper portions of the liver are visualized

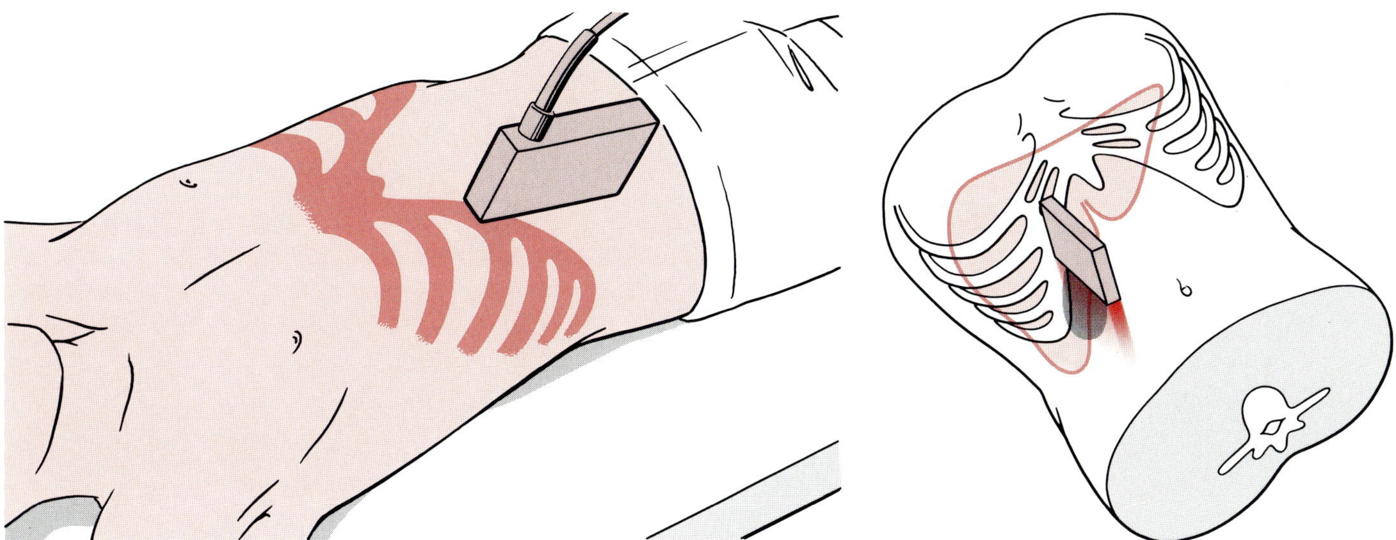

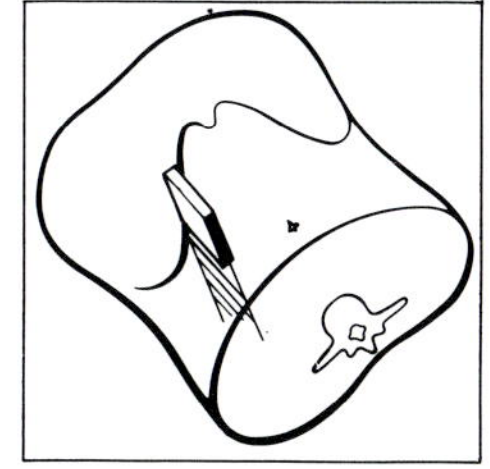

Fig. 2.2. With the transducer head parallel to the axis of the body, longitudinal sections can be obtained. Longitudinal scanning of the right upper abdomen is used to visualize the lower portions of the liver and the gallbladder. When the transducer head is placed directly over the ribs, the abdomen cannot be visualized because of acoustic shadowing from the ribs

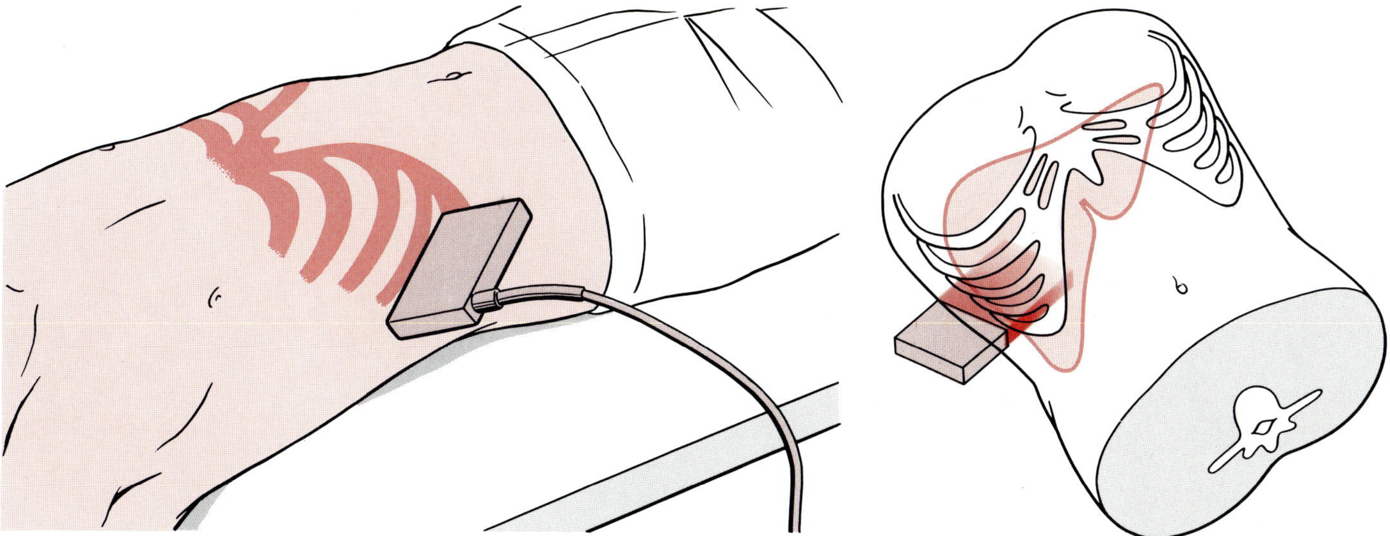

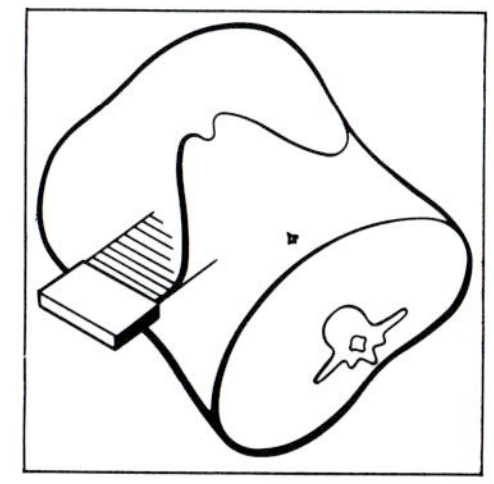

Fig. 2.3. If the transducer head is placed over the intercostal space, the liver is generally well visualized. When the liver is shrunken, this may be the only scanning method with which it is possible to visualize the gallbladder. Scanning through the posterior intercostal spaces is used for observation of the right kidney or adrenal gland

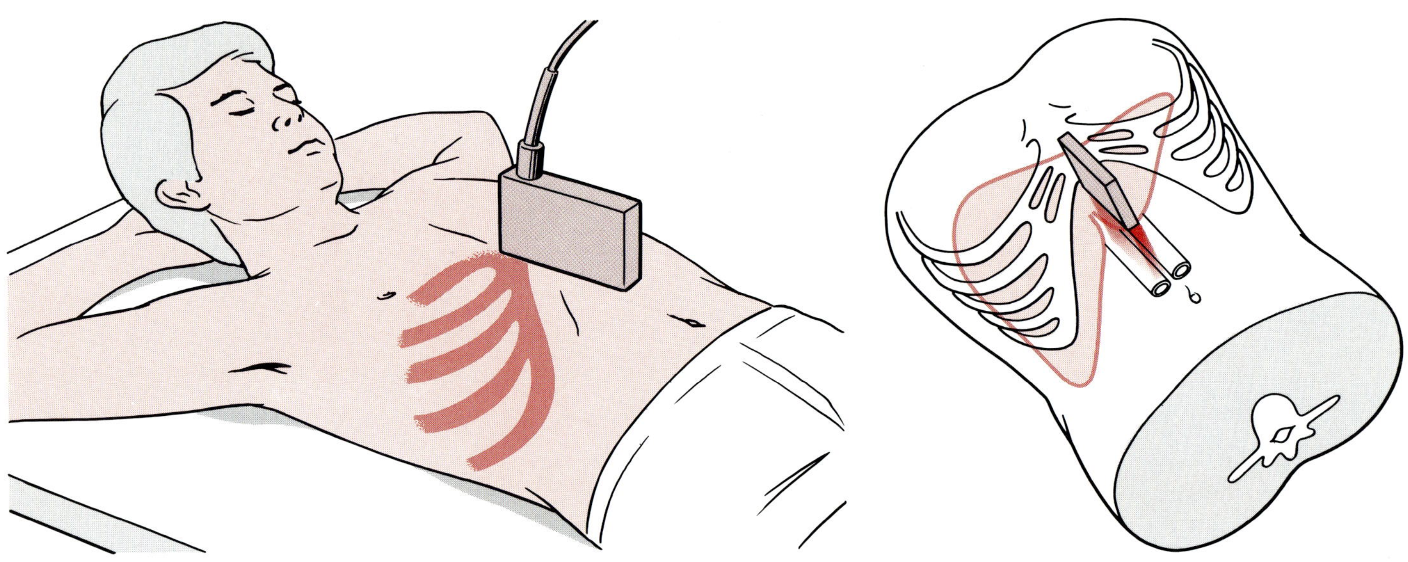

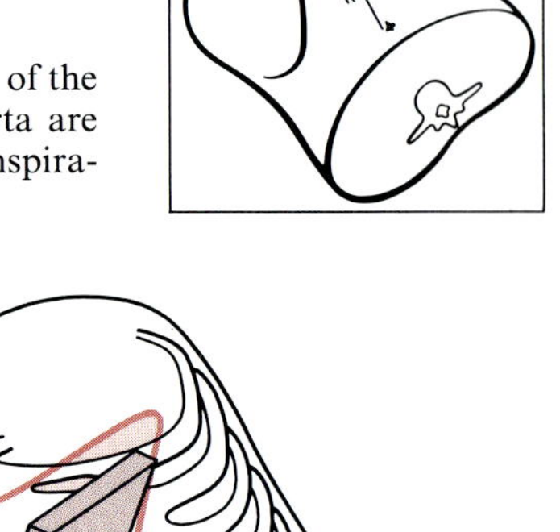

Longitudinal Scanning (Midline)

Fig. 2.4. Longitudinal scanning in the midline visualizes the left lobe of the liver and the pancreas. The inferior vena cava and abdominal aorta are visualized posterior to the liver. Scanning should be done in deep inspiration so that the liver is not hidden behind the rib cage

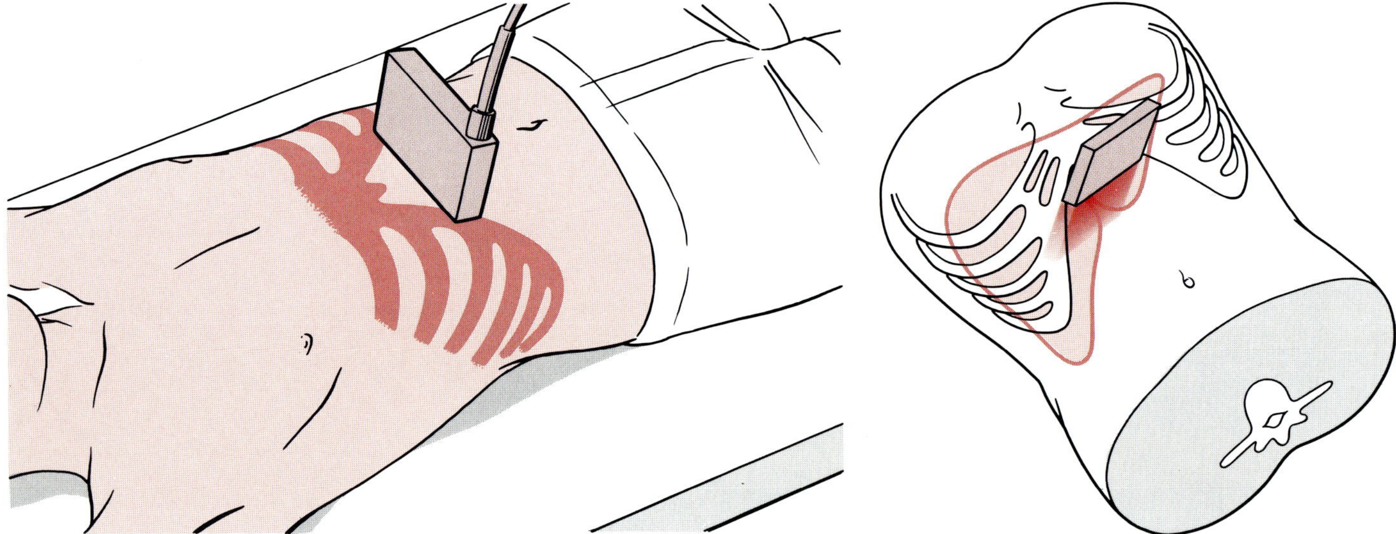

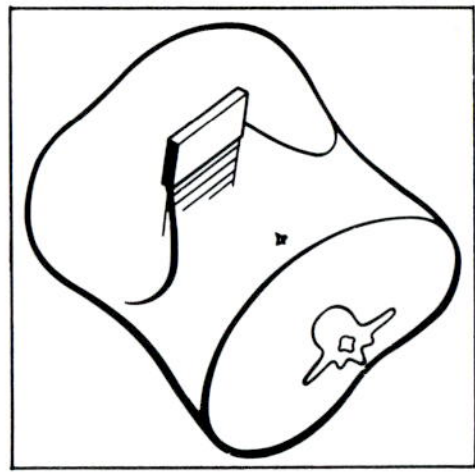

Transverse Scanning

Fig. 2.5. In the midline, the left lobe of the liver and the pancreas are visualized. The gallbladder is also visualized when transverse scanning is performed from a right subcostal location

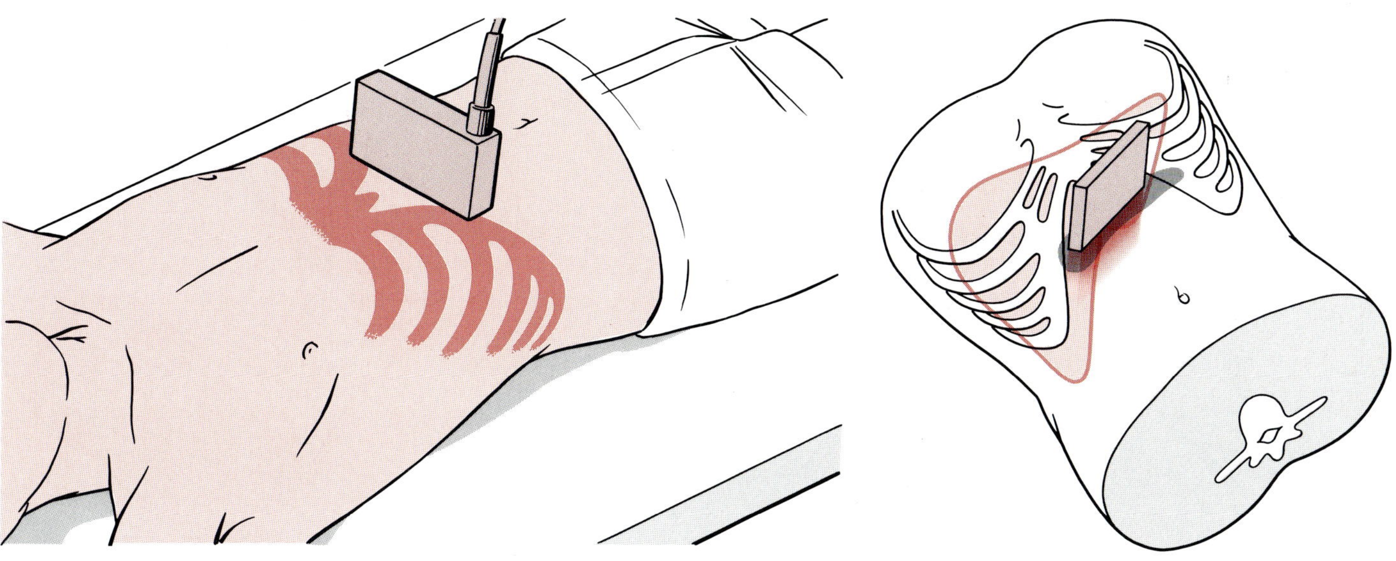

Oblique Scanning

Fig. 2.6. When the transducer head is slightly tilted from the transverse scanning position, the pancreatic head and the body are visualized simultaneously as the head is 2−4 cm caudal to the body of the pancreas

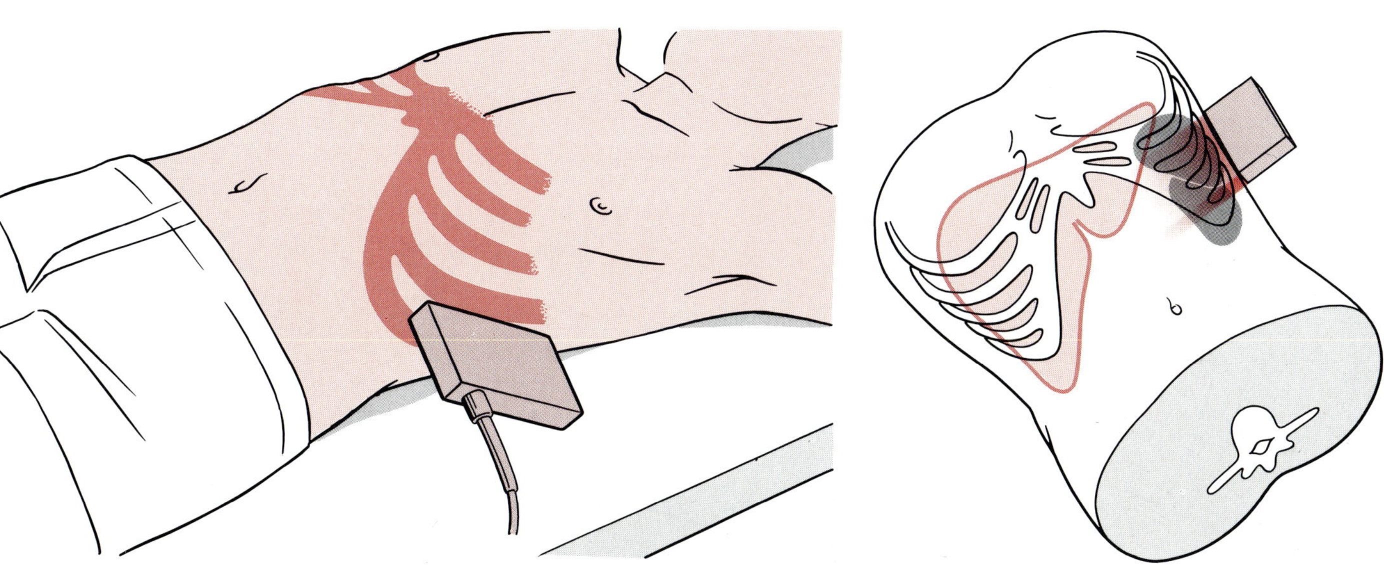

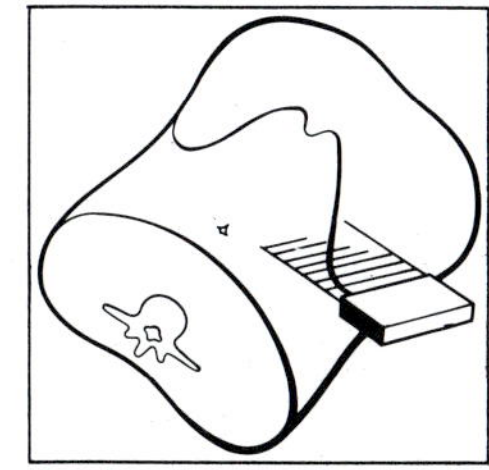

Intercostal Scanning (Left Side)

Fig. 2.7. Intercostal scanning on the left side of the abdomen is used to examine the spleen. Splenic examination may be performed with the patient in a right posterior oblique or decubitus position

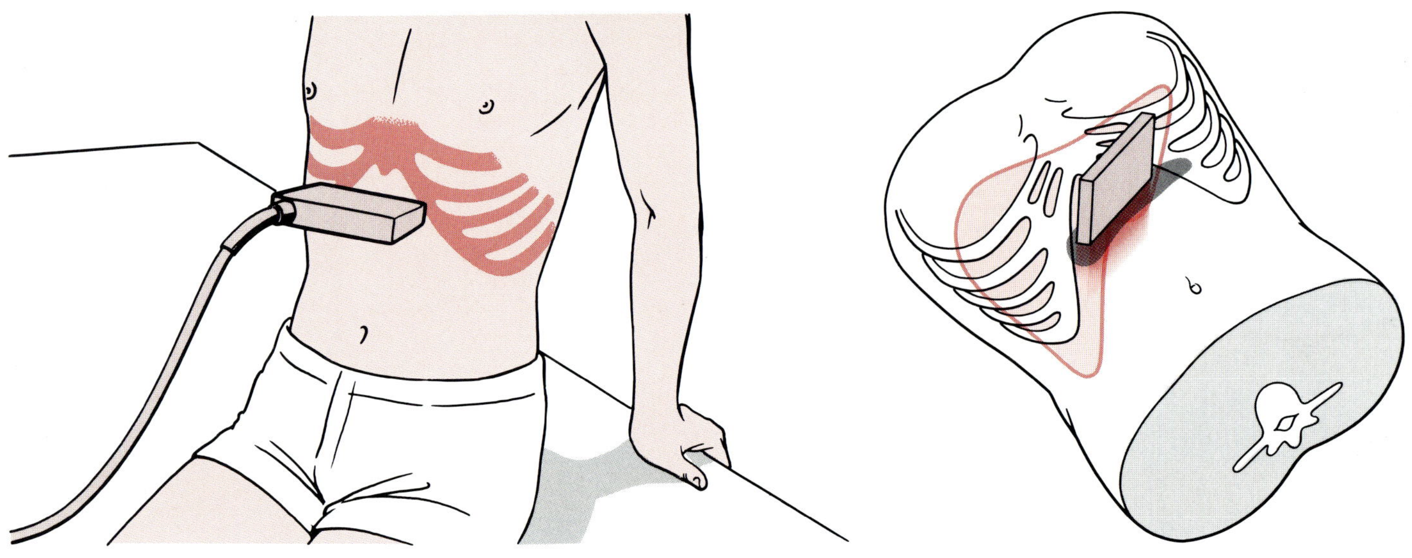

**Scanning
in the Erect (Sitting) Position**

Fig. 2.8. The sitting position can be used for examination of the pancreas. It is most comfortable for the patient to sit with legs dangling over the side of the bed. With oral administration of water, this position is more effective

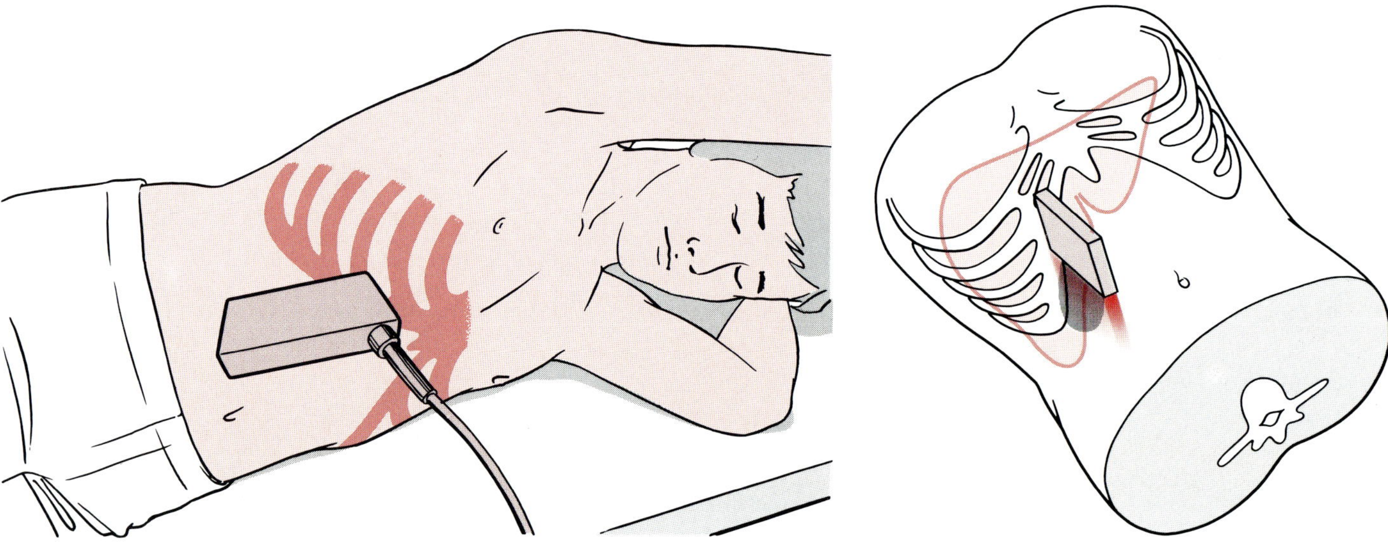

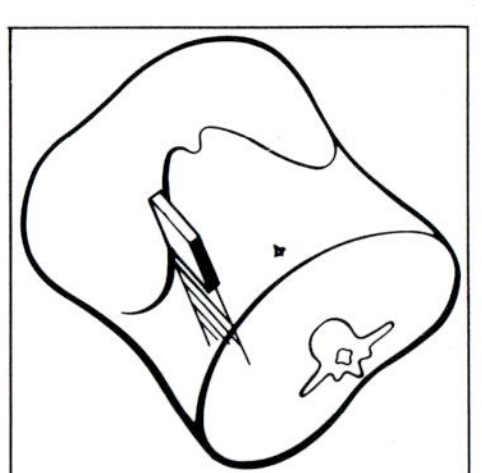

**Scanning
in the Left Decubitus Position**

Fig. 2.9. The extrahepatic bile duct is well visualized in the left decubitus position. The gallbladder may also be well visualized with less overlapping of intestinal gas. Mobility of a gallstone can be observed as the patient moves from the supine to the decubitus position. Finally, this position provides a wider visual field to evaluate the upper portion of the liver

Orientation of Ultrasonographic Images

To facilitate interpretation, image orientation in ultrasonography should be consistent. Widely used conventions are described below.

1. The orientation of transverse sections is the same as in CT in which the images are obtained as though the viewer were positioned at the patient's feet and looking up. The patient's left side is projected on the right side of the image. The oblique section of the pancreas should follow this convention (Fig. 2.10 A, C).
2. The longitudinal section is obtained with the patient's head to the left, feet to the right (Fig. 2.10 A, C).
3. Longitudinal sections of the kidneys with the patient prone are obtained with the same conventions in 2., with the feet to the right. However, on transverse sections of the kidneys with the patient prone, the patient's right is projected on the right side of the image (Fig. 2.10 C).
4. Right-sided intercostal images are obtained with the right side of the image closest to the patient's umbilicus (Fig. 2.10 A).
5. The left-hand side of a left intercostal scan, for example, in images of the left kidney or spleen, is toward the umbilicus (Fig. 2.10 B).

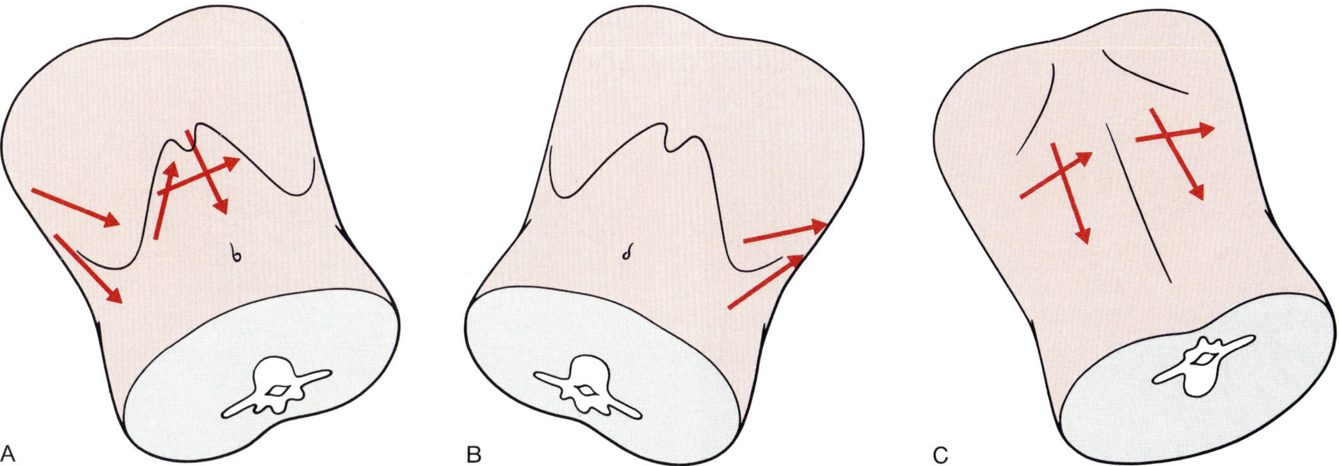

Fig. 2.10 A–C. Conventional orientation of ultrasonographic images. The *heads of the arrows* should be on the right side of the monitor and the film

Patient Preparation

Fasting

The patient should fast for 8–12 h before an ultrasonographic examination of the abdomen. Following food intake, the gallbladder contracts and becomes difficult to visualize. Also, air in the gastrointestinal tract, swallowed at the time of food intake, makes visualization of the abdominal organs difficult. If the purpose of the examination is only to rule out neoplastic lesions of the liver or simply to visualize the size and shape of the kidneys and spleen, fasting is not necessary. In order to rule out gallstones in a patient with acute abdominal pain, ultrasonographic examination should be attempted even if the patient has recently had a meal. Large gallstones or acute cholecystitis can be diagnosed even after a recent meal. If there is inadequate visualization because of intestinal gas, a repeat study could be obtained after fasting.

Distention of the Urinary Bladder

The urinary bladder should be distended when an ultrasonographic examination of the pelvis is performed, especially when the uterus (Fig. 2.11), ovaries, prostate, or urinary bladder are being examined. With an empty urinary bladder, these pelvic organs cannot be well visualized because of interference by gas-containing intestinal loops. In order to ensure a full bladder, patients should be asked to drink large amounts of water 1–2 h before the examination and they must be instructed not to urinate. In examinations of the uterus in the third trimester, a full bladder may not be necessary to visualize the fetus as the enlarged uterus displaces the intestinal loops allowing adequate visualization.

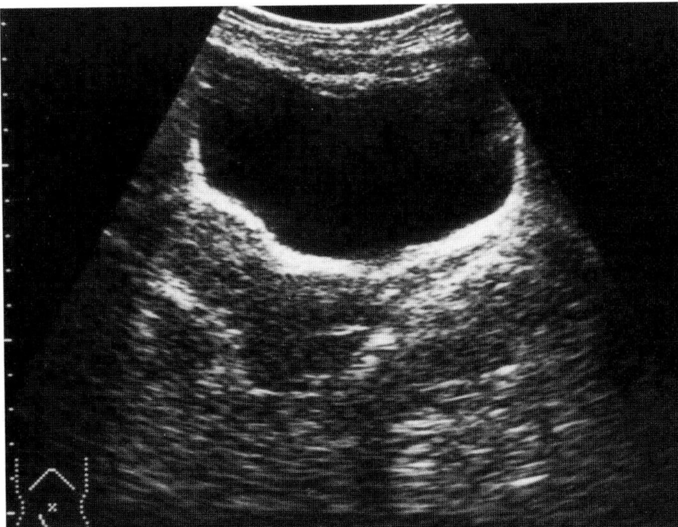
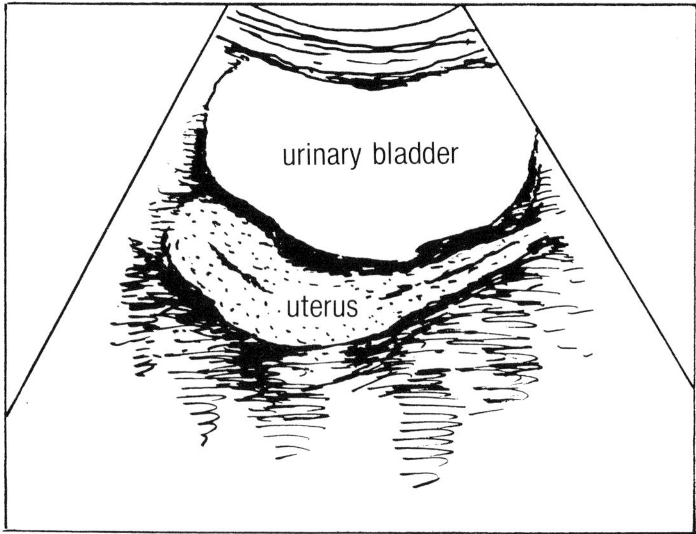

Fig. 2.11. Normal uterus visualized through the full bladder

Elimination of Gas

In some institutions, laxatives are given to patients before ultrasonographic examinations in order to reduce the amount of feces and gas within the colon. However, the effectiveness of laxatives is doubtful as they cannot totally eliminate gas within the colon even though they can reduce the amount of stool. For the same reason, medication for reducing intestinal gas is not effective.

Contact Media

Before an ultrasonographic examination, water-soluble gel or olive oil is applied widely to the skin surface in order to eliminate air between the skin and the probe, allowing for better penetration of the ultrasound beam at the skin surface. These agents are referred to as contact media or coupling media.

Examination Methods

Position

Ultrasonographic examination of the abdomen is performed with the patient in a supine position with the arms either under the head or crossed on the chest. The decubitus or the erect position may be used as needed.

Respiratory Control

Optimal respiration during an ultrasonographic examination of the upper abdomen is important for adequate visualization. Blind spots in the liver, spleen, and kidneys due to overlapping ribs can be eliminated by changing the respiratory phase. The costal cartilages may cause distortion of the liver, spleen, and the right kidney due to refraction of the ultrasound beam obscuring small lesions in these organs. This can be avoided by careful respiratory control. A larger portion of the liver can be visualized by subcostal scanning during deep inspiration.

In inspiration, the liver, which covers the pancreas, can be used as an acoustic window (see below). However, in obese patients or patients with a small left lobe of the liver, the liver cannot be used as an acoustic window. In these situations, the pancreas is better visualized on expiration; interference from intestinal gas will be less. Also, the abdomen expands on inspiration, and the pancreas is then further away from the transducer head. Usually, a larger portion of the spleen is visualized during expiration.

Acoustic Window

The abdominal organs which have intestine interposed between them and the abdominal wall cannot be visualized because gas within the intestine will reflect most of the ultrasound beam. On the other hand, solid organs, such as the liver, spleen, and kidneys, and the fluid-filled urinary bladder cause little attenuation of the ultrasound beam, resulting in good visualization of the structures deep to these organs. These organs which serve as good pathways of ultrasound are called "acoustic windows". When utilizing a sector probe, a large area can be examined with only a small acoustic window.

Routine Examination of the Upper Abdomen

Fig. 2.12. *Note:* the schemata illustrate standard patterns and do not necessarily correspond to the ultrasonographic images

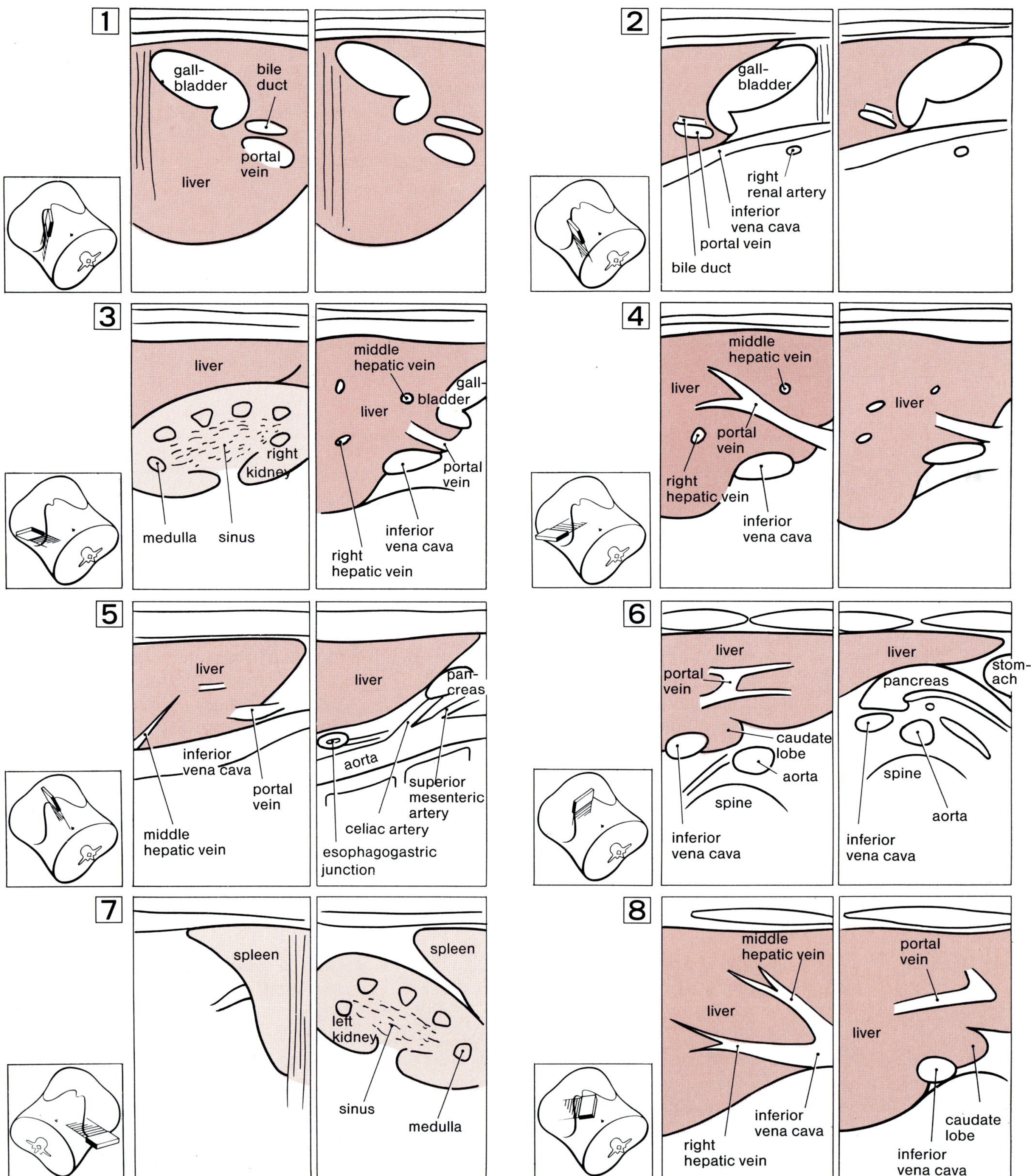

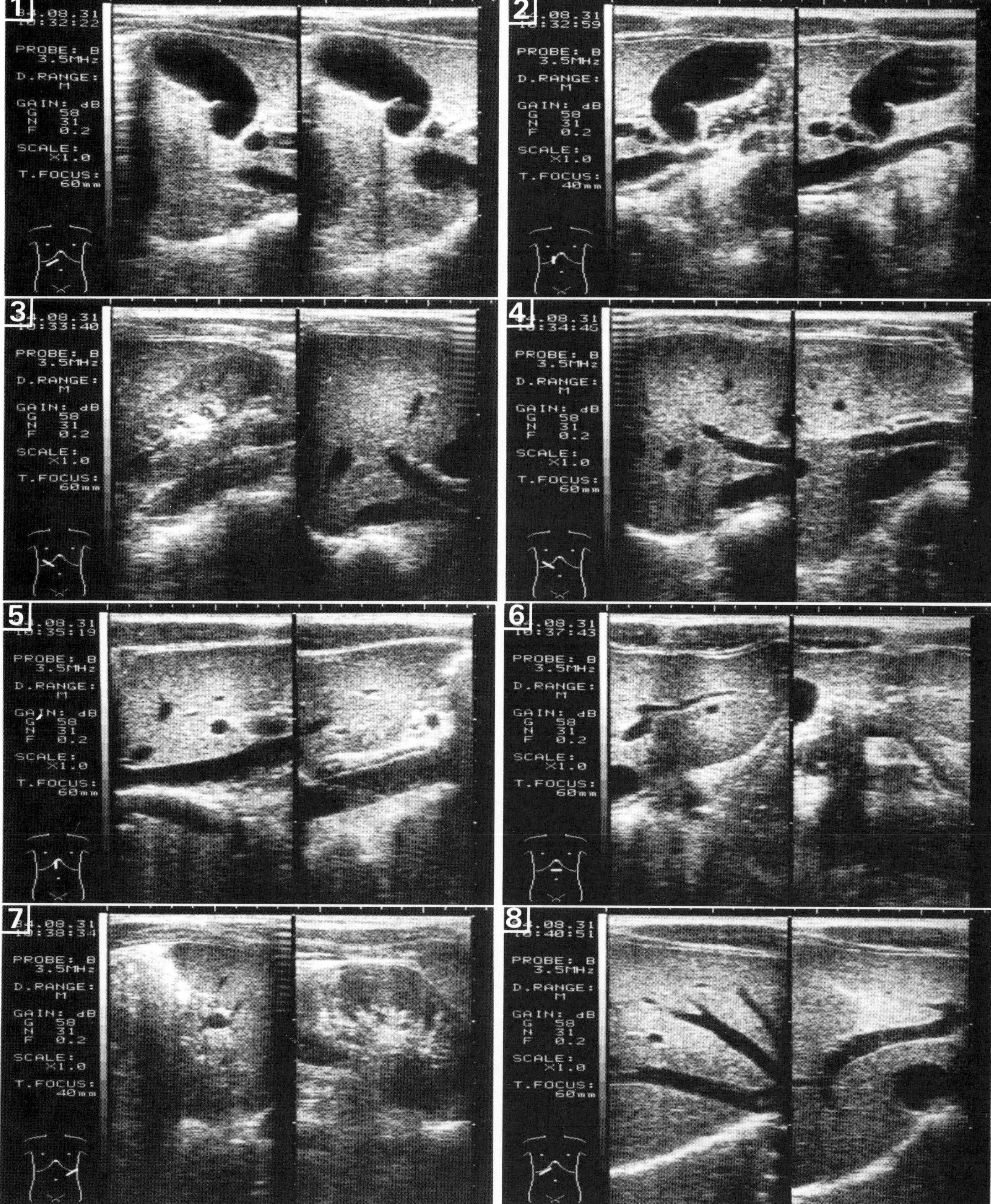

Sectional Anatomy

Although it is a great advantage that an ultrasonographic examination can be done in transverse, sagittal, coronal, and oblique planes, it is at the same time a disadvantage because it may make interpretation more complex and difficult. An understanding of anatomy is essential to obtaining the appropriate ultrasonographic images and in their interpretation.

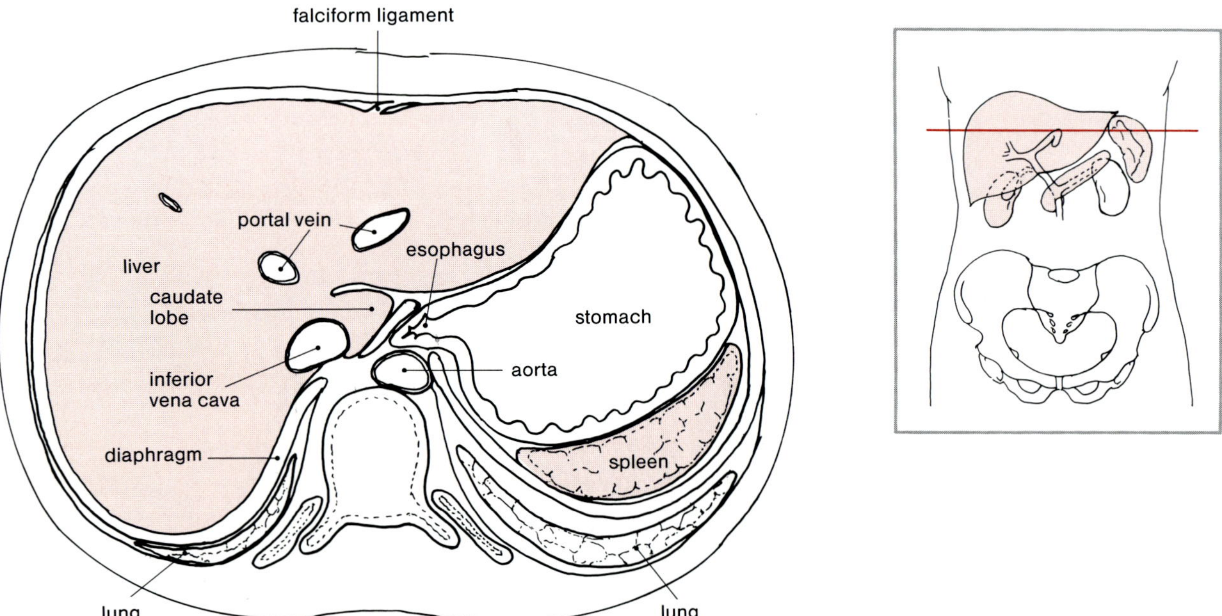

Fig. 2.13. *Transverse image at T10.* Note the relationship between the caudate lobe and the inferior vena cava, aorta and esophagus, stomach and spleen, and spleen and the left lower lobe of the lung

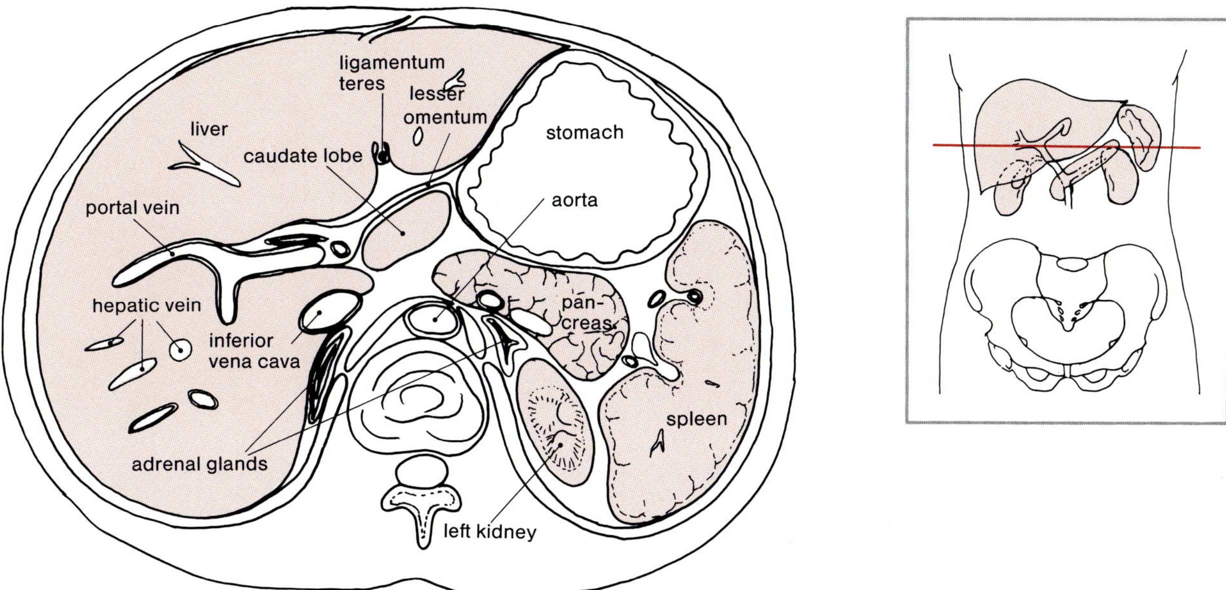

Fig. 2.14. *Transverse image at the thoracolumbar junction.* Note the relative positions of the tail of the pancreas, upper pole of the left kidney, spleen, and stomach

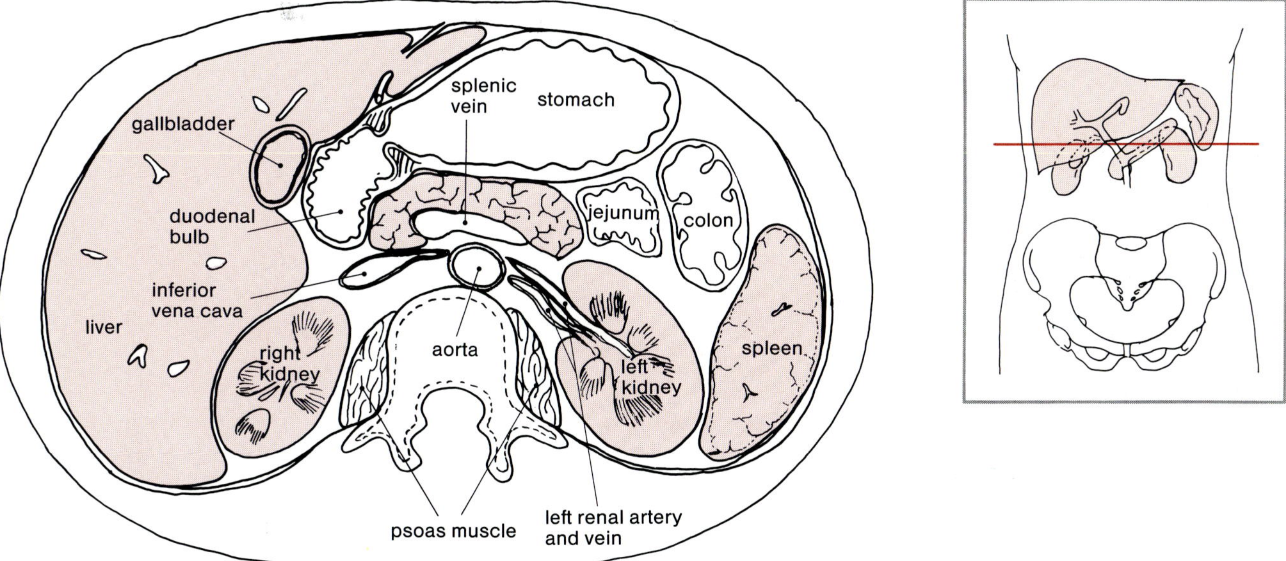

Fig. 2.15. *Transverse image at L2.* Note the relative position of the gallbladder, duodenal bulb, and the pancreatic head. Also note the relationship of the liver and right kidney, kidneys and psoas muscles, and left kidney and the spleen

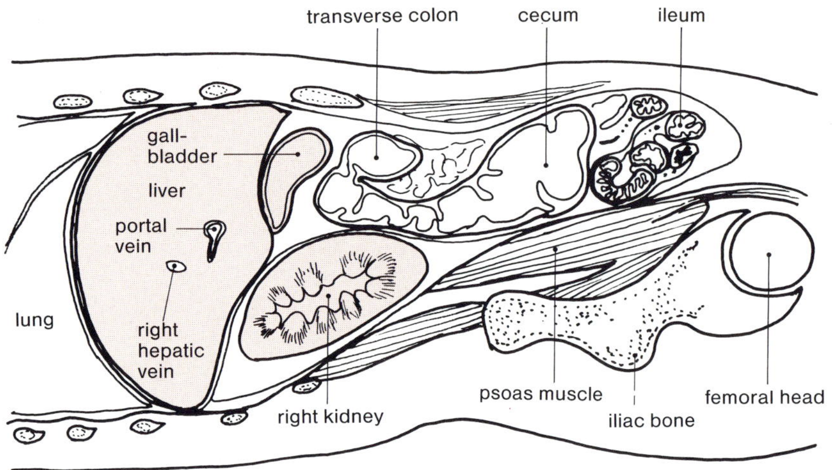

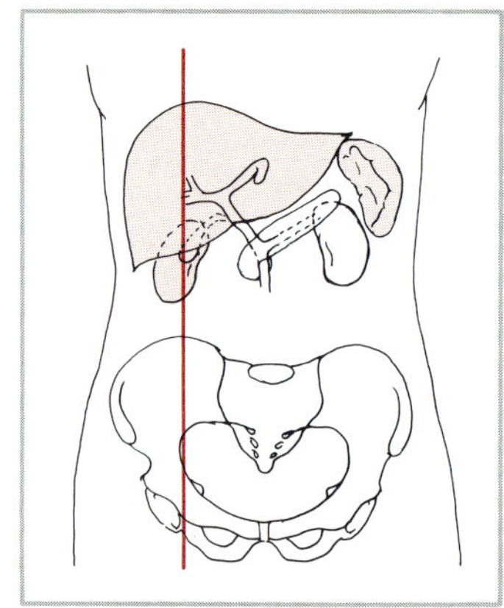

Figs. 2.16–2.21. Continuous sagittal images of the abdomen

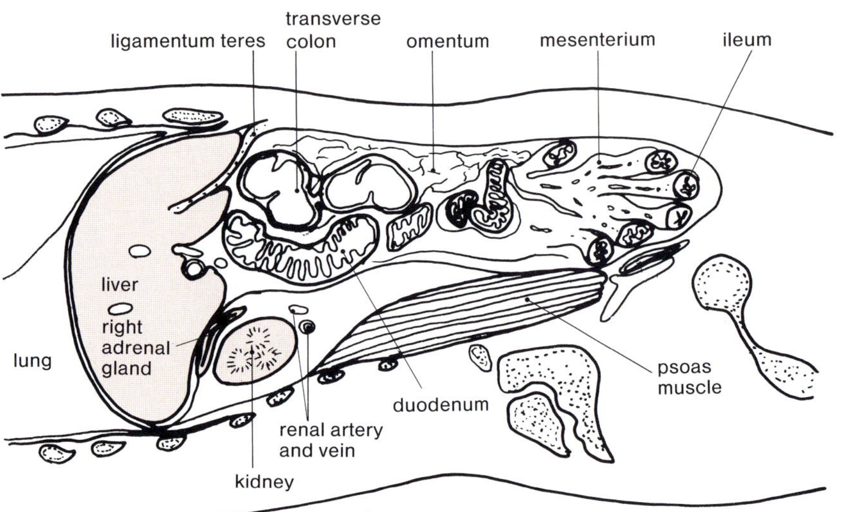

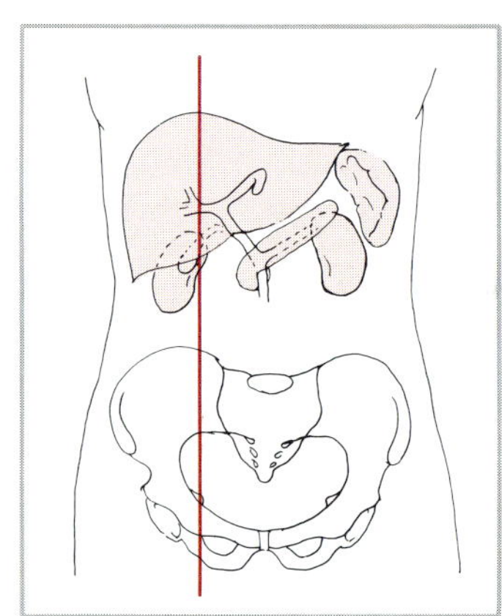

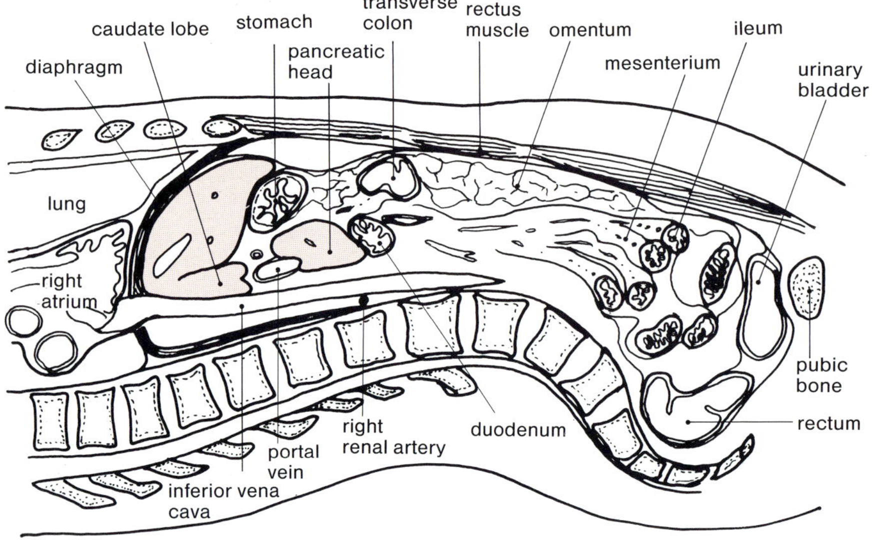

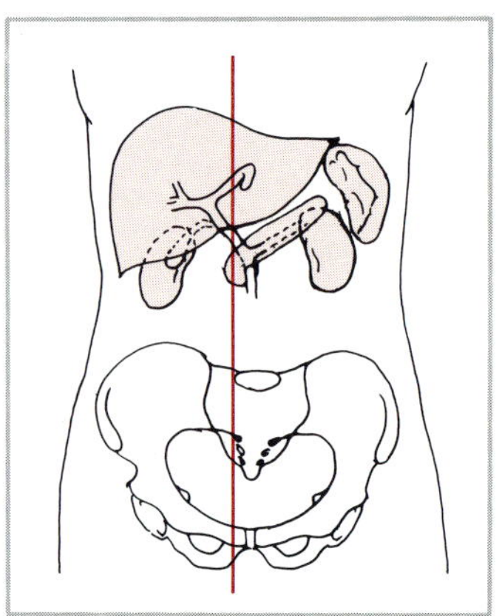

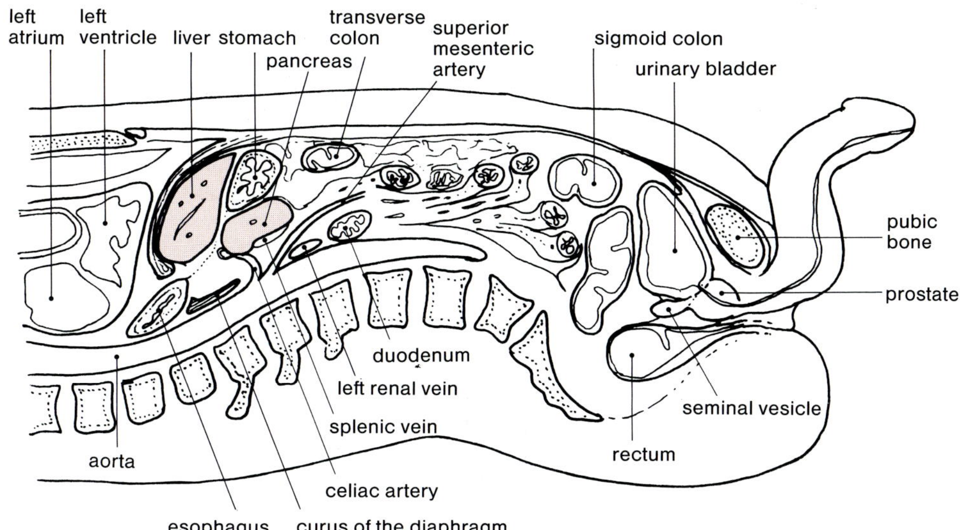

left atrium
left ventricle
liver
stomach
pancreas
transverse colon
superior mesenteric artery
sigmoid colon
urinary bladder
pubic bone
prostate
seminal vesicle
rectum
duodenum
left renal vein
splenic vein
celiac artery
aorta
esophagus
curus of the diaphragm

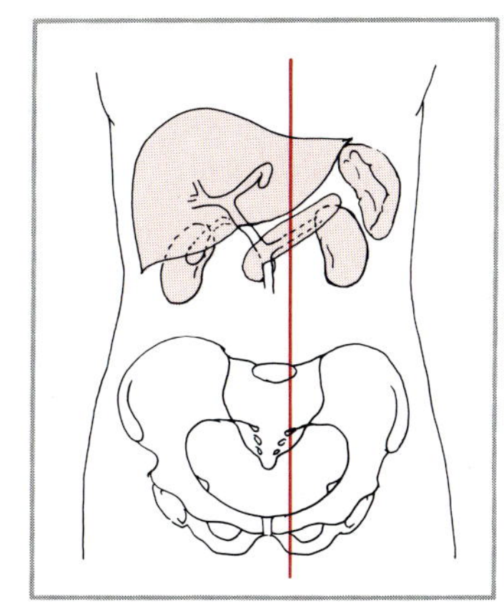
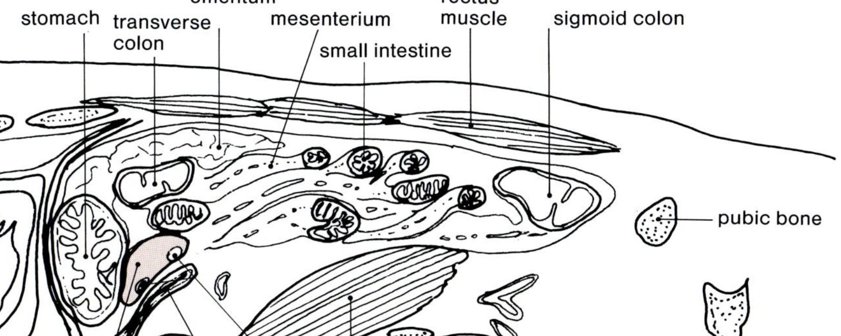

stomach
transverse colon
omentum
mesenterium
small intestine
rectus muscle
sigmoid colon
pubic bone
psoas muscle
splenic artery and vein
adrenal gland
pancreas
left kidney

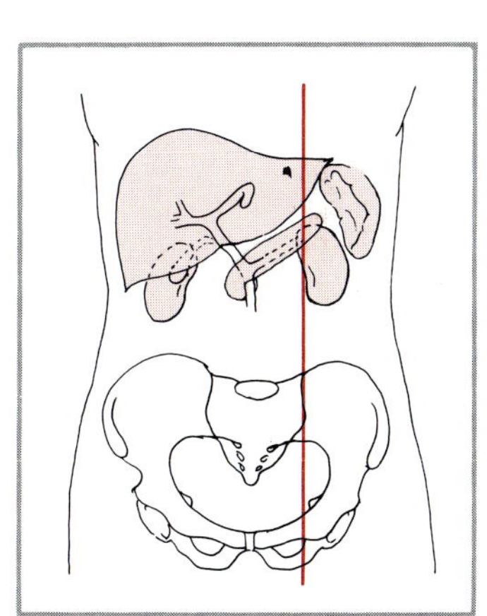
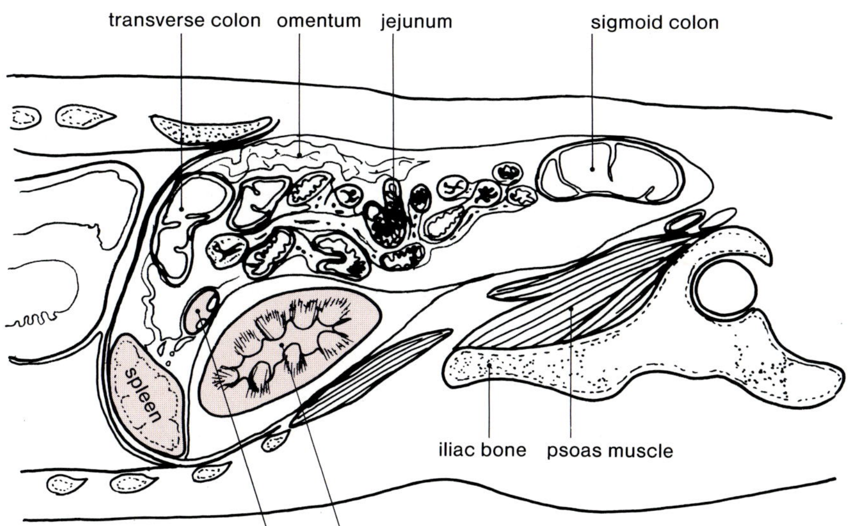

transverse colon
omentum
jejunum
sigmoid colon
spleen
iliac bone
psoas muscle
pancreas
left kidney

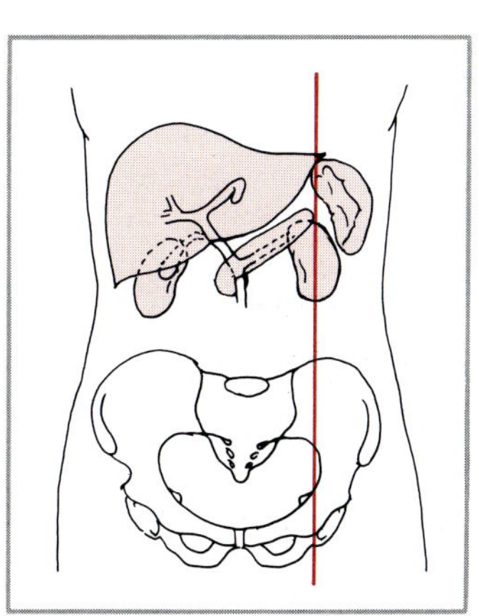

Normal Ultrasonogram of the Upper Abdomen

Fig. 2.22 A–F. For a better understanding of the entire upper abdomen, images obtained with a contact compound scanner are shown. **A–D** Transverse images 2 cm apart. The portal vein and hepatic veins are clearly visualized within the liver. The left upper quadrant is not clearly visualized because of gas-containing structures such as the stomach, and small and large intestine. **E** Subcostal scan showing the right and middle hepatic veins. A cross-section of the anterior segmental branch of the right portal vein is visualized between these two. **F** Longitudinal section along the abdominal aorta. The pancreas is seen posterior to the liver. The origins of the celiac artery and the superior mesenteric artery are visualized

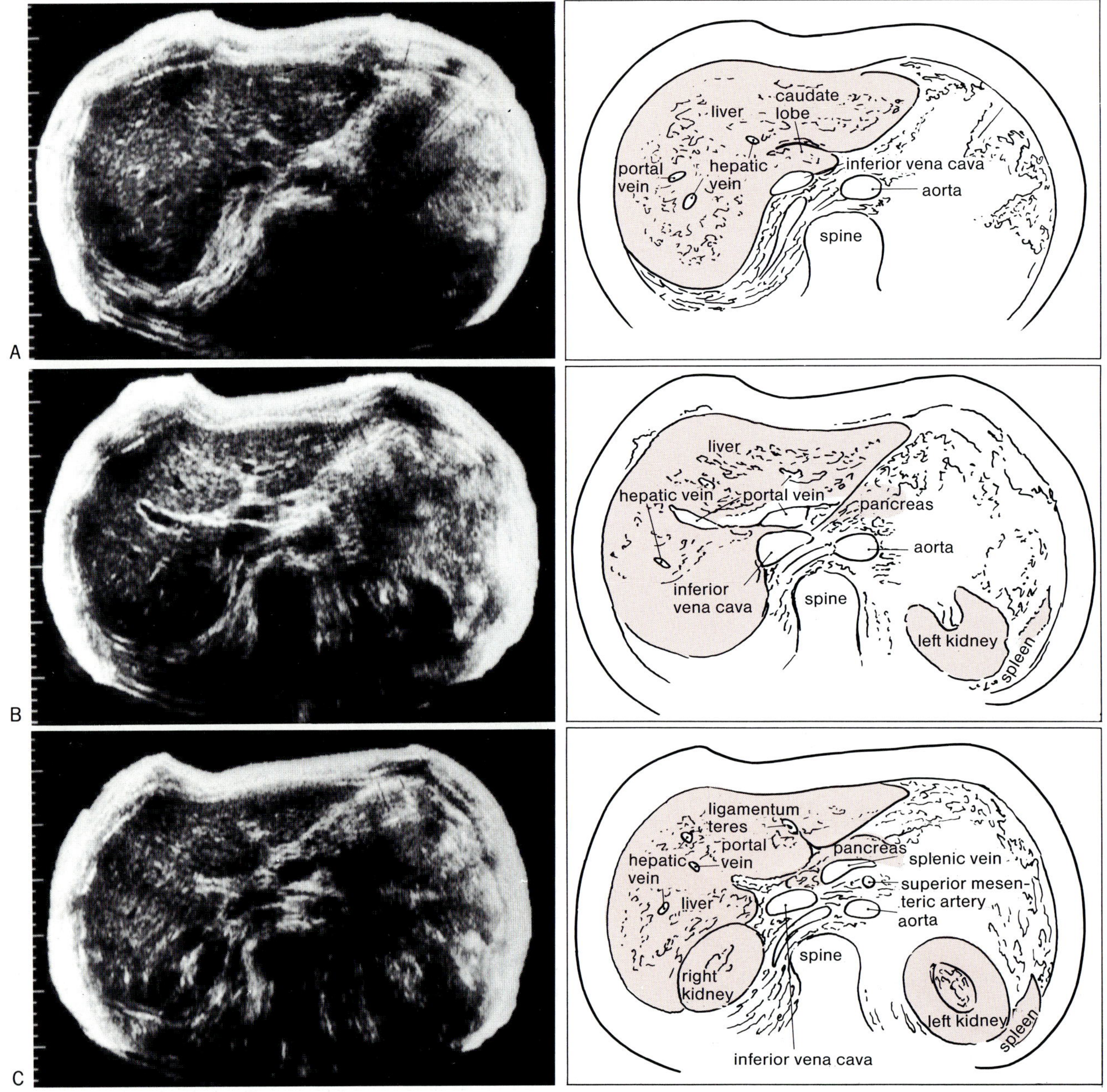

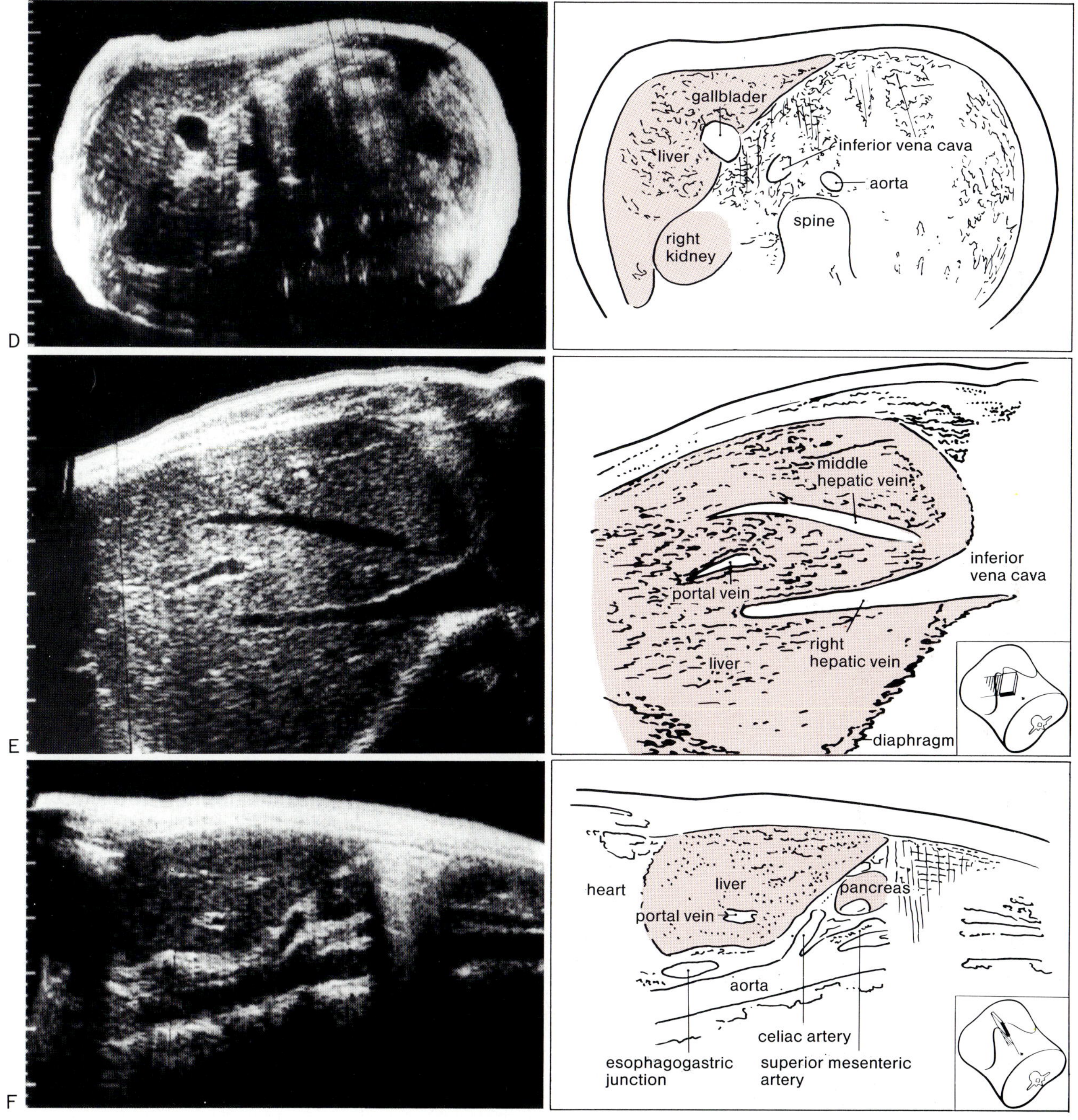
gallblader
liver
inferior vena cava
aorta
spine
right
kidney
middle
hepatic vein
inferior
vena cava
portal vein
right
hepatic vein
liver
diaphragm
heart
liver
pancreas
portal vein
aorta
celiac artery
esophagogastric
junction
superior mesenteric
artery
D
E
F

3 Liver

Anatomy of the Liver

The liver is divided into the right and left lobes by the main lobar fissure. The right lobe is further divided into an anterior and a posterior segment, and the left lobe is divided into a medial and a lateral segment. The main lobar fissure is in a plane which can be approximated by drawing a line connecting the gallbladder bed and the inferior vena cava (Cantlie line). The middle hepatic vein courses within the main lobar fissure. The right hepatic vein runs between the anterior and the posterior segments of the right lobe. The falciform ligament, which contains the ligamentum teres, separates the medial from the lateral segment of the left lobe.

Ultrasonographically, each segment of the liver can be identified by recognizing the associated hepatic portal venous structures. However, since membranous structures, such as the interlobar pleura of the lungs, do not exist between the segments of the liver, the planes between the segments cannot be visualized, and the segments appear contiguous. If an abnormality (e.g., tumor) is a distance from the main vascular structures, it can be difficult to determine the segment in which the abnormality exists.

The anterior and posterior segments of the right lobe and the lateral segment of the left lobe are further divided into superior and inferior subsegments. The caudate lobe should be considered as a structure separate from the left and right lobes. It is bounded posteriorly by the fossa of the inferior vena cava and anteriorly by the fissure of the ligamentum venosum. In this way, the liver is divided into subsegments which are numbered 1 to 8 (Fig. 3.1).

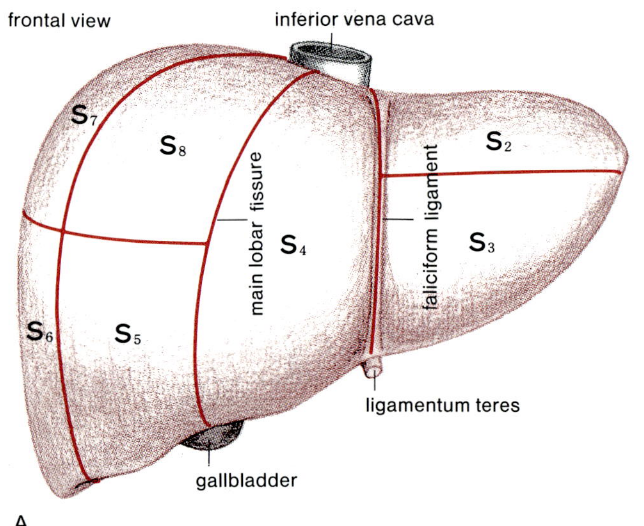

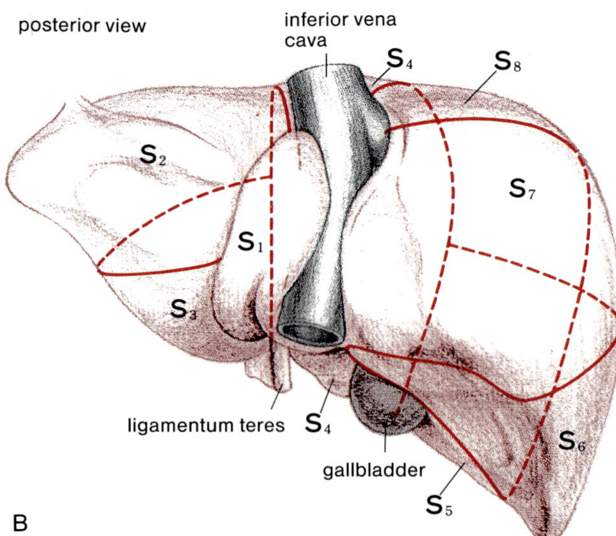

Fig. 3.1 A, B. *Hepatic segments according to Couinaud.* **A** Frontal view with main lobar fissure; **B** posterior view. S_1, caudate lobe; S_2, lateral superior segment; S_3, lateral inferior segment; S_4, medial segment; S_5, anterior inferior segment; S_6, posterior inferior segment; S_7, posterior superior segment; S_8, anterior superior segment

Intrahepatic Tubular Structures

There are four types of tubular structures in the liver: hepatic arteries, hepatic veins, portal veins, and bile ducts. Only the hepatic and portal veins are visualized on ultrasonography. The bile ducts are visualized only when dilated. The hepatic arteries are not visualized in the liver because of their small size.

There are three major hepatic veins which converge and enter the inferior vena cava as it penetrates the diaphragm. The hepatic veins and the portal veins can be easily differentiated on ultrasonography as they have different courses within the liver which criss-cross each other. Another important differentiating point is that portal veins have echogenic walls, whereas the hepatic veins do not.

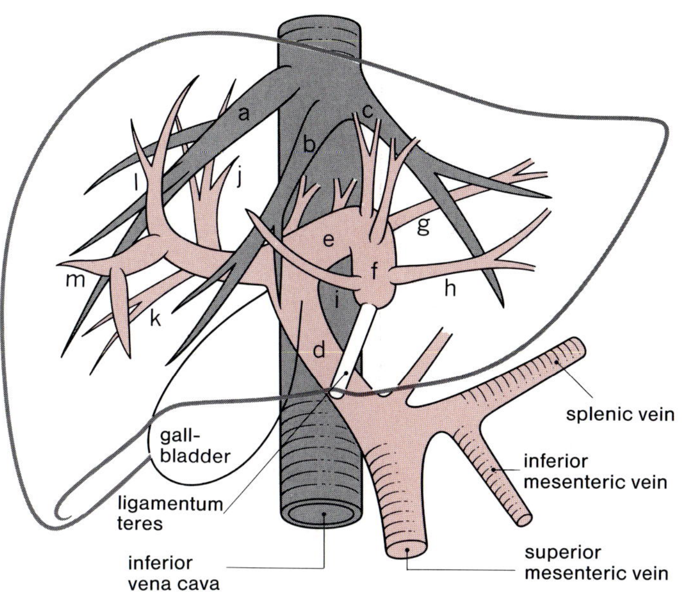

Fig. 3.2. *Intrahepatic portal vein and hepatic vein. a*, right heptic vein; *b*, middle hepatic vein; *c*, left hepatic vein; *d*, main portal vein; *e*, horizontal portion of left portal vein; *f*, umbilical portion of left portal vein; *g*, branch to the lateral superior segment of the left lobe; *h*, branch to the lateral inferior segment of the left lobe; *i*, branch to the medial segment of the left lobe; *j*, branch to the posterior superior segment of the right lobe; *k*, branch to the posterior inferior segment of the right lobe; *l*, branch to the anterior superior segment of the right lobe; *m*, branch to the anterior inferior segment of the right lobe

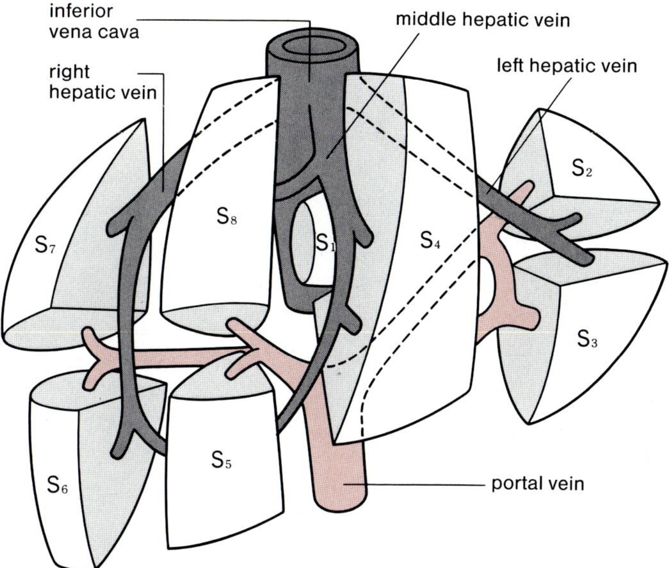

Fig. 3.3 *Hepatic segments and hepatic veins.* Each hepatic subsegment is illustrated as a separate structure. Note that the right and middle hepatic veins run between the hepatic segments, whereas the major branches of the portal vein are distributed in the center of the hepatic segments

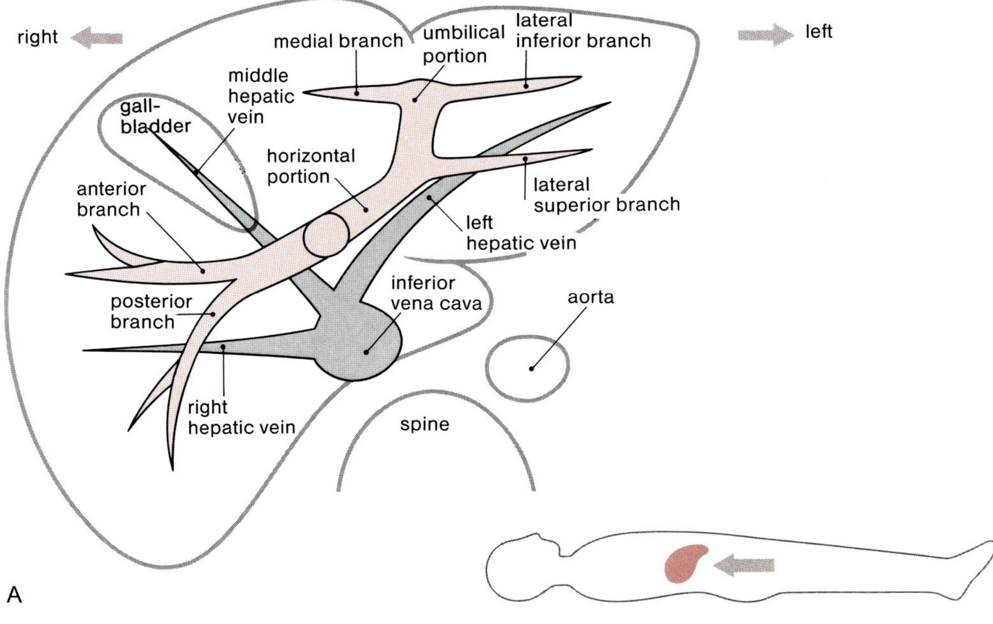

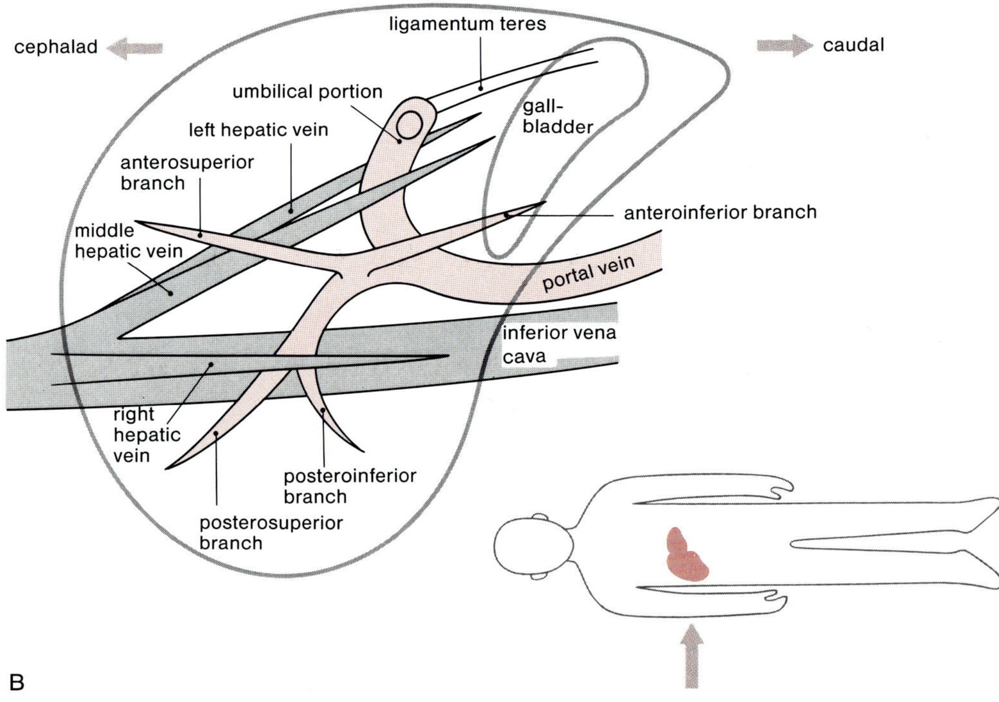

Fig. 3.4 A, B. *Vascular structures in the liver*. **A** Vascular structures seen from below. A craniocaudal radiograph of a cadaver torso with contrast material in the vessels would look like this. **B** Intrahepatic vessels observed from the right side. This would be similar to a lateral radiograph of the abdomen with contrast material in the vascular structures

Scanning Techniques and Intrahepatic Vessels

Intercostal or subcostal scanning of the liver is employed because the liver is surrounded by ribs. The relationship between the vascular structures which are visualized by these methods and the direction of the ultrasound beam is shown in Figs. 3.5–3.9. The portal veins are depicted in red and the hepatic veins in blue. Dark red designates the portal branches that are in the scanning plane (the ultrasonographic plane is depicted in yellow). Similarly, dark blue designates the hepatic veins which are in the scanning plane. On each figure, the image of the scanning plane seen from the reverse side is drawn as it would be seen on the monitor of the ultrasonographic equipment.

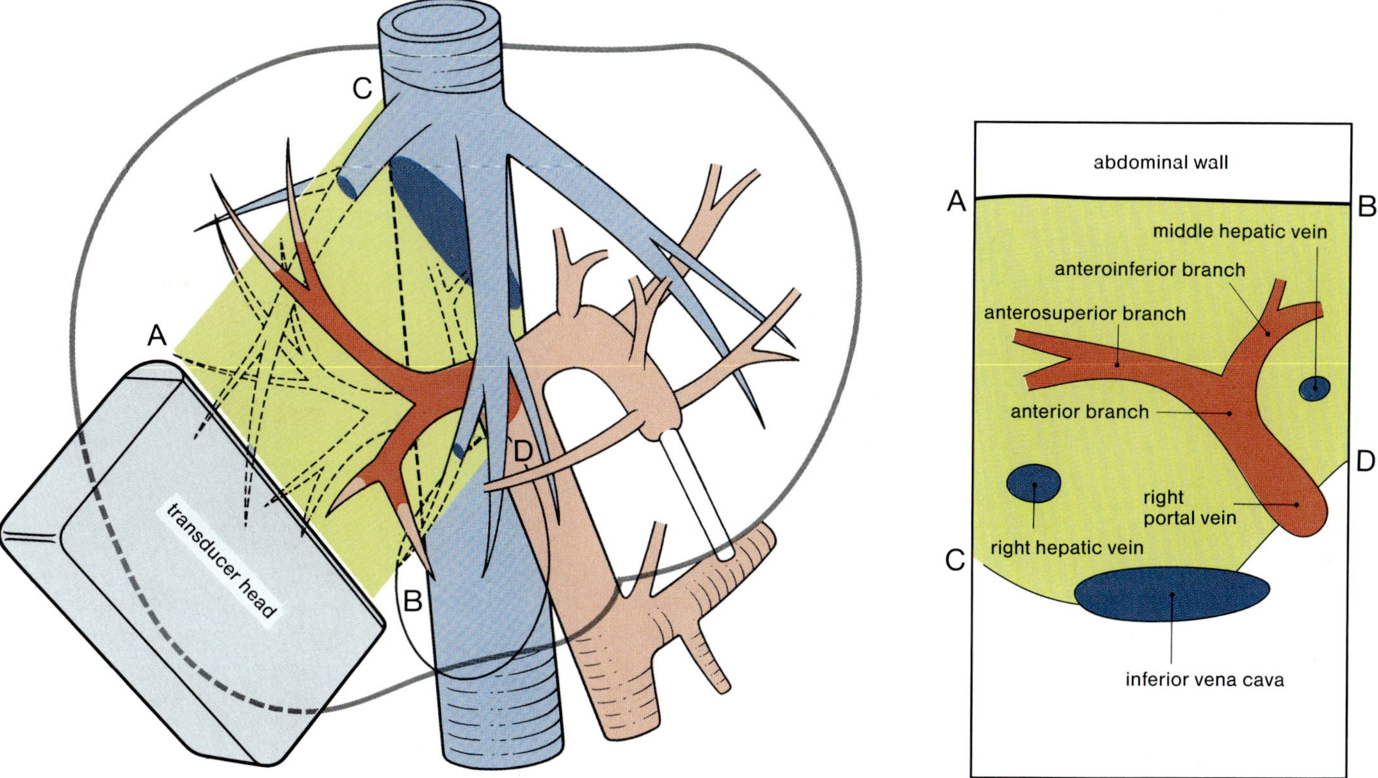

Fig. 3.5. Intercostal scan from the patient's right side. The portal branches depicted in *dark red* in the scanning plane as shown on the left will be visualized on the monitor as shown on the right

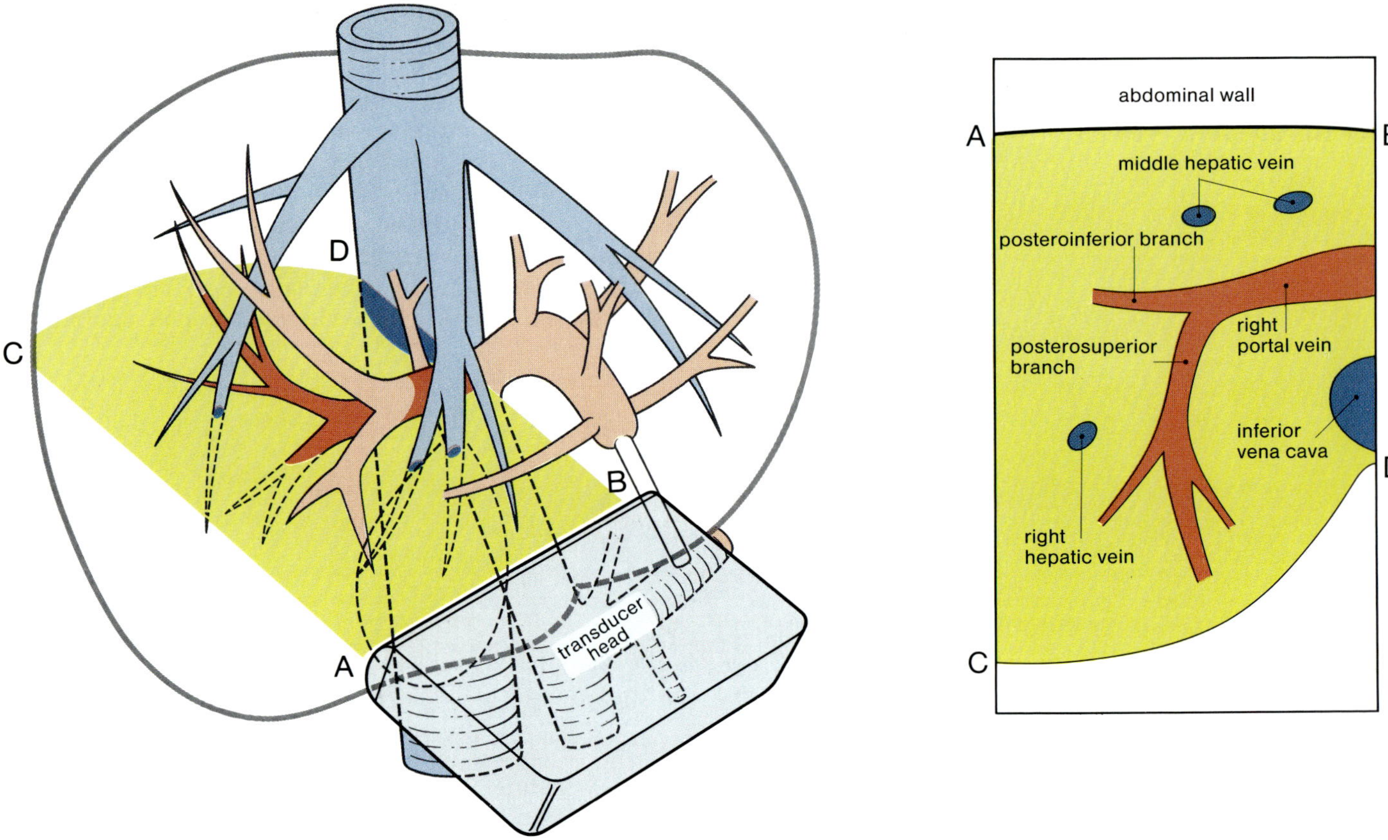

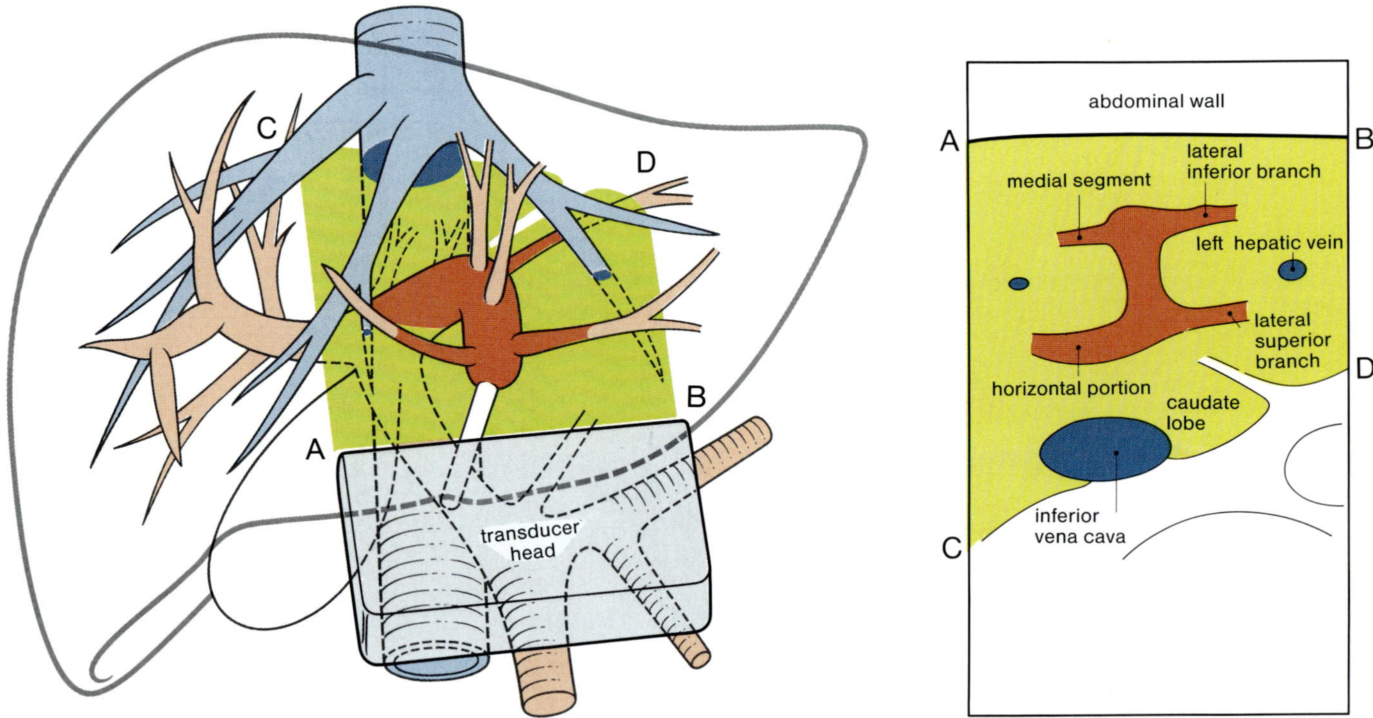

Fig. 3.6. Portal branches in a plane obtained with subcostal scanning

Fig. 3.7. How the horizontal portion of the left portal vein, the umbilical portion and its branches, is visualized as an "H" lying on its side on transverse scanning performed in the midline of upper abdomen

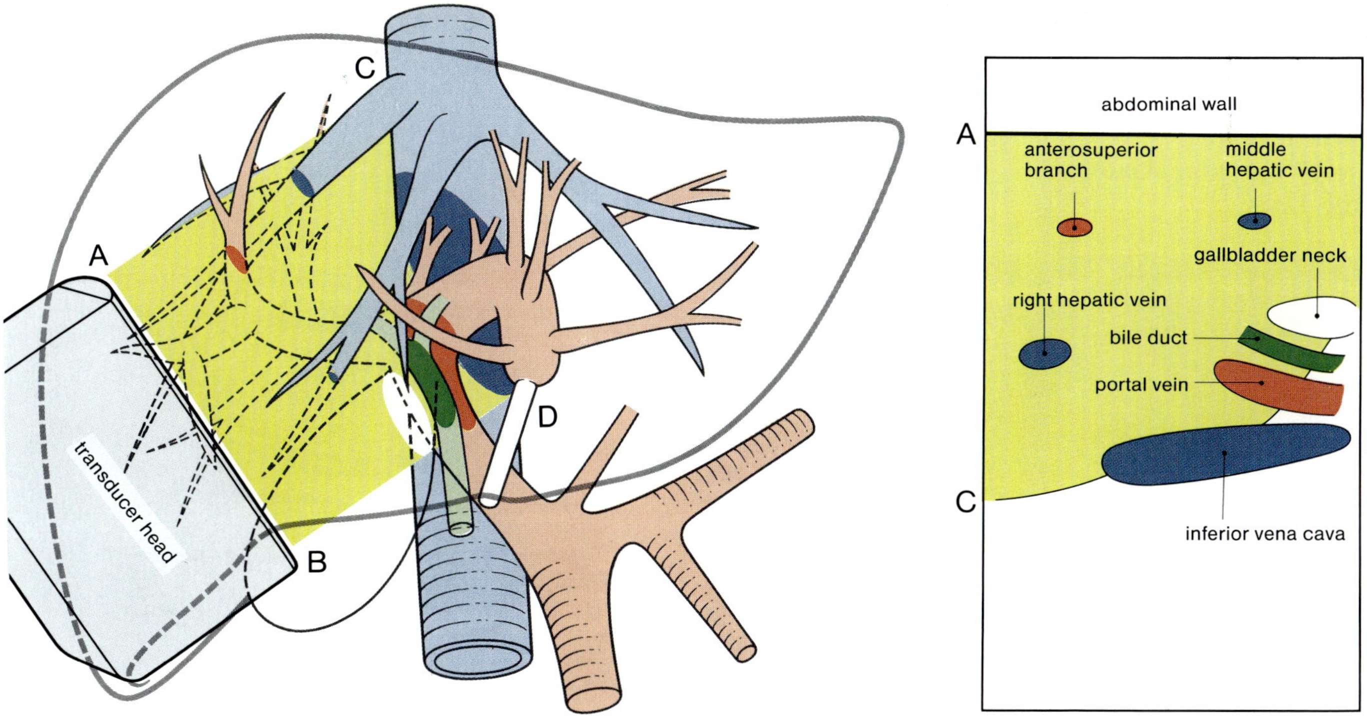

Fig. 3.8. Vascular structures as visualized in the region of the porta hepatis on intercostal scanning

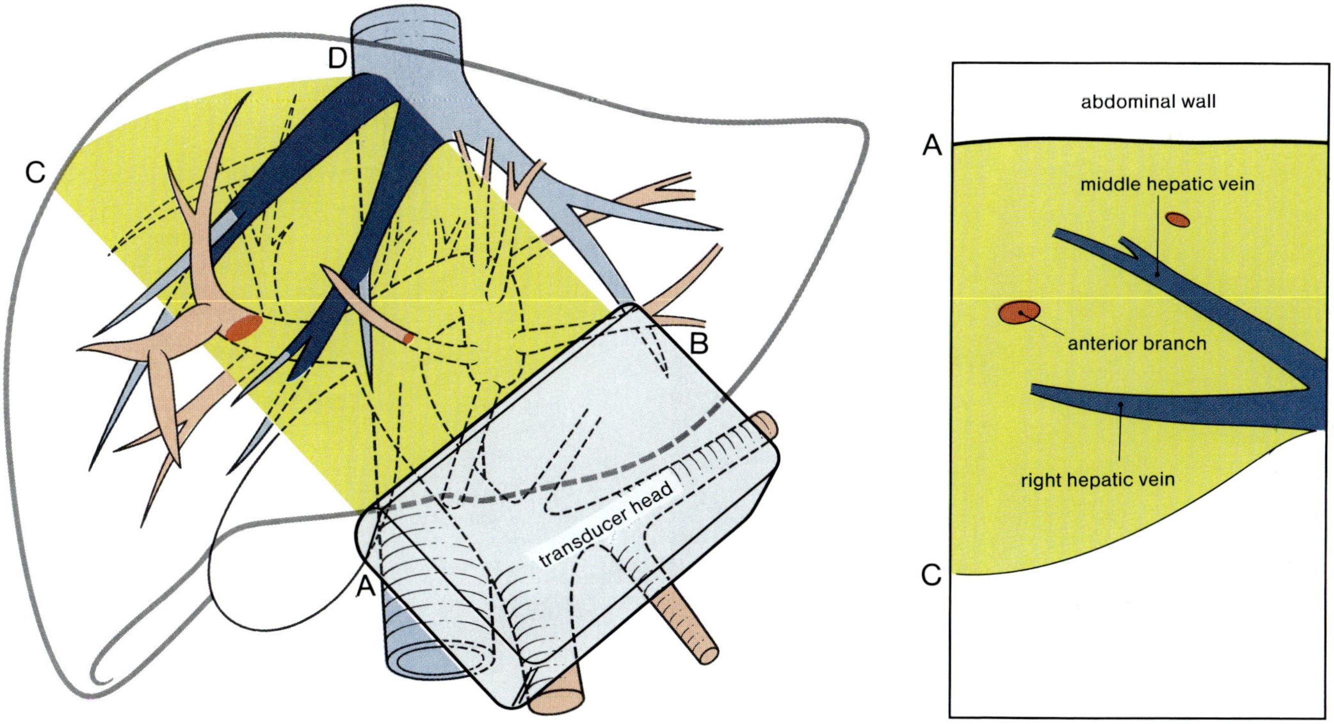

Fig. 3.9. Right and middle hepatic veins as visualized on subcostal scanning

Ultrasonographic Appearance of Normal Vascular Anatomy of the Liver

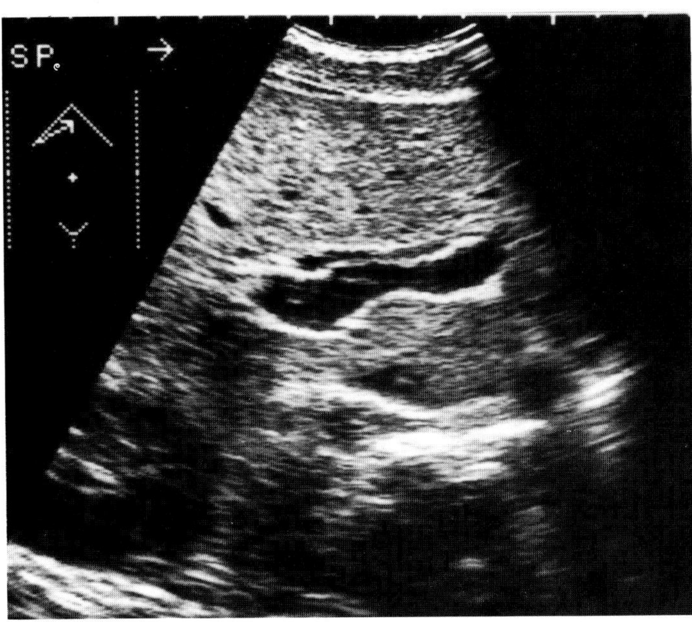

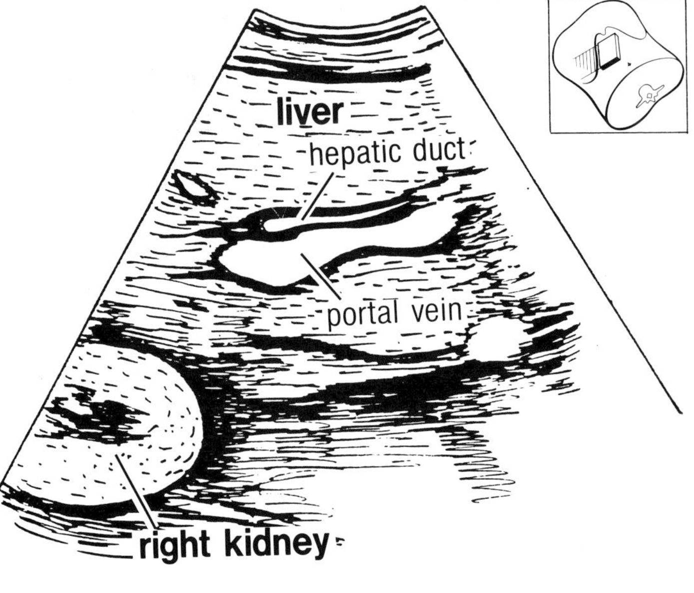

Fig. 3.10. *The horizontal portion of the portal vein and the hepatic duct.* The horizontal segment of the left portal vein is clearly visualized. The small tubular structure anterior to it is the hepatic duct (primary branch of the intrahepatic bile duct). Normally, the intrahepatic bile duct is visualized only to this level, and more peripheral branches are not seen unless they are dilated

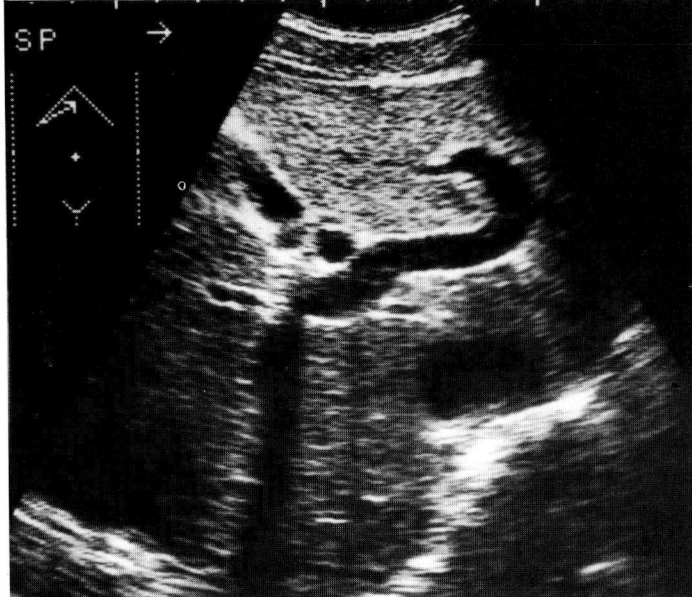

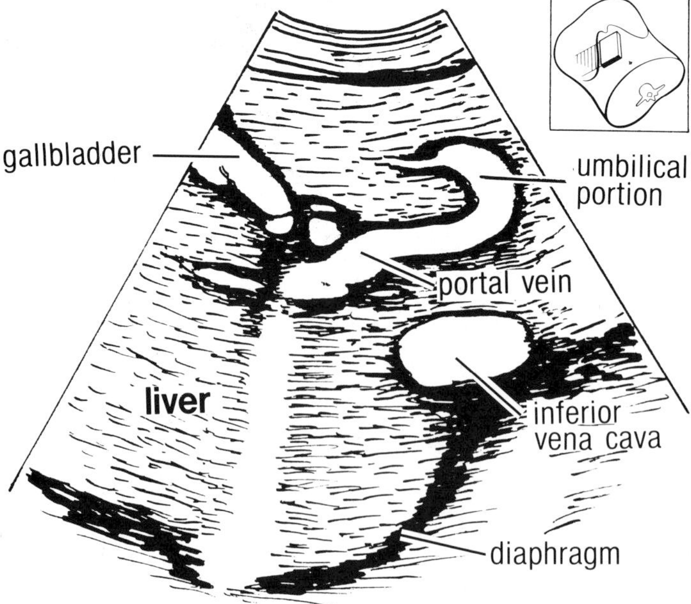

Fig. 3.11. *The horizontal and umbilical portions of the portal vein.* Same case as in Fig. 3.10. While visualization of the hepatic duct was the intent of the image in Fig. 3.10, on this image, the left portal vein is well visualized. Slight changes in angulation of the transducer head greatly changes the appearance of the vessels in the liver

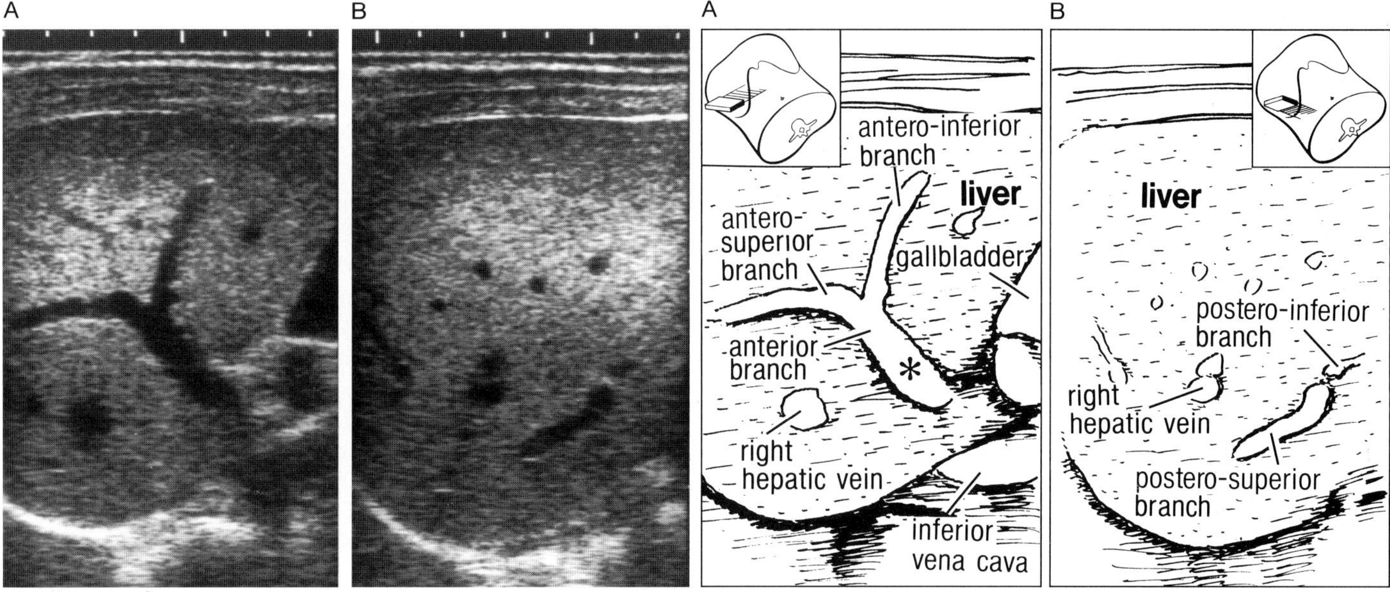

Fig. 3.12 A, B. *Anterior and posterior segmental branches of the portal system.* An intercostal scan of the intrahepatic portal veins. Division of the anterior segmental branch into the anterosuperior and the anteroinferior segmental branches is shown in **A**. **B** Branching of the posterior segmental branch is seen as imaged from the intercostal space one below the image in **A**. This posterior segmental branch originated from the portion of the vessel labeled with an asterisk on the sketch in **A**

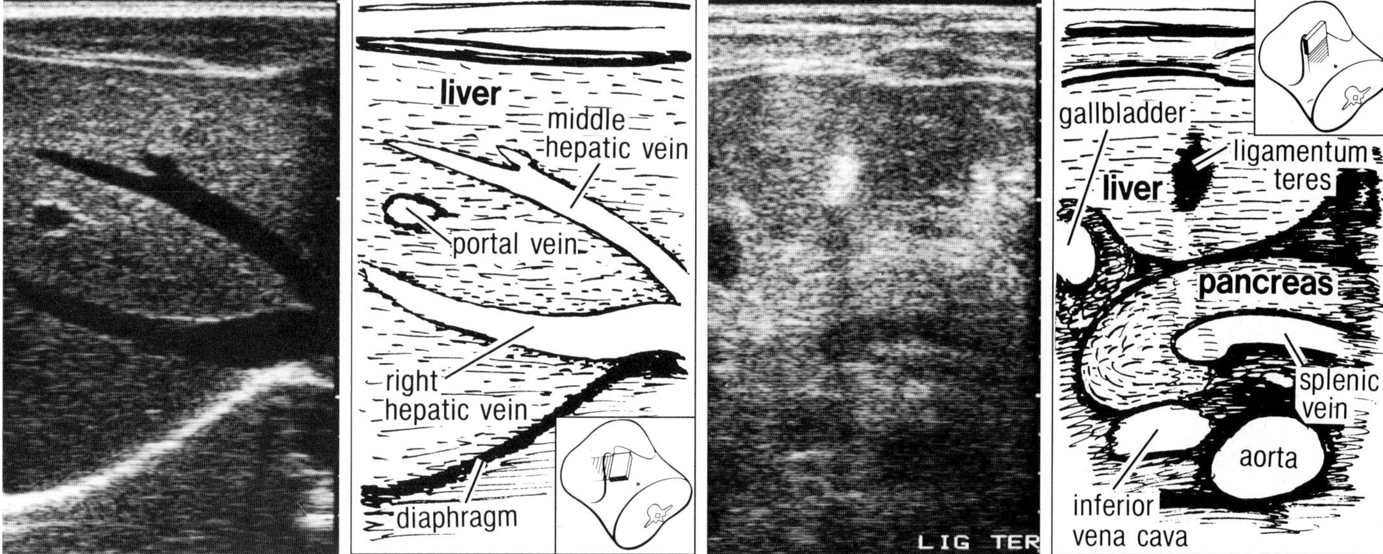

Fig. 3.13. *Right and middle hepatic veins.* On this subcostal scan, the right and middle hepatic veins are visualized on a single plane. Between these veins is a section of the anterior segmental branch of the portal vein

Fig. 3.14. *The ligamentum teres.* A transverse image in the midline of the epigastrium. The hyperechoic focus accompanied by acoustic shadowing is the ligamentum teres. It is the adipose tissue around the ligamentum teres which produces such a strong echo

Hepatic Tumors

Echo Pattern

Hepatic tumors can be divided into the following eight ultrasonographic patterns:

1. *Hyperechoic mass* (Fig. 3.15): tumor with greater echogenicity than the surrounding normal liver parenchyma. Hemangiomas are the most common tumors of this type. Tumors with degeneration, necrosis, or fat may also have this appearance.
2. *Hypoechoic mass* (Fig. 3.16): tumors with less echogenicity than normal liver tissue. Tumors consisting of homogeneous substances have this appearance. Small hepatocellular carcinomas are typical of this group.
3. *Bull's eye or target sign* (Fig. 3.17): tumors which are isoechoic to, or slightly more hyperechoic than normal liver tissue and are surrounded by a hypoechoic rim (halo). The rim may be thick (3–5 mm), relative to the size of the tumor, or thin (1–2 mm). The former is often seen with metastatic tumors and is called a bull's eye. The latter is seen with hepatocellular carcinomas having expansile growth.
4. *Mass of mixed echogenicity* (Fig. 3.18): heterogeneous tumors with mixed hyper- and hypoechoic areas. This pattern is seen when hypoechoic areas develop secondary to bleeding or degeneration in an initially hyperechoic tumor.
5. *Mosaic pattern* (Fig. 3.19): mosaic pattern, also called "tumor in a tumor", exhibits hypoechoic septal structures and is seen only in tumors of at least 4 cm in size. This pattern is said to be typical of hepatocellular carcinoma; however, it is not often seen. Metastases may also demonstrate this pattern.

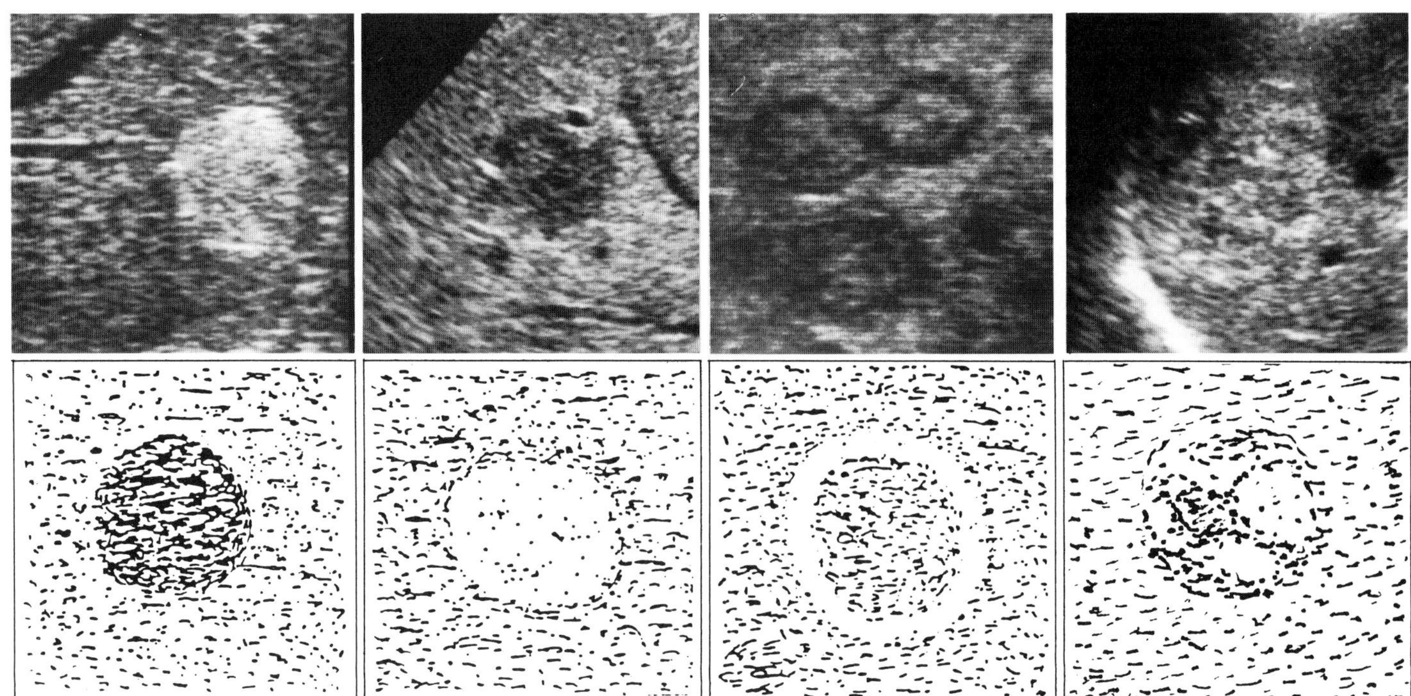

Fig. 3.15. Hyperechoic mass   **Fig. 3.16.** Hypoechoic mass   **Fig. 3.17.** Bull's eye or target sign   **Fig. 3.18.** Mixed echogenicity

6. *Central necrosis pattern* (Fig. 3.20): as a tumor such as hepatocellular carcinoma or metastatic tumor grows, a central anechoic area develops secondary to liquefactive necrosis. Metastatic tumors, especially from malignancies of the female reproductive system, often demonstrate this pattern.

7. *Calcification* (Fig. 3.21): calcified tumors are uncommon, but can be seen in metastatic tumors from mucin-producing carcinomas of the colon or stomach. Ultrasonographically, calcifications demonstrate strong echoes with acoustic shadowing.

8. *Diffuse infiltrative growth* (Fig. 3.22): this pattern is seen when a multinodular hepatocellular carcinoma enlarges and becomes coalescent, and in the case of a tumor with diffusely infiltrating growth. The contour of the lesion is indistinct.

The echo pattern of hepatic tumors is basically divided as above. Some investigators describe further classifications of hepatic tumors and try to correlate these echo patterns with various types of hepatic tumors (hepatocellular carcinoma, metastatic tumor, cholangiocarcinoma, cavernous hemangioma, hepatic adenoma, focal nodular hyperplasia, etc.). Although there is some statistical correlation, it is often difficult to determine the nature of the tumor in any given case based only on the ultrasonographic examination.

Other imaging modalities (such as CT or angiography), biochemical data (including alpha-fetoprotein and carcinoembryonic antigen), and clinical history should also be considered. In certain cases, a follow-up examination may be necessary. When the tumor is small, final diagnosis has to be made by biopsy; however, biopsy cannot always determine the histologic diagnosis.

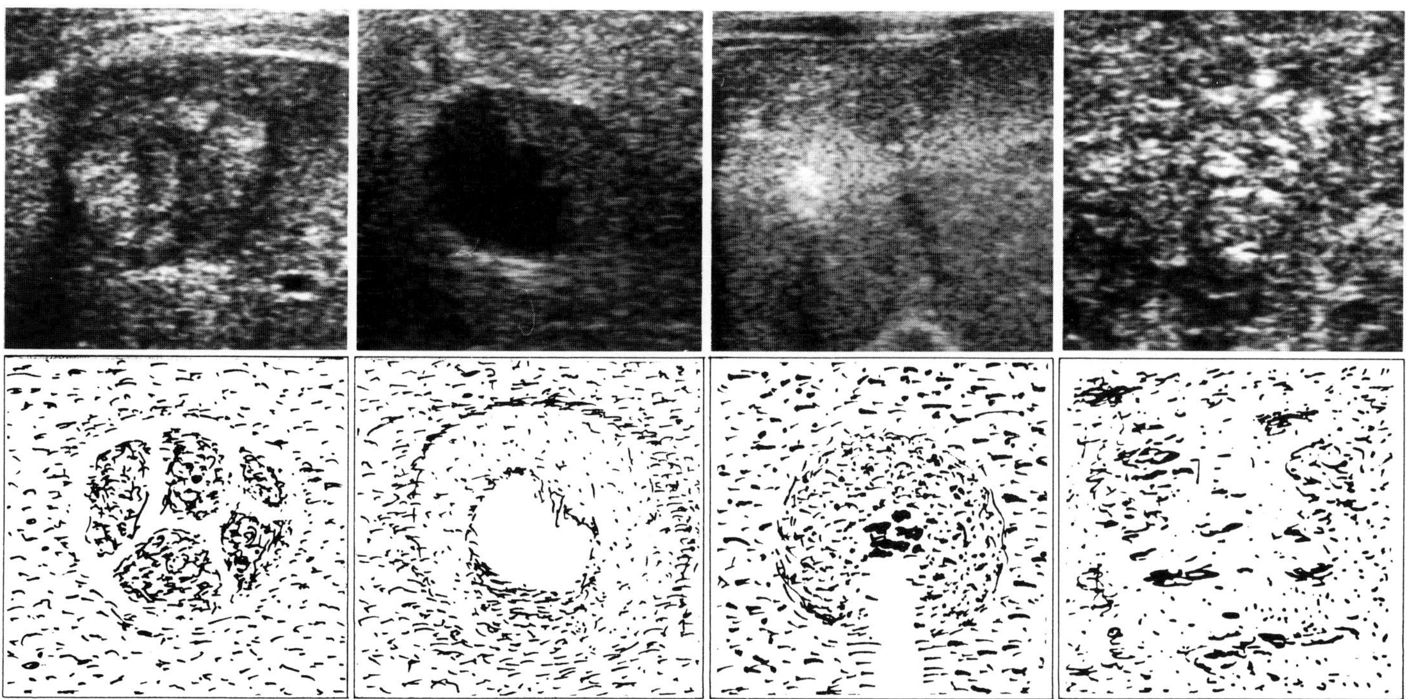

Fig. 3.19. Mosaic pattern   **Fig. 3.20.** Central necrosis   **Fig. 3.21.** Calcification   **Fig. 3.22.** Diffuse infiltrative growth

Findings to Be Investigated in Each Case of Hepatic Tumor

1. *Size of the tumor:* it is relatively easy to measure the size of a hepatic tumor on an ultrasonographic study. There is a relationship between the size and the echo pattern of the tumor, i.e., the echo pattern may change as the size changes (see Fig. 3.23).

2. *Overall echogenicity of the tumor:* the echogenicity is important in determining the nature of a hepatic tumor. For example, most of the primary hepatocellular carcinomas which are 2 cm or less in diameter are hypoechoic, whereas the majority of small cavernous hemangiomas of about 2 cm are hyperechoic. Metastatic tumors from the colon are frequently hyperechoic. Calcified tumors have strong central echoes with acoustic shadowing. Strong echoes suggesting gas production may be seen within a tumor following therapeutic arterial embolization.

3. *Internal echo texture of the tumor:* It is important to determine if the internal echo texture is homogeneous or heterogeneous. For example, a nodular pattern inside a tumor is called a mosaic pattern or "tumor in a tumor", and this is thought to be characteristic of primary hepatocellular carcinoma. The cut surface of a macroscopic specimen of hepatocellular carcinoma commonly shows nodularity, and each nodule can have a different consistency and color. Distinct septations may be observed between the nodules. Any tumor which develops necrosis, degeneration, or bleeding as it enlarges will also demonstrate a heterogeneous echo texture.

4. *Margin of the tumor:* the margin of the tumor can be smooth or irregular. In certain cases, the nature of the margin may be difficult to determine. A marginal halo is an interesting finding. A halo is observed when there is a thin layer of homogeneous material, such as a capsule, surrounding the mass. This may be seen in primary or metastatic tumors.

5. *Presence of refractive shadowing:* a refractive shadow (Fig. 3.24) may be observed arising from the lateral aspects of the tumor, directed posteriorly. This phenomenon is seen only when the surface of the tumor is smooth. Encapsulated hepatocellular carcinomas with expansile growth frequently exhibit this finding. Some of the metastatic tumors and many of the hepatic cysts also demonstrate this phenomenon.

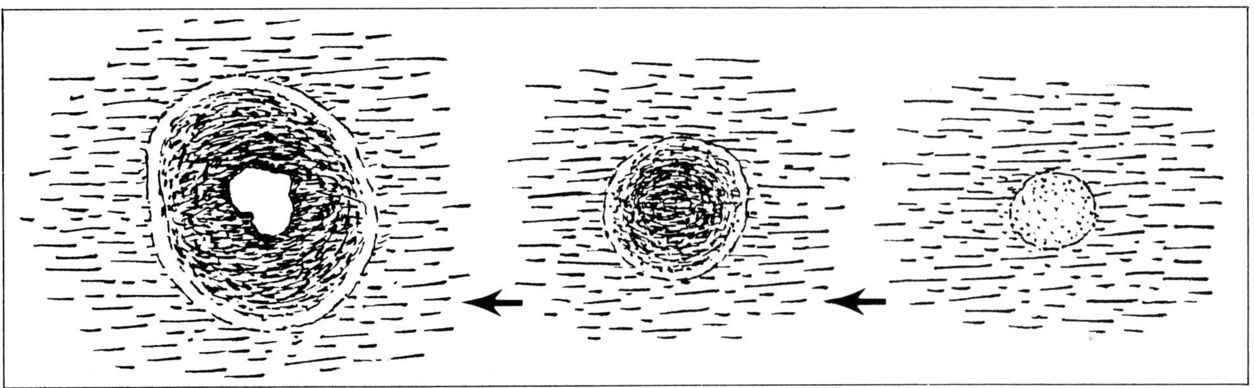

Fig. 3.23. *Tumor size and echo pattern.* As in the case of hepatocellular carcinoma, most of the small tumors of 2 cm or less are hypoechoic, but as the tumor enlarges, it becomes hyperechoic, and a surrounding halo appears. As the tumor enlarges still further, central necrosis develops

6. *Increased echoes posterior to the tumor:* increased echoes posterior to a tumor may or may not be present. This observation occurs for one of two reasons: (a) owing to a relative decrease of attenuation of the ultrasound beam through a tumor, enhanced through-transmission occurs and is observed as increased echoes posterior to the tumor; (b) an alternative cause of increased echoes posterior to a tumor is a reverberation artifact. Reverberation within the tumor produces a false image posterior to the tumor.

7. *Number of tumors:* in general, a solitary intrahepatic tumor is likely to be a hepatocellular carcinoma, whereas multiple tumors are likely to be metastases. However, multifocal hepatocellular carcinomas are not uncommon. When only one tumor is visualized on the ultrasonographic examination, CT or angiography may identify additional tumors in the liver.

8. *Tumor thrombus in the portal vein:* although differentiation between diffuse infiltrating hepatocellular carcinoma and advanced hepatic cirrhosis is difficult, hepatocellular carcinoma can be diagnosed with confidence when there is tumor thrombus in the portal vein. It should be noted that, rarely, metastases can cause tumor thrombus.

9. *Shape of the liver and the spleen:* hepatocellular carcinoma may be secondary to hepatic cirrhosis. With cirrhosis, the liver and the spleen have characteristic changes in shape, and some of these are clearly visualized ultrasonographically. A solid hepatic tumor in a patient who has ultrasonographic evidence of hepatic cirrhosis is strongly suggestive of hepatocellular carcinoma.

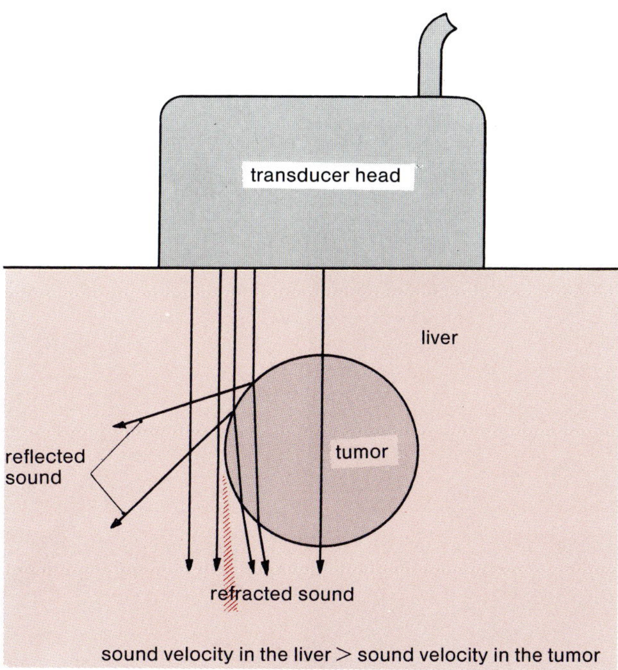

Fig. 3.24. *Principle of refractive shadowing.* When the ultrasound beam passes the outer portion of a mass with a smooth surface, it is refracted according to Snell's law. There is therefore no ultrasound beam in the *shaded area,* resulting in a type of acoustic shadowing. This is called refractive shadowing

Hepatocellular Carcinoma

Correlation between size and echo pattern is often seen in hepatocellular carcinoma. Small hepatocellular carcinomas, less than 2 cm in size, are almost always visualized as hypoechoic lesions, whereas intermediate-sized tumors of 3–4 cm often exhibit anechoic rims or a mosaic pattern. Relatively large tumors of 5 cm or greater demonstrate mixed patterns with echogenic and anechoic areas.

These findings can be explained by differences in the homogeneity of the tumor tissue. Hepatocellular carcinomas smaller than 2 cm in size produce less reflection of ultrasound because of dense and homogeneous distribution of cancer cells. As the tumor becomes larger, it undergoes mild degeneration and becomes less homogeneous. As a result, there is more reflection of the ultrasound beam, and the lesion becomes iso- or hyperechoic. However, at this stage, there are tumor cells without degeneration in the peripheral portion creating a peripheral anechoic area which is called a halo. When an expanding tumor has a distinct capsule, this is also visualized as a halo. As the tumor grows further, areas of hemorrhage or necrosis occur inside the tumor, appearing as anechoic regions.

It is the infiltrating type of hepatocellular carcinoma that is apt to be overlooked. This is especially true when the visualized field is totally occupied by tumor. It is important to be familiar with the normal ultrasonographic pattern of the liver with each ultrasonographic scanner employed.

Small Hepatocellular Carcinoma

As a result of improved ultrasonographic equipment, it is not uncommon to identify small tumors of around 2 cm in size. In a patient with hepatic cirrhosis, however, it is not easy to differentiate a small tumor from a regenerating nodule. This differentiation is almost impossible when the lesion is less than 1 cm in size.

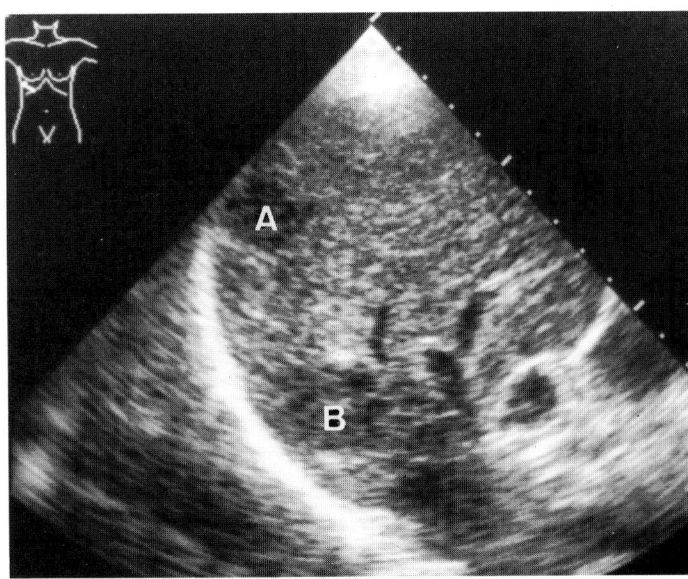

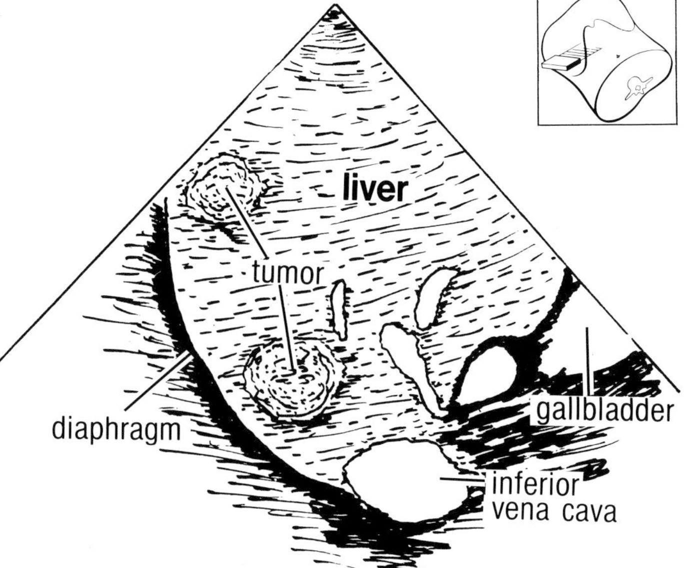

Fig. 3.25. *Case 1*. There are two hypoechoic masses of about 2 cm in size in the right lobe of the liver, just under the diaphragm. Lesion *A* could not have been visualized with a linear scanner. A sector scanner must be used so as not to miss small lesions in this location

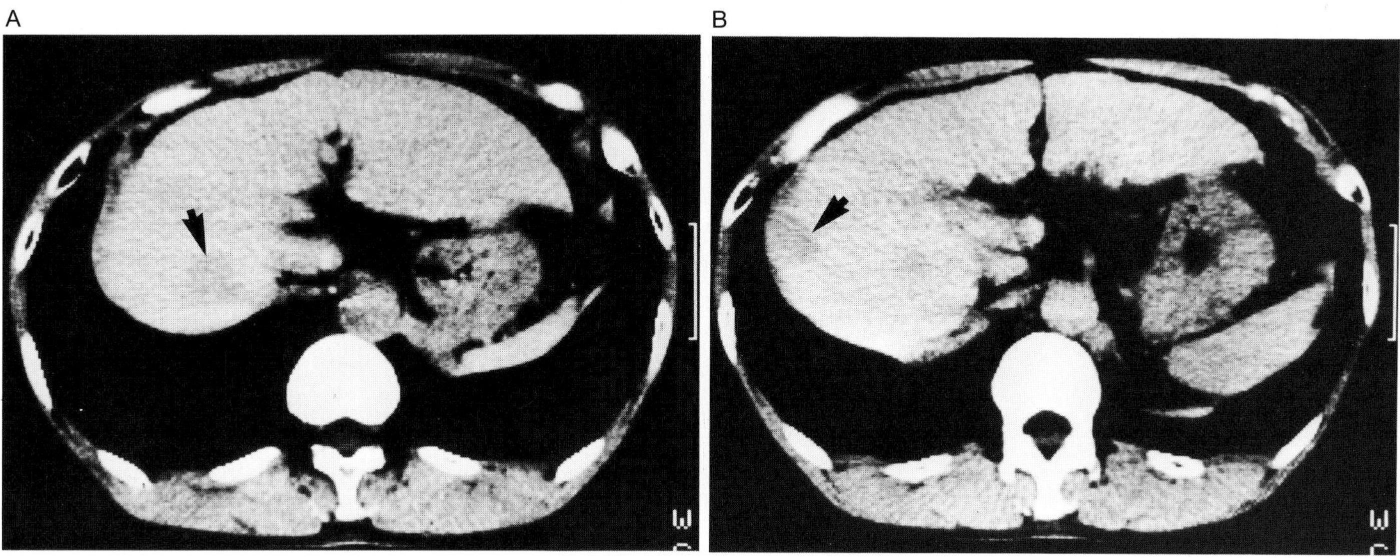

Fig. 3.26 A, B. *Case 1, CT scans.* The *arrow* in **A** indicates mass *B* in Fig. 3.25. The *arrow* in **B** indicates mass *A* in Fig. 3.25

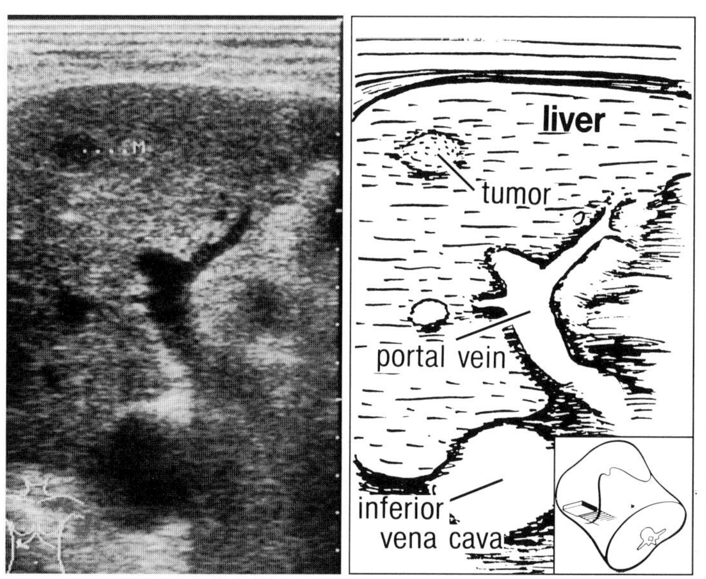

Fig. 3.27. *Case 2.* There is a 12-mm hypoechoic mass in the anterosuperior aspect of the right lobe of the liver. There were several other smaller lesions in this case (not shown). Irregularity of the surface of the liver and splenomegaly (not shown) strongly suggested that this lesion was a hepatocellular carcinoma

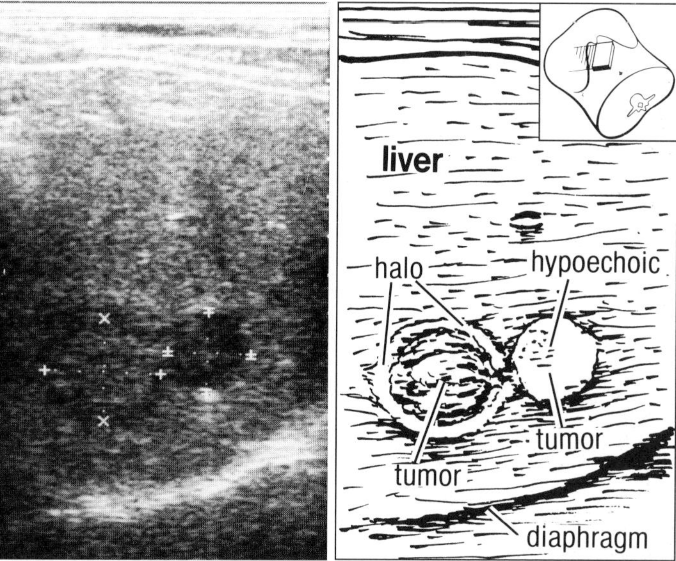

Fig. 3.28. *Case 3.* In the right lobe of the liver, there are two solid lesions of 2 and 3 cm next to each other. The smaller mass is hypoechoic. The larger mass has a peripheral anechoic area (halo). When there is more than one lesion, as in this case, different echo patterns are often seen

Intermediate-Sized Hepatocellular Carcinoma

Most of the tumors of less than 2 cm in diameter are homogeneously hypoechoic, but larger tumors of 5 cm or more typically demonstrate generalized hyperechogenicity or a mixed pattern with anechoic areas suggesting hemorrhage or necrosis. Tumors with expansile growth may exhibit a distinct halo which is sometimes associated with refractive shadowing.

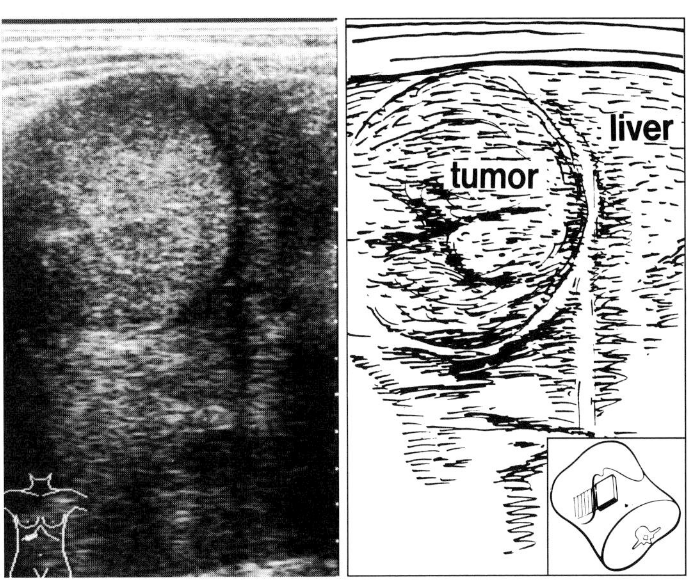

Fig. 3.29. *Case 1.* In the anteroinferior aspect of the right lobe of the liver, there is a 6-cm hyperechoic mass demonstrating a distinct halo and a refractive shadow. There were many other solid tumors in the liver in this case (not shown)

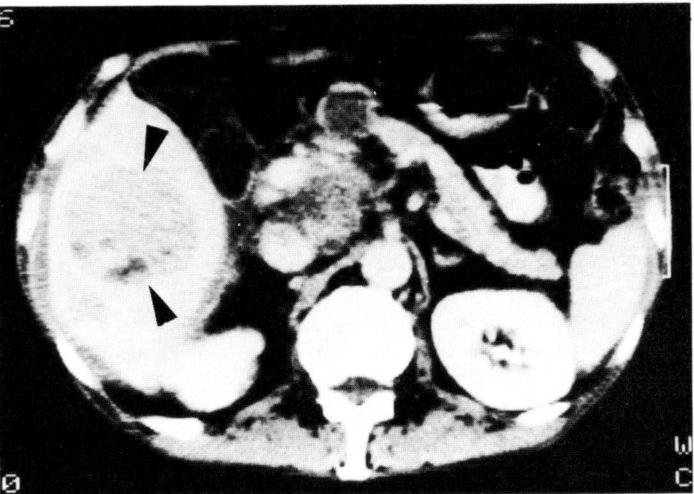

Fig. 3.30. *Case 1, CT scan.* There is a 6-cm low-attenuation mass with central areas of even lower attenuation (*arrows*)

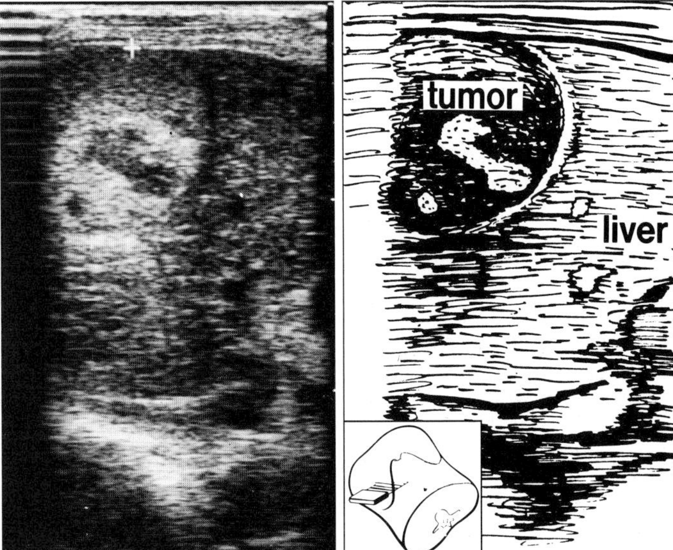

Fig. 3.31. *Case 2.* This image shows a 5-cm hyperechoic mass with scattered hypoechoic areas within it, suggesting degeneration

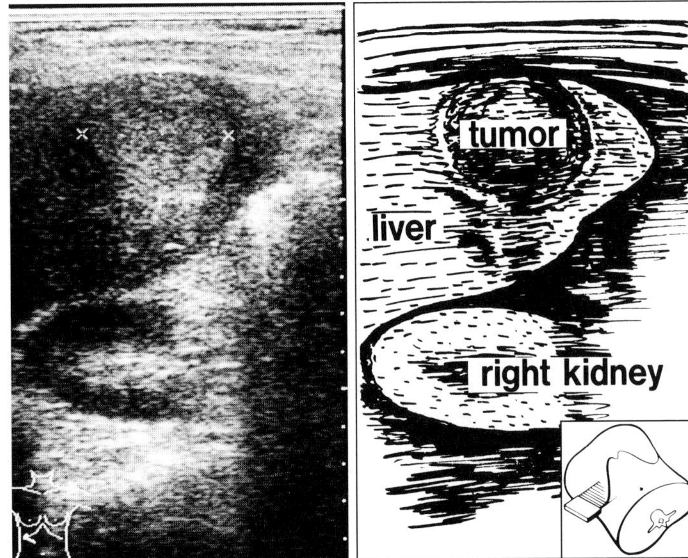

Fig. 3.32. *Case 3.* The tumor is visualized as a hyperechoic lesion. Note the presence of posterior enhancement

*Hepatocellular Carcinoma
with Exophytic Growth*

Some hepatocellular carcinomas show exophytic growth outside the liver. If the tumor grows superiorly, this is visualized as an abnormal bulging of the diaphragm on the chest X-ray. It is not easy to visualize this type of tumor ultrasonographically as it is surrounded by air in the lung. Tumors arising from the inferior portion of the liver and growing inferiorly or to the left can mimic tumors originating from other organs.

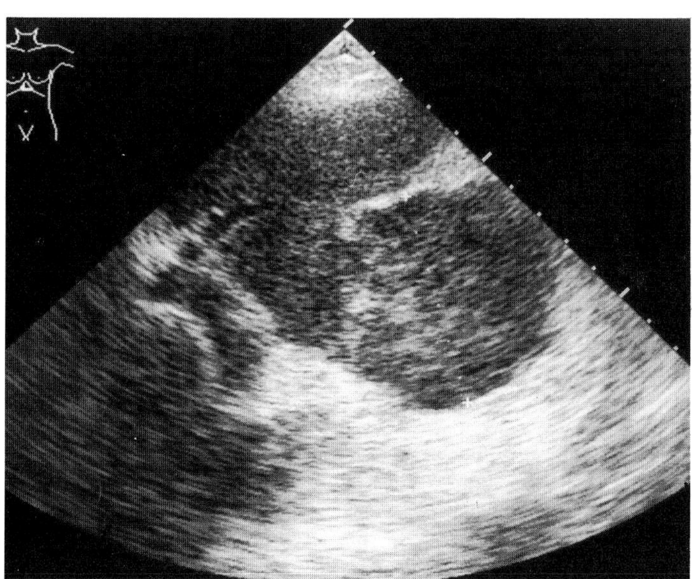

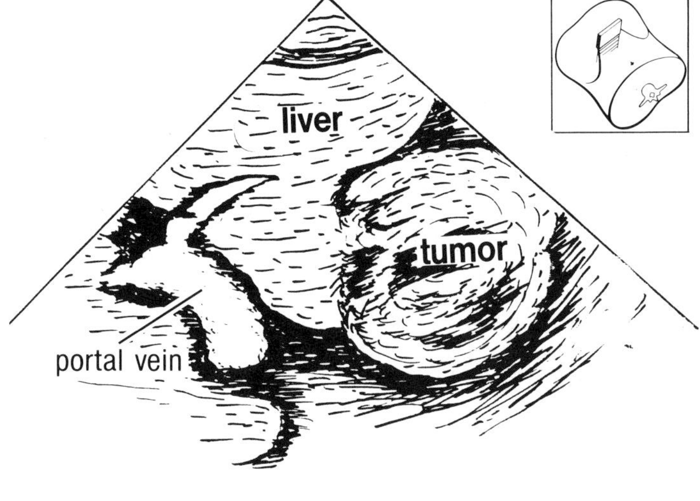

Fig. 3.33. *Case 1.* A 6-cm hepatocellular carcinoma arising from the lateral segment of the left lobe of the liver with exophytic growth toward the left. An upper gastrointestinal study showed extrinsic compression on the lesser curvature of the stomach

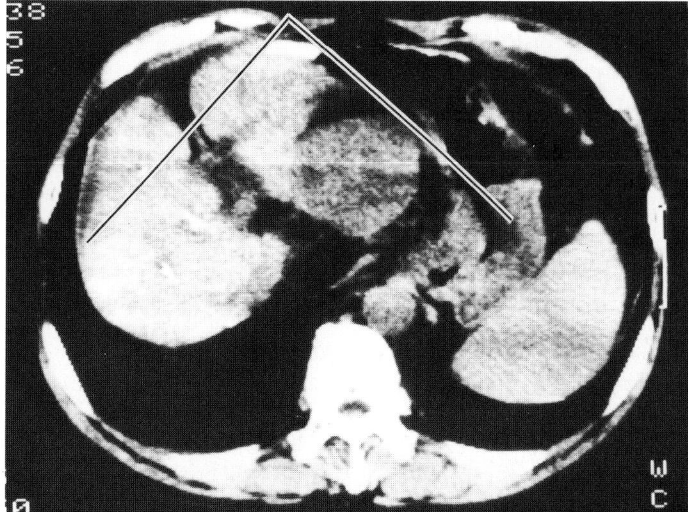

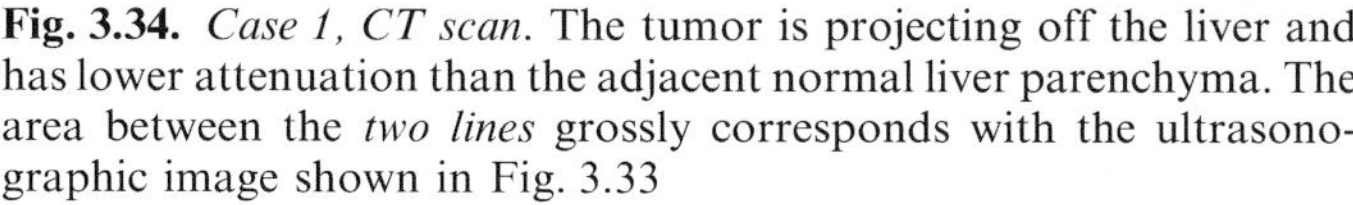

Fig. 3.34. *Case 1, CT scan.* The tumor is projecting off the liver and has lower attenuation than the adjacent normal liver parenchyma. The area between the *two lines* grossly corresponds with the ultrasonographic image shown in Fig. 3.33

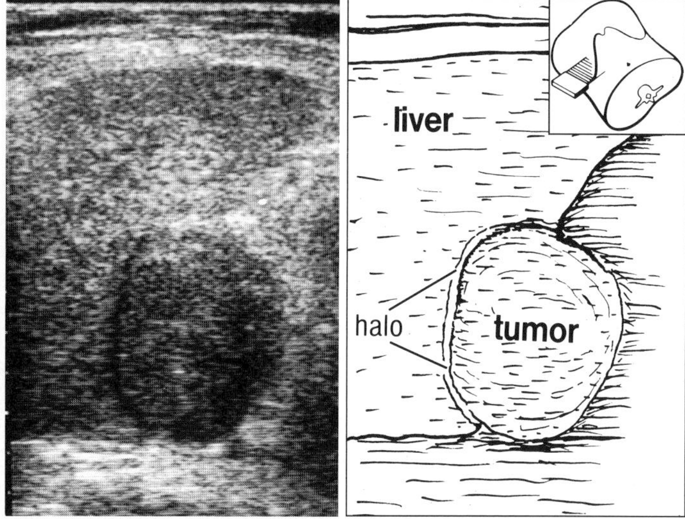

Fig. 3.35. *Case 2.* Exophytic tumor arising from the posterior surface of the right lobe of the liver. On closer inspection, there is a halo between the tumor and the normal liver parenchyma

Diffuse Infiltrating Hepatocellular Carcinoma

There is a type of hepatocellular carcinoma which infiltrates diffusely without forming a well-defined mass. This type can be difficult to detect ultrasonographically since there is no distinct border. It is also difficult to differentiate this type of hepatocellular carcinoma from advanced hepatic cirrhosis which similarly demonstrates a heterogeneous echo pattern. Diffuse infiltrating tumors often extend into the portal vein. Note that the multinodular type of hepatocellular carcinoma may coalesce and thereby mimic the diffusely infiltrating type.

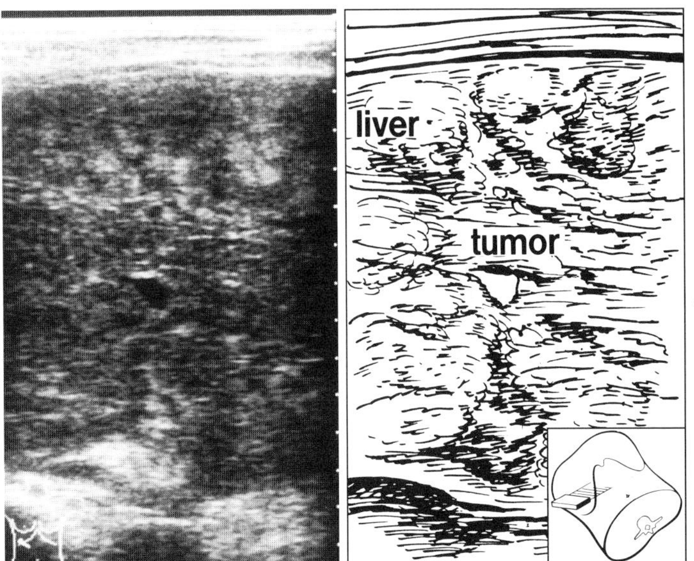

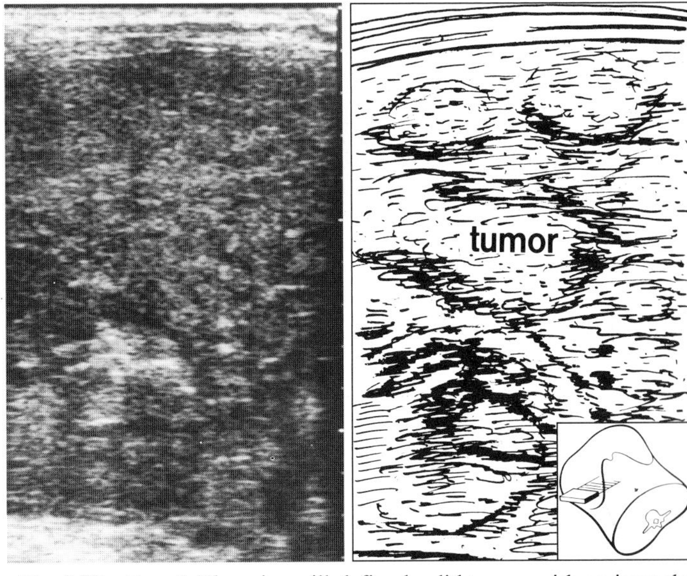

Fig. 3.36. *Case 1.* The surface of the liver is irregular, and the echo texture of the parenchyma is markedly heterogeneous. The lumen of the portal vein in the left lobe is obscured due to tumor involvement. Carcinoma is present throughout the visualized field

Fig. 3.37. *Case 2.* There is an ill-defined solid tumor with an irregular echo texture in the right lobe of the liver. The portal vein could not be identified within the region of the tumor

Ultrasonographic "Blind Spots" of the Liver

There are several areas in the liver which are difficult to visualize ultrasonographically. The superior portion of the right lobe of the liver, often referred to as the dome of the liver, cannot be adequately examined with a linear scanner as it is surrounded by air in the lungs. A lesion in this location can be impossible to visualize even when a tumor is known to be present by CT or angiography. This area can be visualized with either a sector or convex scanner.

It is difficult to visualize small lesions in the superficial portions of the liver since reverberation artifacts from the musculature or fatty layers of the abdominal wall can obscure ultrasonographic information in the near field. Cystic lesions may be overlooked as they do not appear anechoic.

Lesions in the deep portion of the liver may be difficult to detect as well. The posterosuperior portion of the liver is examined with the transducer head on the anterior surface of the abdomen in order to avoid traversing air in the lungs. Tumors in this location may not be adequately visualized owing to decreased resolution secondary to the distance from the transducer head. The lateral segment of the left lobe can be large and may be interposed between the left hemidiaphragm and the spleen. A tumor in this location may be overlooked.

It is generally difficult to obtain adequate ultrasonographic examinations in patients with severe hepatic cirrhosis who have small shrunken livers, in patients with thick subcutaneous or peritoneal fatty layers, and in patients who have undergone partial hepatic resection.

*Portal Thrombosis
by Hepatocellular Carcinoma*

Hepatocellular carcinoma, particularly the diffusely infiltrating type, tends to extend into the portal vein. If there is tumor involvement of the portal vein, it is almost always a hepatocellular carcinoma. This finding is quite rare in a metastatic tumor. Careful observation is necessary to identify the portal vein when the portal vein is filled with tumor thrombus as it may have a similar echogenicity to the surrounding liver parenchyma.

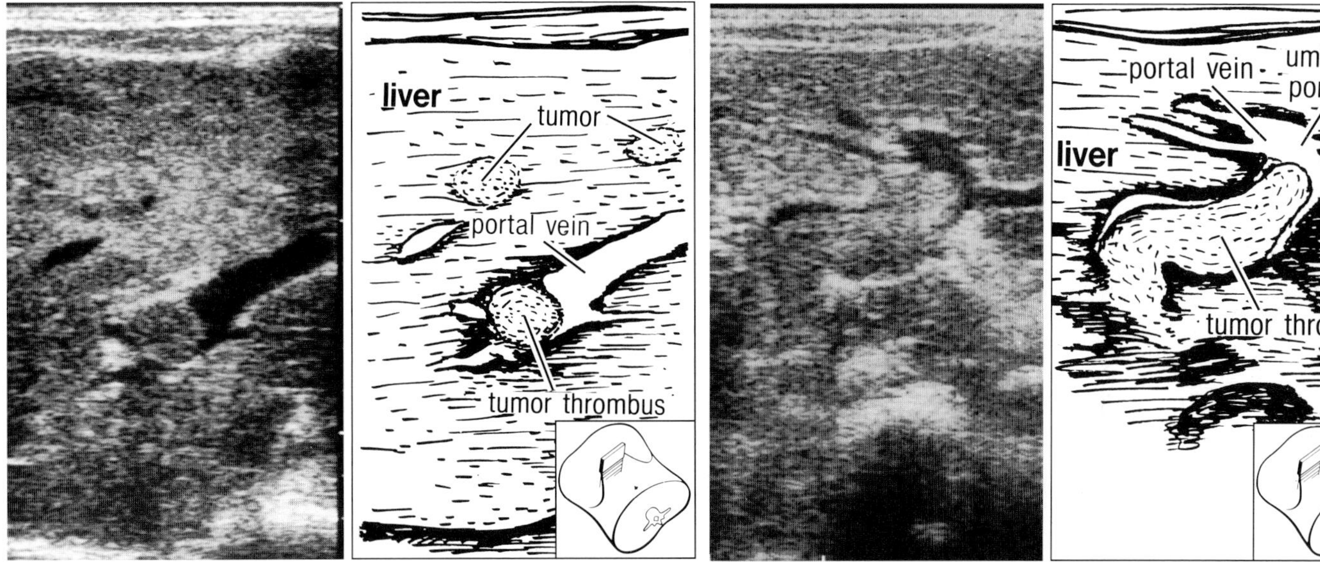

Fig. 3.38. *Case 1*. The transverse portion of the left branch of the intrahepatic portal vein is visualized, demonstrating a round tumor thrombus within it. This tumor thrombus originated in the right portal vein and extended retrogradely to the confluence of the right and left portal veins

Fig. 3.39. *Case 2*. There is tumor thrombus in the transverse and umbilical portions of the portal vein

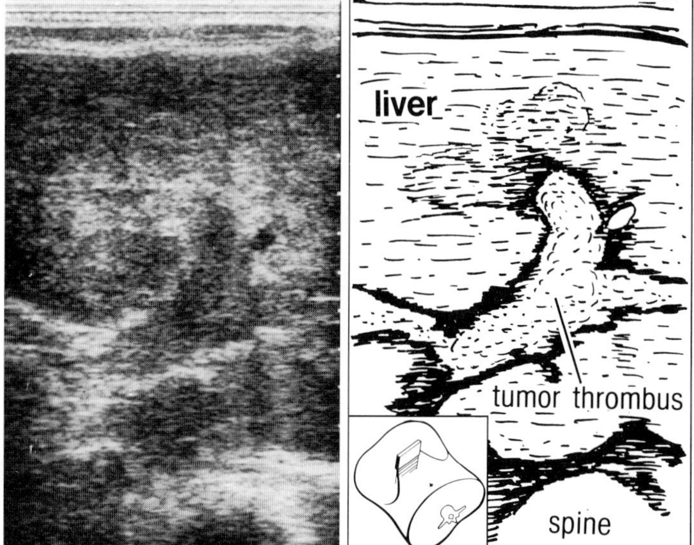

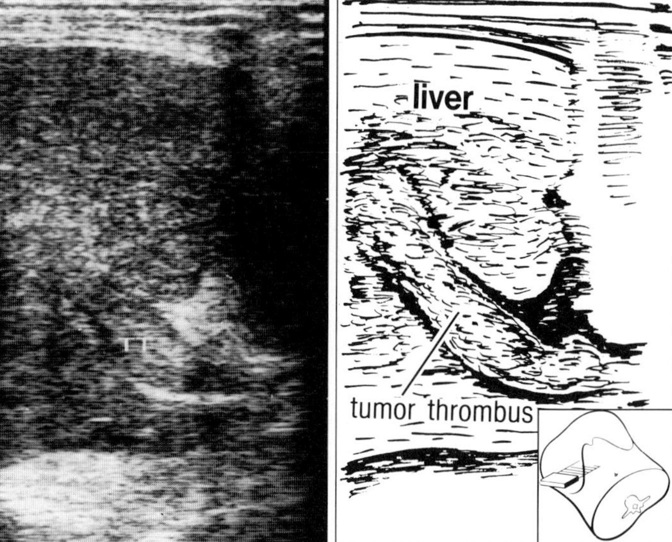

Fig. 3.40. *Case 3*. The transverse and umbilical portions of the left branch of the portal vein are filled with tumor. Tumor thrombus is also seen in the portal branch that supplies the lateral segment of the left lobe

Fig. 3.41. *Case 4*. Intercostal image of the right lobe of the liver. The right branch of the portal vein is filled with tumor

Superficially located hepatocellular carcinoma can rupture and cause massive intraperitoneal bleeding. This is particularly frequent in tumors with exophytic growth. Rupture can occur without a significant external force. In a patient with a superficially located hepatic tumor, sudden onset of severe abdominal pain, severe anemia, and an ascites-like anechoic space in the peritoneal cavity on ultrasonographic examination strongly suggest rupture.

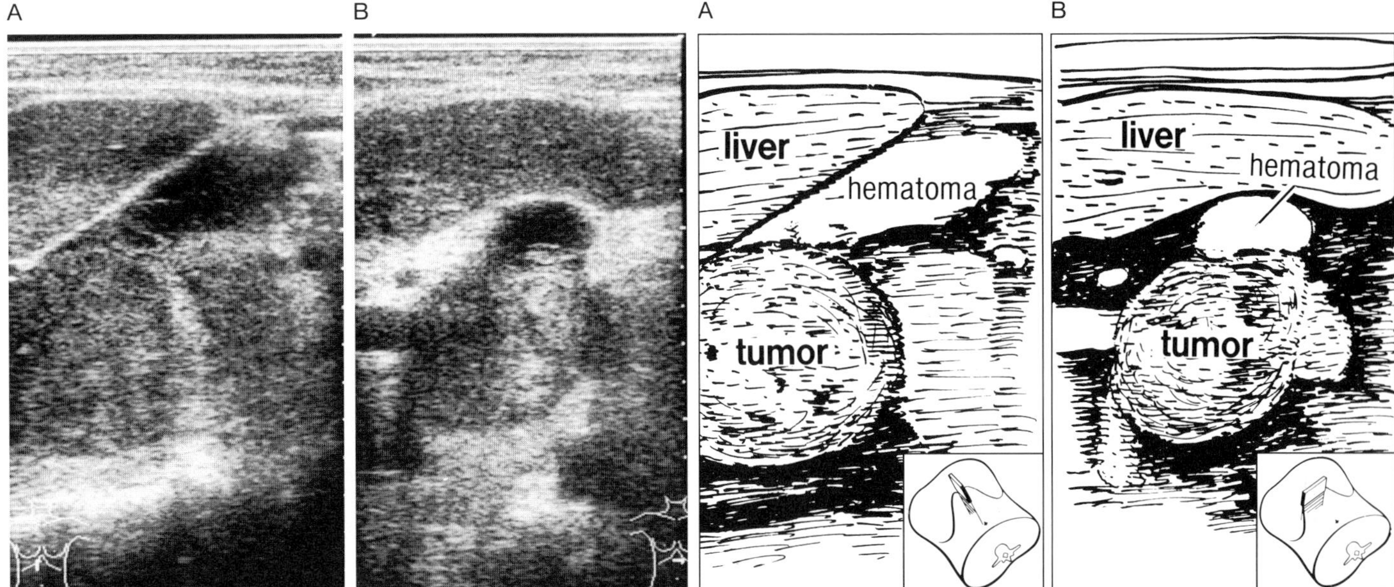

Fig. 3.42 A, B. *Case 1.* There is a large tumor in the caudate lobe. An anechoic space, similar in appearance to the gallbladder, is seen between the caudate lobe and the left lobe. The gallbladder is visualized in its normal location. This patient had experienced sudden onset of upper abdominal pain, hypotension, and anemia 2 months earlier. Considering this history, this anechoic space is thought to be an old hematoma

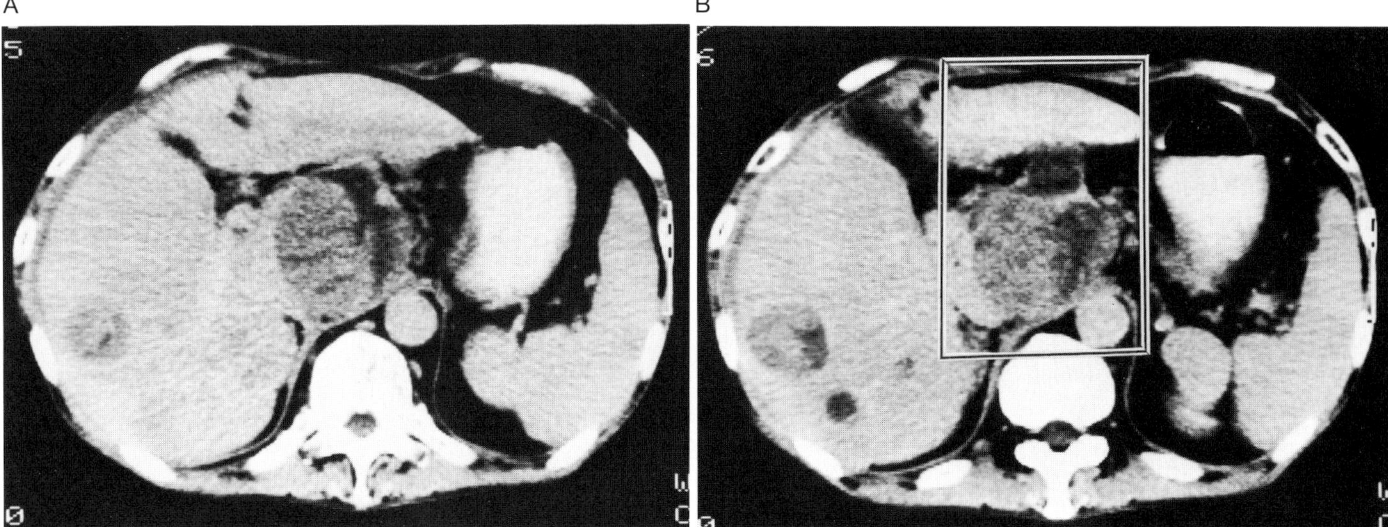

Fig. 3.43 A, B. *Case 1, CT scans.* **A** A section 1 cm caudal to the image in **B**. There is a large low-density mass in the caudate lobe. The area of lower density extending from this tumor toward the left lobe represents a hematoma. The area within the *square* (**B**) roughly corresponds to the ultrasonographic image in Fig. 3.42. Multiple tumors are present in other portions of the liver

Effect
of Therapeutic Embolization

Transcatheter arterial embolization (TAE) is commonly used to treat hepatocellular carcinoma. Three to five days after TAE, strong echoes indicating gas within the tumor appear and then typically disappear within 2 weeks. Subsequently, the tumor size gradually diminishes. Following TAE, many of the hypoechoic tumors become hyperechoic, and some develop weak acoustic shadowing.

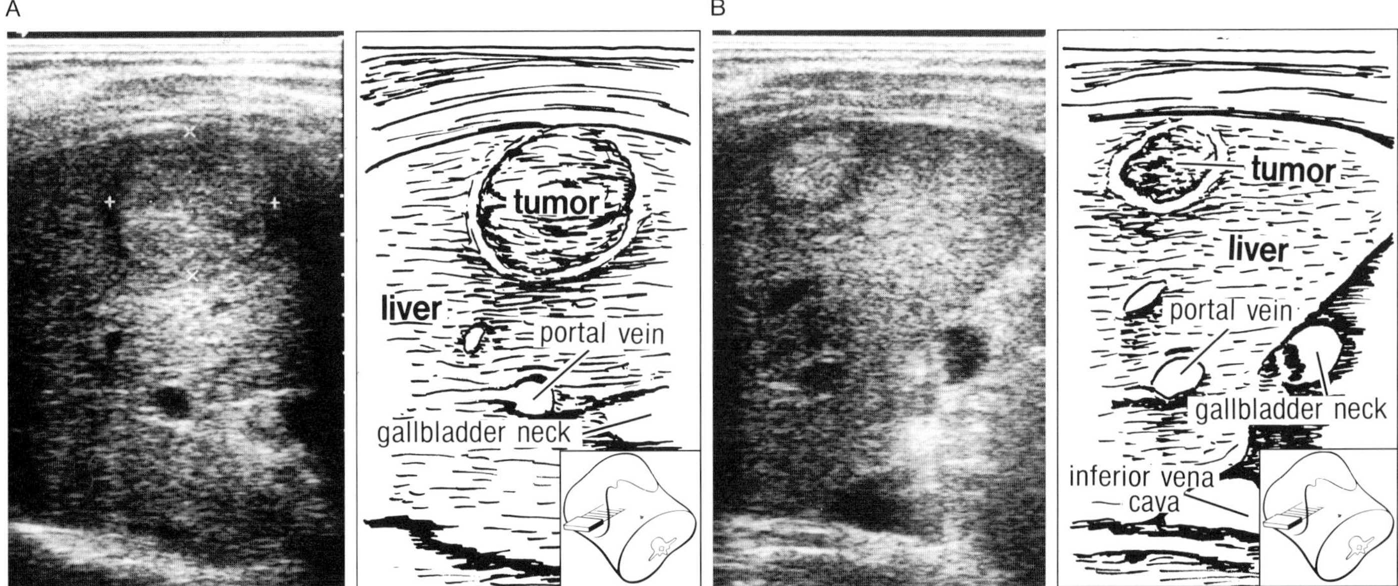

Fig. 3.44 A, B. *Case 1*. **A** A 4-cm solid mass in the right lobe. **B** The same tumor 70 days after TAE. It is significantly smaller (2.6 cm) and has become hyperechoic when compared to the pre-TAE image

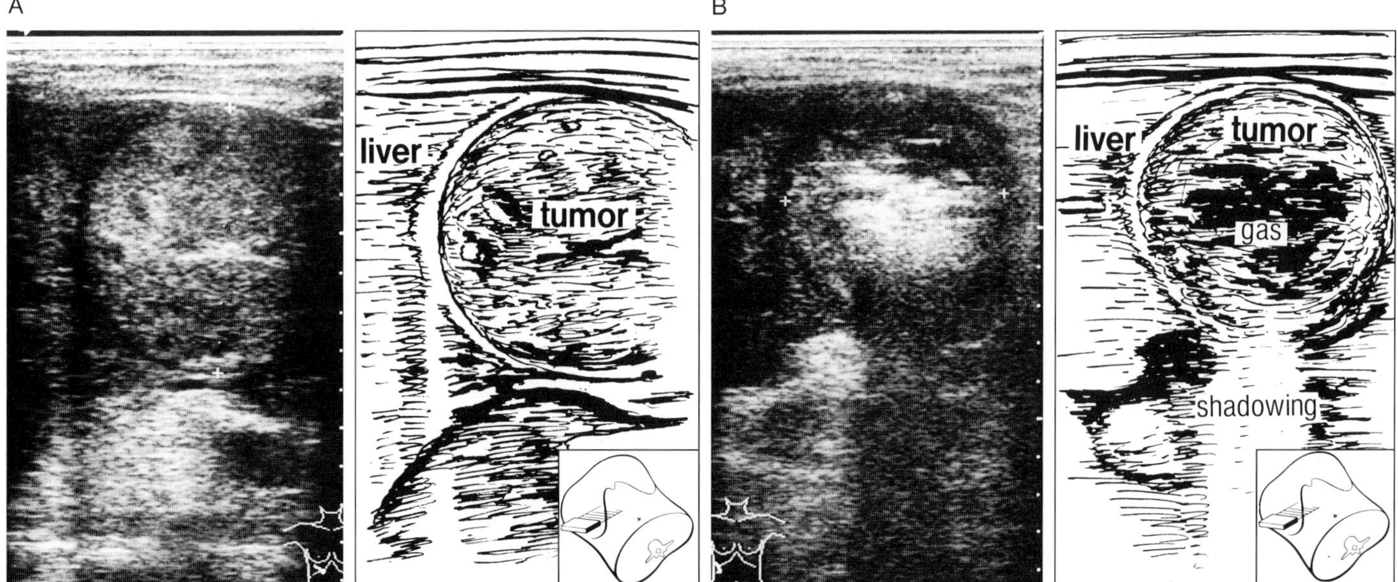

Fig. 3.45 A, B. *Case 2*. **A** The intercostal scan shows a solid tumor, 6.8 cm in diameter. **B** The same tumor 40 days after TAE. It has become slightly smaller. The center is hyperechoic with associated acoustic shadowing indicating gas production

Metastatic Liver Tumors

There is wide variation in the ultrasonographic appearance of metastatic liver tumors, including hyper- and hypoechoic, and heterogeneous patterns. There are no absolute relationships between primary sites and echo patterns of metastatic deposits, but some correlation does exist. Most metastatic liver tumors are multiple, but the multiplicity of lesions alone cannot differentiate a metastatic from a primary tumor as multinodular hepatocellular carcinomas are not uncommon.

Tumors with Peripheral Anechoic Areas

The bull's eye sign is frequently seen with metastases from lung and gastric carcinomas.

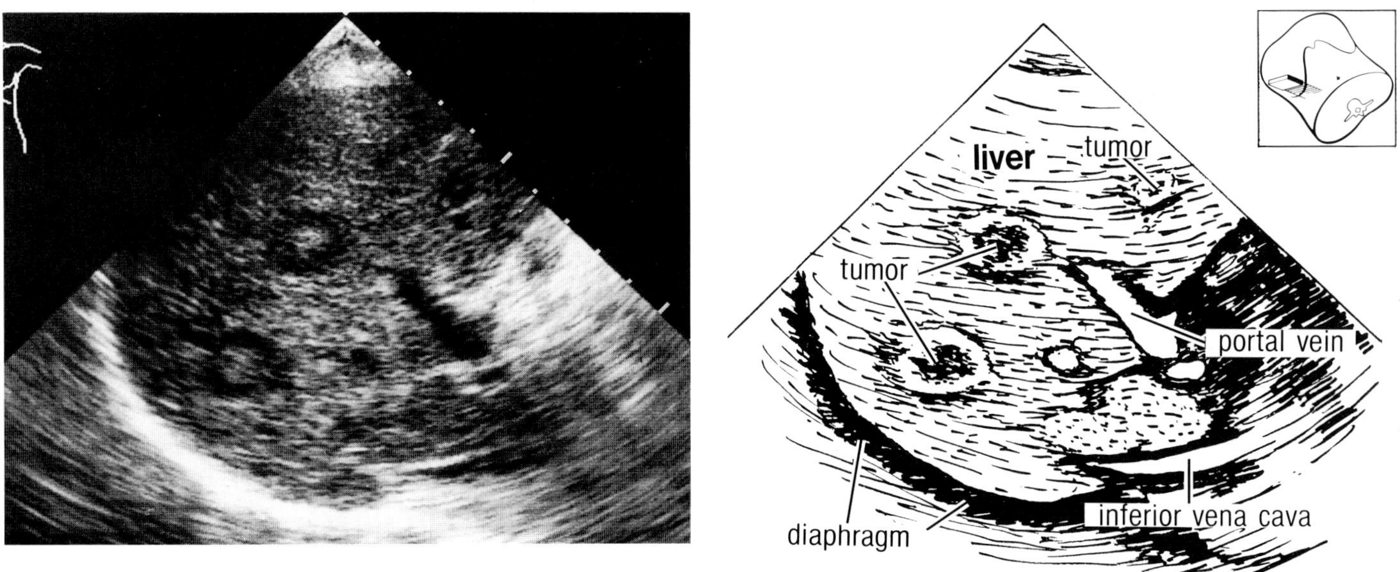

Fig. 3.46. *Case 1.* There are multiple tumors with peripheral anechoic areas in both lobes of the liver. The primary tumor was not detected

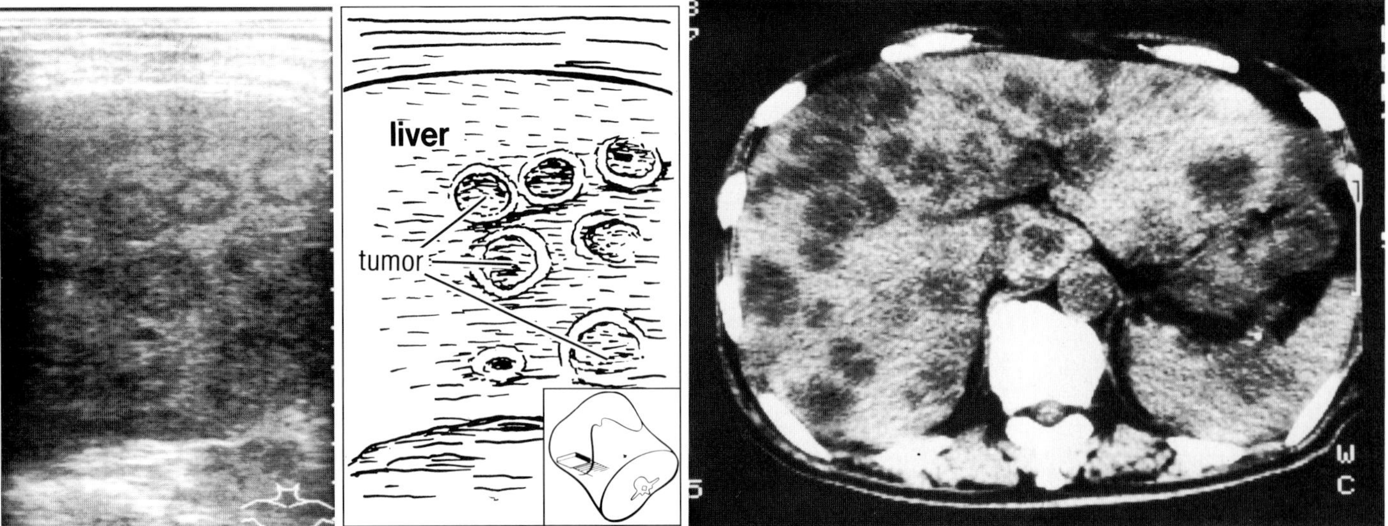

Fig. 3.47. *Case 2.* Metastases from gastric carcinoma. There are multiple tumors, about 2 cm in size, with haloes

Fig. 3.48. *Case 2, CT scan.* There is hepatomegaly associated with multiple low-density masses

Hyperechoic Tumors

Metastases from colonic or gastric carcinomas are frequently hyperechoic, even when small in size. This is because these tumors tend to degenerate even when the tumor is small. If there are hyperechoic masses in the liver, gastrointestinal studies should be performed in search of the primary site. Note that hepatocellular carcinomas frequently become hyperechoic after TAE therapy.

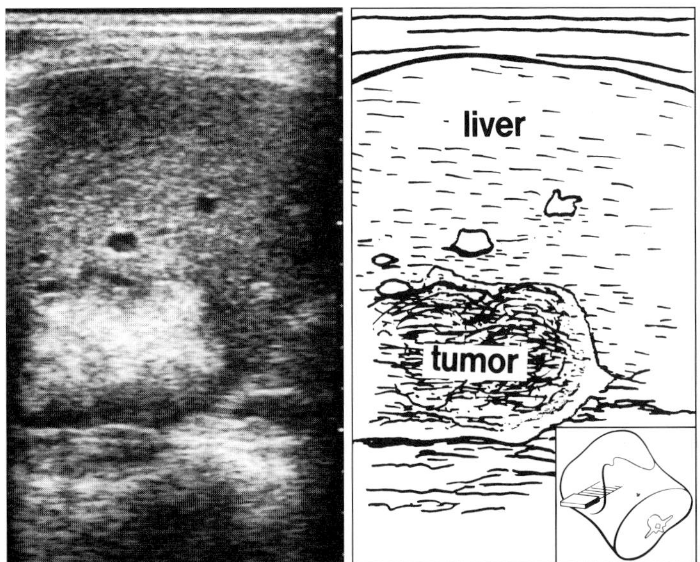

Fig. 3.49. *Case 1*. There is a 4 × 6-cm hyperechoic mass with an irregular border in the posterior portion of the right lobe of the liver. The peripheral portion of this mass is hypoechoic. This is a metastatic tumor from rectal carcinoma

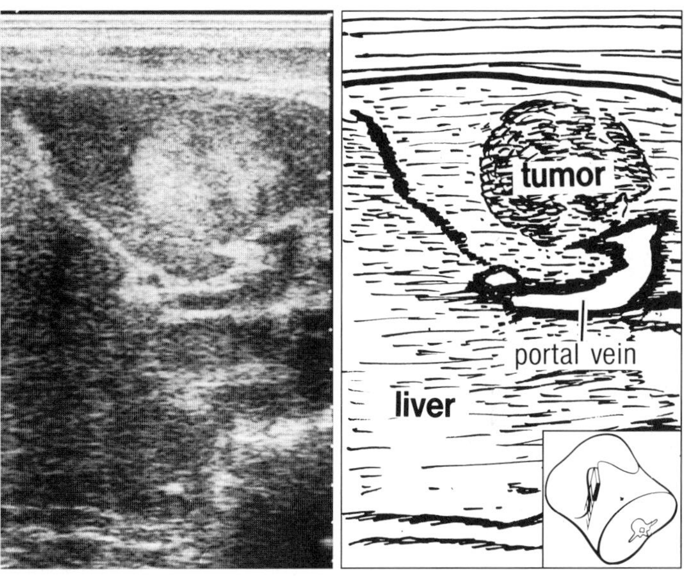

Fig. 3.50. *Case 2*. There is a 4-cm hyperechoic mass in the lateral segment of the left lobe of the liver. Hypoechoic areas are also seen within the mass. This patient had had gastrectomy for carcinoma 3 months earlier

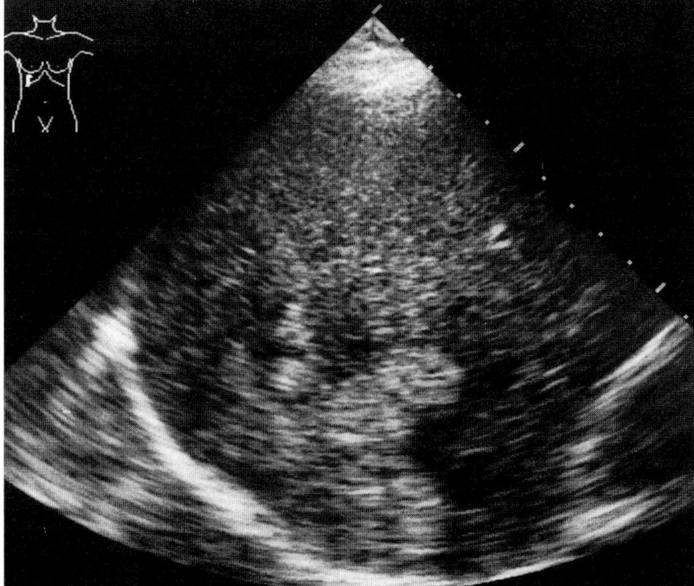

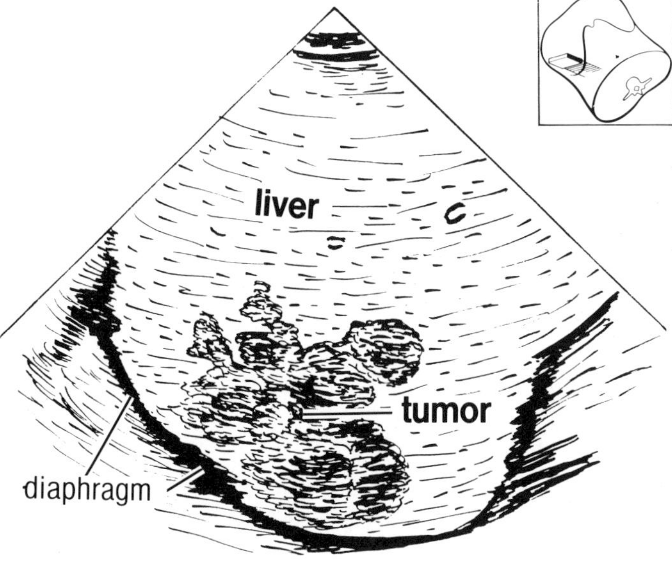

Fig. 3.51. *Case 3*. There is a lobulated hyperechoic mass in the posterior segment of the right lobe. This patient had had a sigmoidectomy for carcinoma 3 years earlier amd had had a recent elevation in his carcinoembryonic antigen level

Hypoechoic Tumors   Metastases from sarcomas are characteristically hypoechoic. Metastases from malignant melanoma or pancreatic carcinoma are frequently hypoechoic.

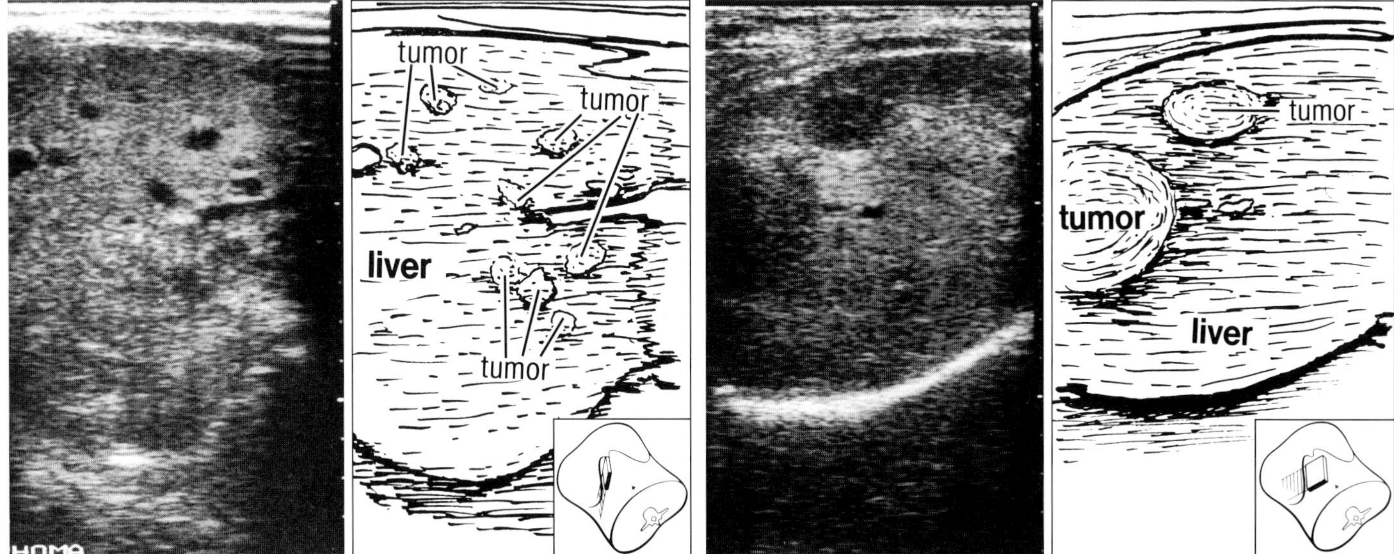

Fig. 3.52. *Case 1.* Metastatic melanoma. There are multiple hypoechoic masses of approximately 1 cm in size scattered throughout the liver

Fig. 3.53. *Case 2.* Metastatic pancreatic carcinoma. There are multiple hypoechoic masses of 2–4 cm in diameter

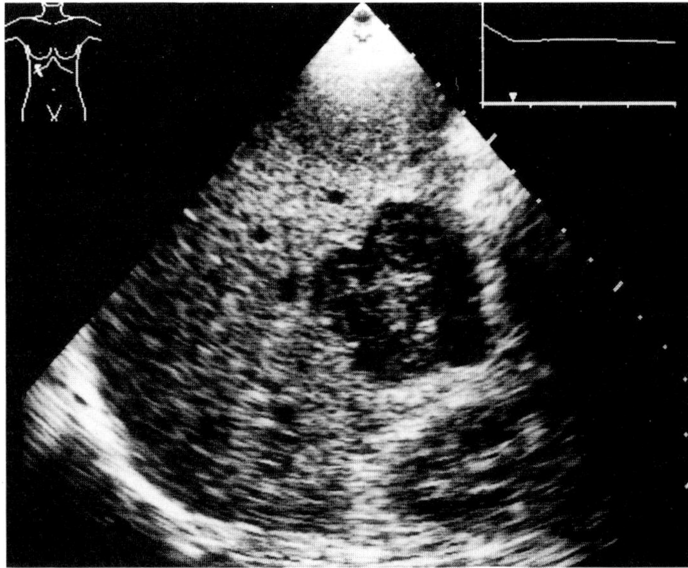

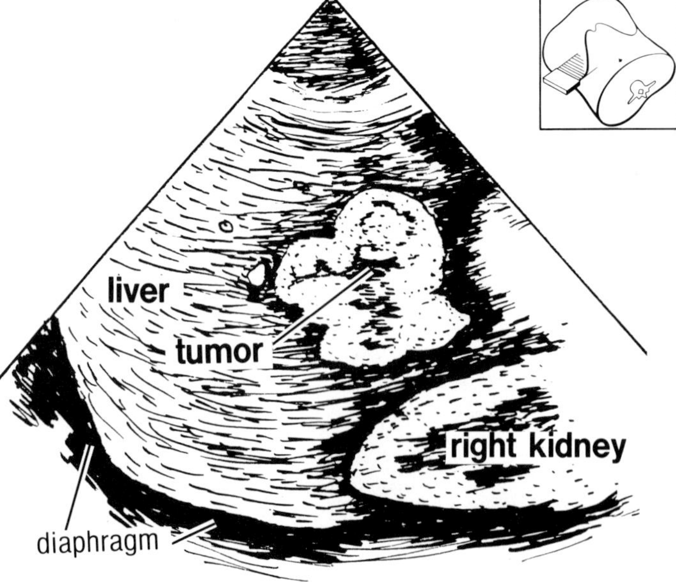

Fig. 3.54. *Case 3.* Metastatic gastric leiomyosarcoma. A hypoechoic 4.5-cm mass with an irregular border and an exophytic component is seen along the inferior surface of the liver. There were several other masses in the liver (not shown)

Central Necrosis

Some metastatic liver tumors develop central necrosis. A tumor with a large central anechoic space is almost always metastatic since this finding is quite rare in hepatocellular carcinoma. Gynecologic malignancies are the most frequent primary site of liver metastases displaying this pattern.

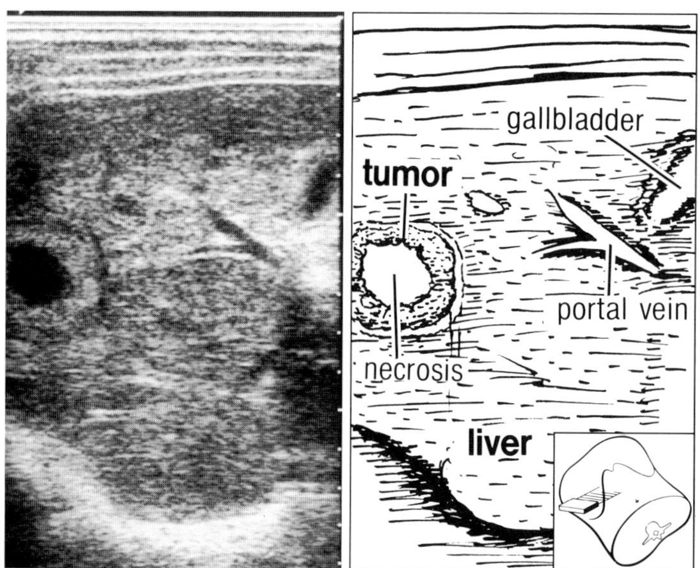

Fig. 3.55. *Case 1*. Metastatic transitional cell carcinoma. There is a 35-mm solid tumor with a central anechoic space of 17 mm in the superior portion of the right lobe of the liver

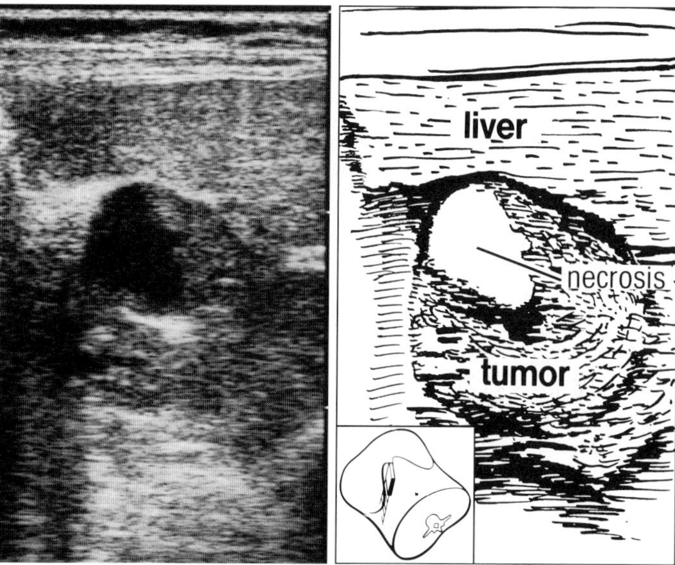

Fig. 3.56. *Case 2*. Metastatic ovarian carcinoma. There is a 6-cm solid tumor near the posterior surface of the right lobe. The tumor is partially necrotic, manifesting as an anechoic region

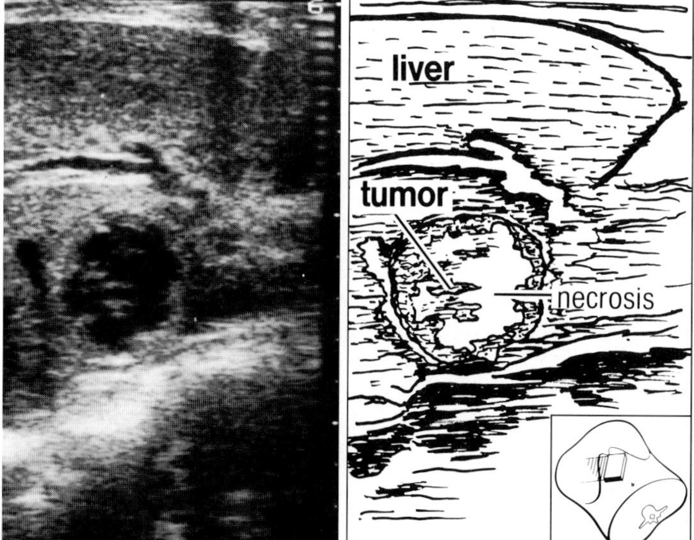

Fig. 3.57. *Case 3*. Metastatic gastric carcinoma. There is a 4-cm mass in the posterior portion of the right lobe of the liver which is predominantly necrotic

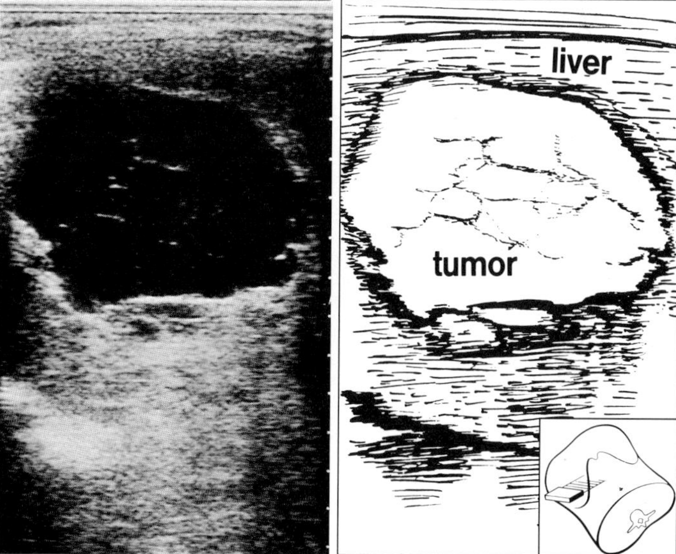

Fig. 3.58. *Case 4*. Metastatic cervical carcinoma. There is a 6–7 cm cystic mass with an irregular border. A network pattern is seen within it

Calcification   Punctate strong echoes with acoustic shadowing within a liver tumor suggest calcification. Metastases from mucin-producing carcinomas of the colon or stomach should be considered when this pattern is present.

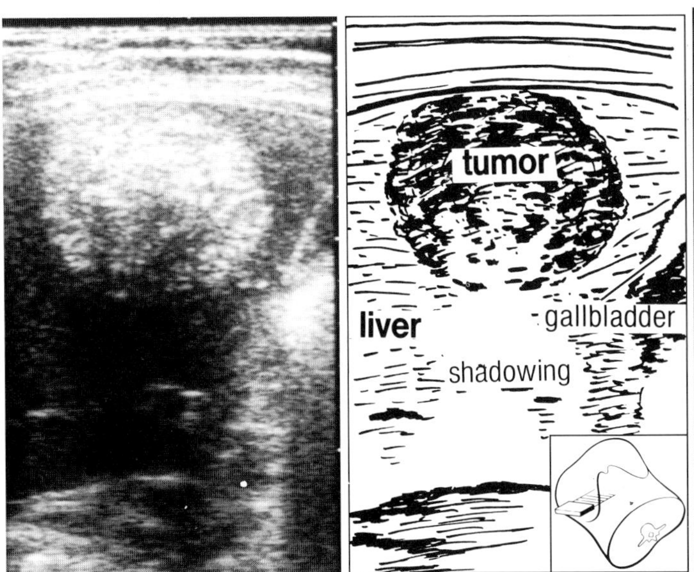

Fig. 3.59. *Case 1.* Metastatic colon carcinoma. There is a 5-cm hyperechoic mass with acoustic shadowing. The posterior border of the mass is not clearly seen because of the shadow

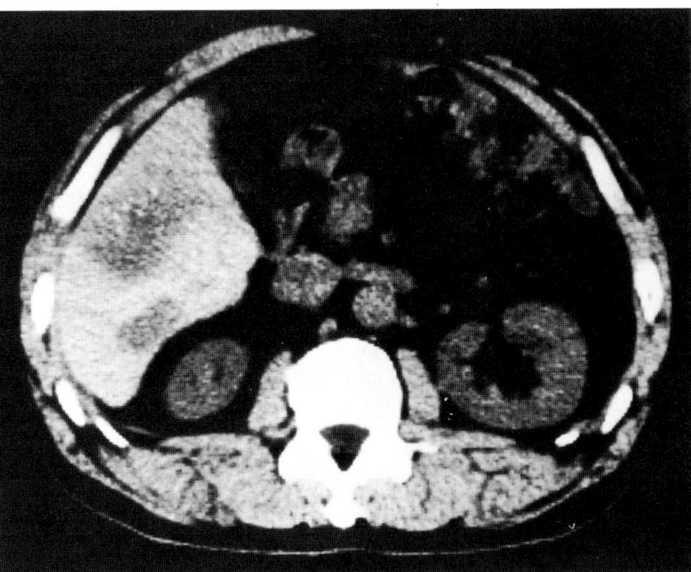

Fig. 3.60. *Case 1, CT scan.* Within the larger low-attenuation mass, there are punctate high-attenuation densities (calcifications). The second low-attenuation mass, near the right kidney, proved to be a hemangioma

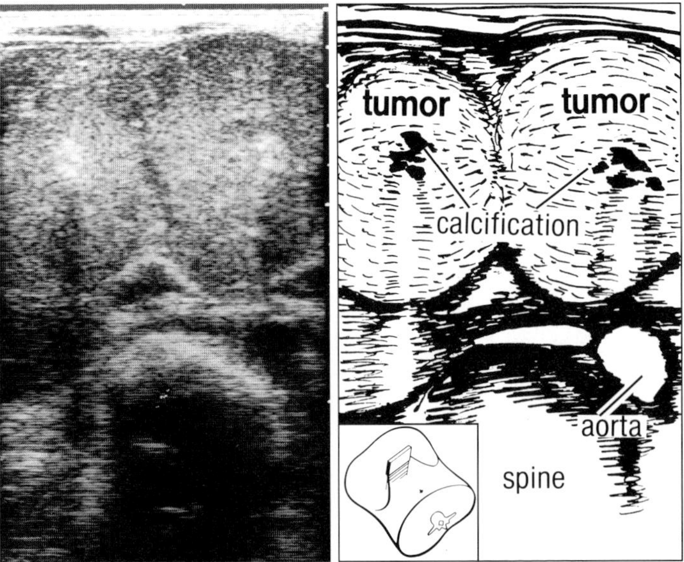

Fig. 3.61. *Case 2.* Metastatic colon carcinoma. There are small, focal, hyperechoic areas with associated acoustic shadowing in the central portions of this 6-cm solid tumor

Cholangiocarcinoma

Cholangiocarcinoma may be difficult to identify since its echogenicity is similar to that of normal liver parenchyma. Obstruction of a biliary duct with dilatation of peripheral intrahepatic biliary radicles is frequently observed in cases of cholangiocarcinoma. Note that hepatocellular carcinoma may cause segmental dilatation of the biliary tract as well.

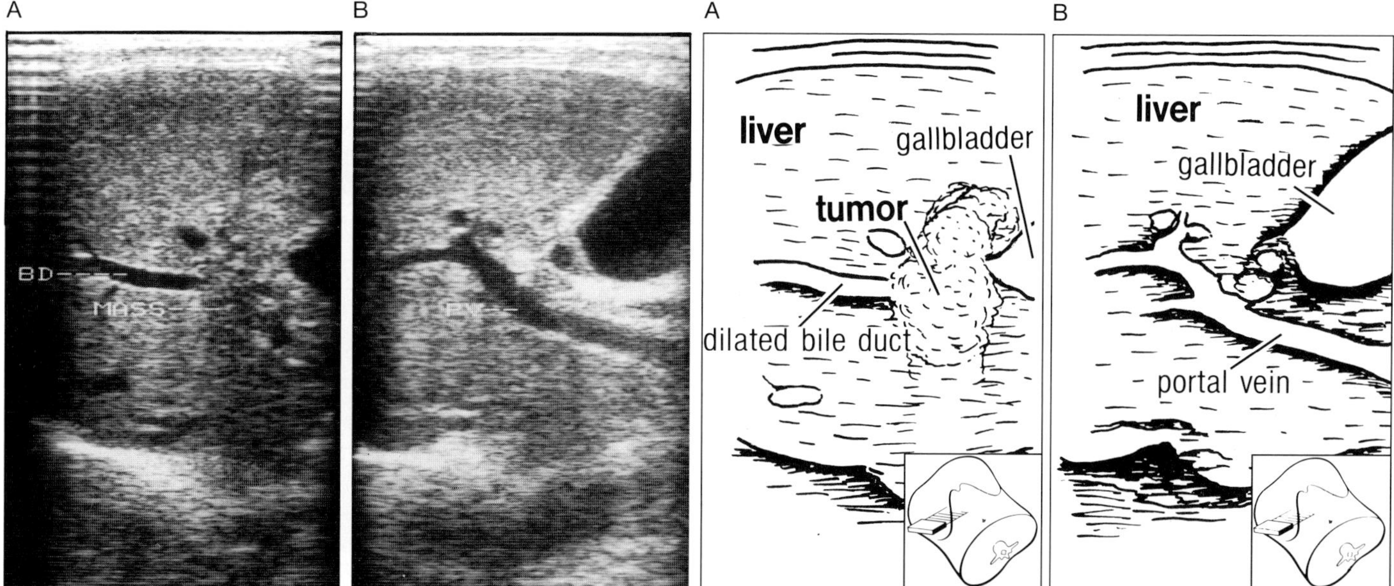

Fig. 3.62 A, B. *Case 1.* The biliary duct is obstructed, and there is mild dilatation of peripheral segments. Careful inspection of the area of obstruction reveals a mass-like lesion with an echo texture which is slightly altered when compared to adjacent liver parenchyma. Image **B** shows the portal vein running parallel to the bile duct. No abnormality is seen in the portal vein

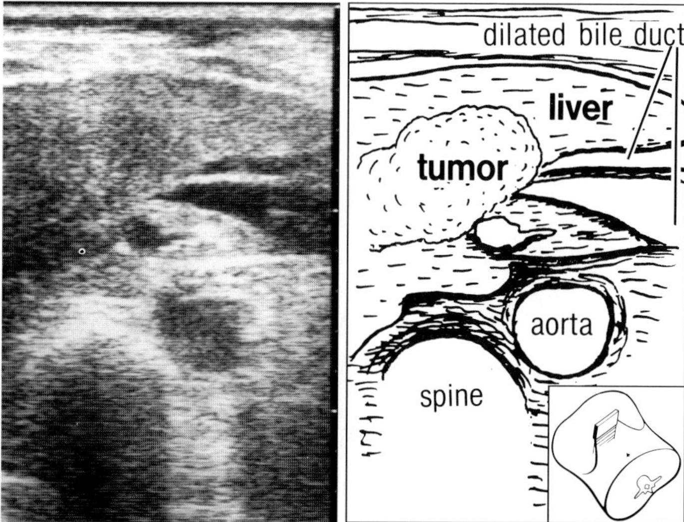

Fig. 3.63. *Case 2.* There is a 3-cm mass in the left hepatic lobe. This has almost the same echogenicity as the normal liver. There is marked dilatation of intrahepatic ducts peripheral to the mass

Cavernous Hemangioma

Small hemangiomas, less than 2 cm in size, are most often visualized as diffuse homogeneous hyperechoic masses without peripheral haloes. Rarely, a small hemangioma is hypoechoic, mimicking a small hepatocellular carcinoma. Slightly larger tumors may have focal hypoechoic areas, and large hemangiomas (larger than 5 cm) typically have mixed hypo- and hyperechoic regions or may be visualized as predominantly hypoechoic masses. Since metastatic disease from colonic or gastric carcinoma can have a similar appearance, it is dangerous to definitely diagnose a small hyperechoic mass as a hemangioma based only on a single ultrasonographic examination.

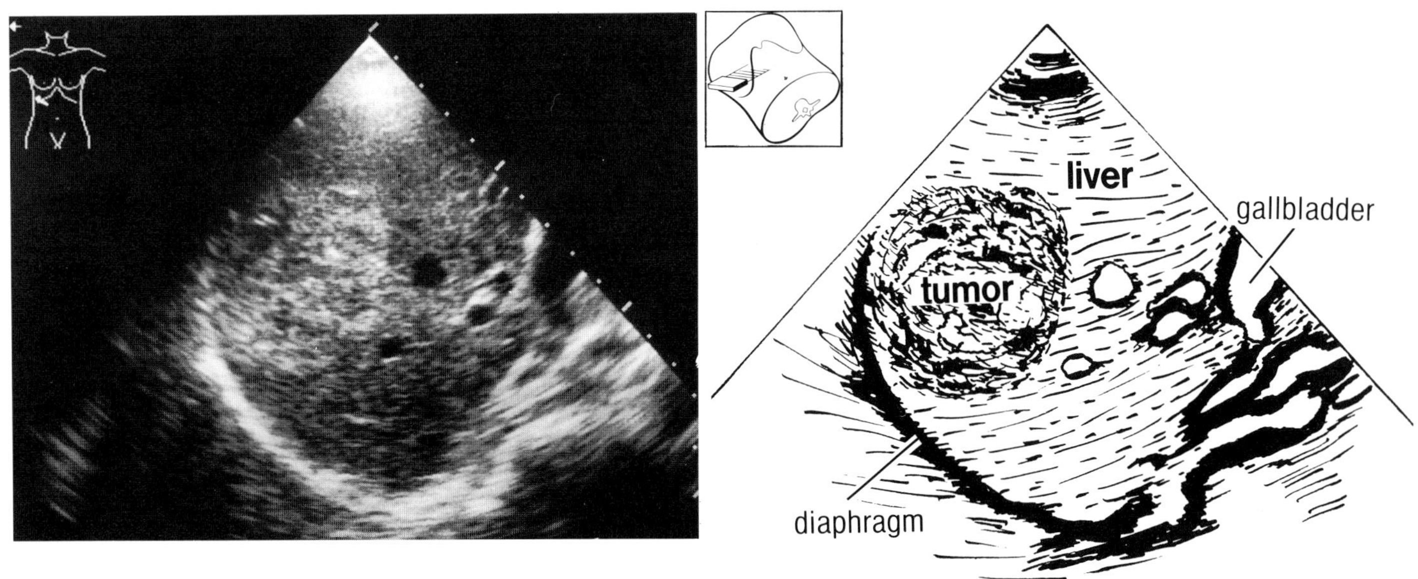

Fig. 3.64. *Case 1.* This hemangioma is large in size (5 cm) and has mixed hyper- and hypoechoic areas

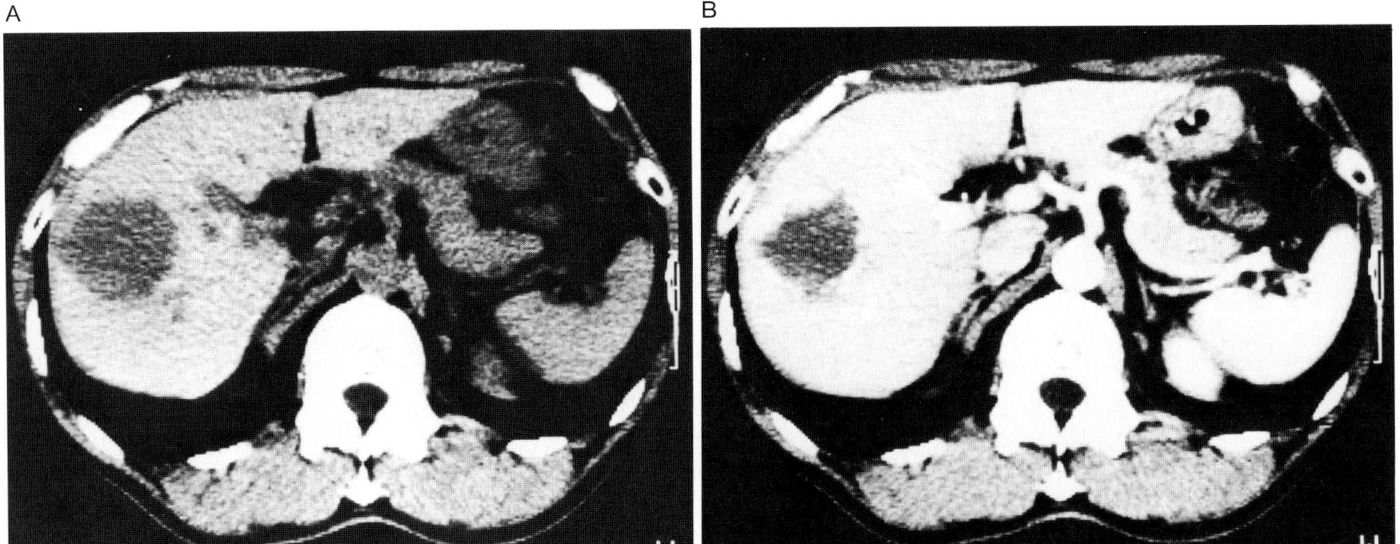

Fig. 3.65 A, B. *Case 1, CT scan.* **A** Before contrast injection. **B** Immediately after bolus injection of contrast material. There is peripheral enhancement which is characteristic of hemangiomas

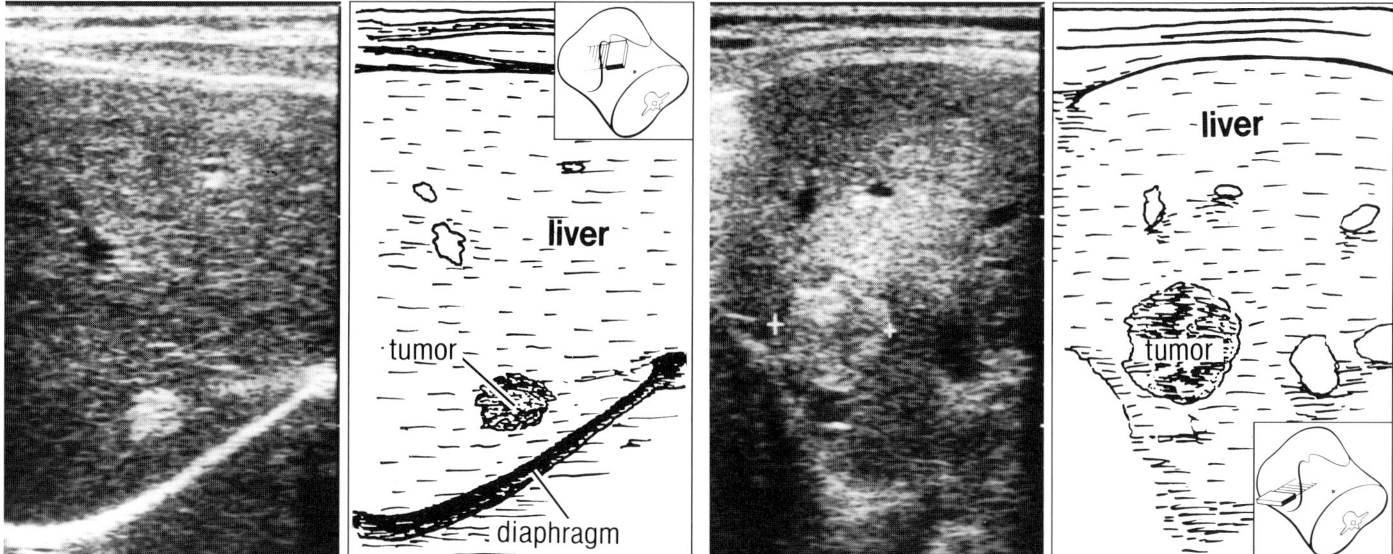

Fig. 3.66. *Case 2.* Typical hyperechoic hemangioma

Fig. 3.67. *Case 3.* A 3-cm hemangioma. Initially, this was diffusely hyperechoic, but after nearly 4 years there was development of small hypoechoic areas within the tumor

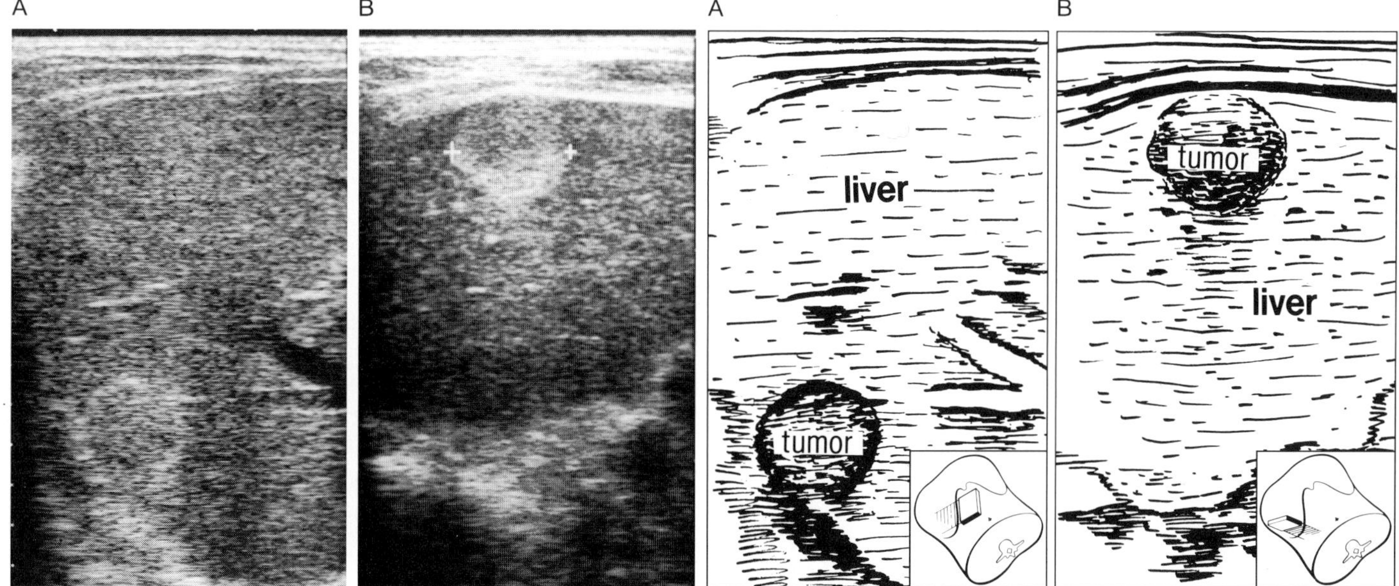

Fig. 3.68 A, B. *Case 4.* A 3-cm hemangioma. **A** Subcostal scan. **B** Intercostal scan. Centrally, the mass is hypoechoic with marginal hyperechoic areas. Note the presence of posterior enhancement. No change in size or echo texture was seen on a follow-up examination 6 months later. These are two images of the same tumor, which differ in appearance due to different scanning directions. This phenomenon is not uncommon on ultrasonographic examinations

Hepatic Cysts

Hepatic cysts are thought to be a congenital abnormality arising from the bile ducts. They are lined by a single layer of epithelium and filled with fluid. Since the advent of ultrasonography and CT, many hepatic cysts are discovered incidentally. Unless they are quite large, they usually need no treatment. Large hepatic cysts may present as an epigastric mass or as a hepatic tumor compressing the stomach on an upper gastrointestinal series of examinations.

It is not difficult to diagnose hepatic cysts of 2 cm or larger in size since they usually have a characteristic cystic pattern (Fig. 3.69). When they are near the surface of the liver, hepatic cysts less than 1 cm in size may be overlooked because of a reverberation

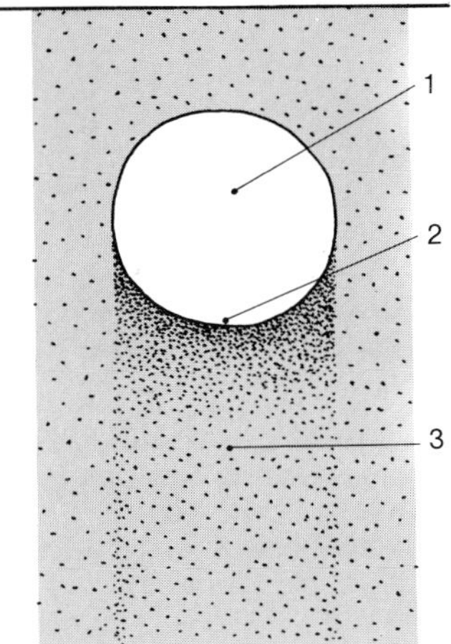

Fig. 3.69. *Cystic pattern.* The designation "cystic pattern" is used when all three of the following conditions are fulfilled (this term is not exclusive for the liver): *1,* there are no internal echoes in the tumor (anechoic); *2,* the posterior wall is distinct; *3,* there is posterior enhancement

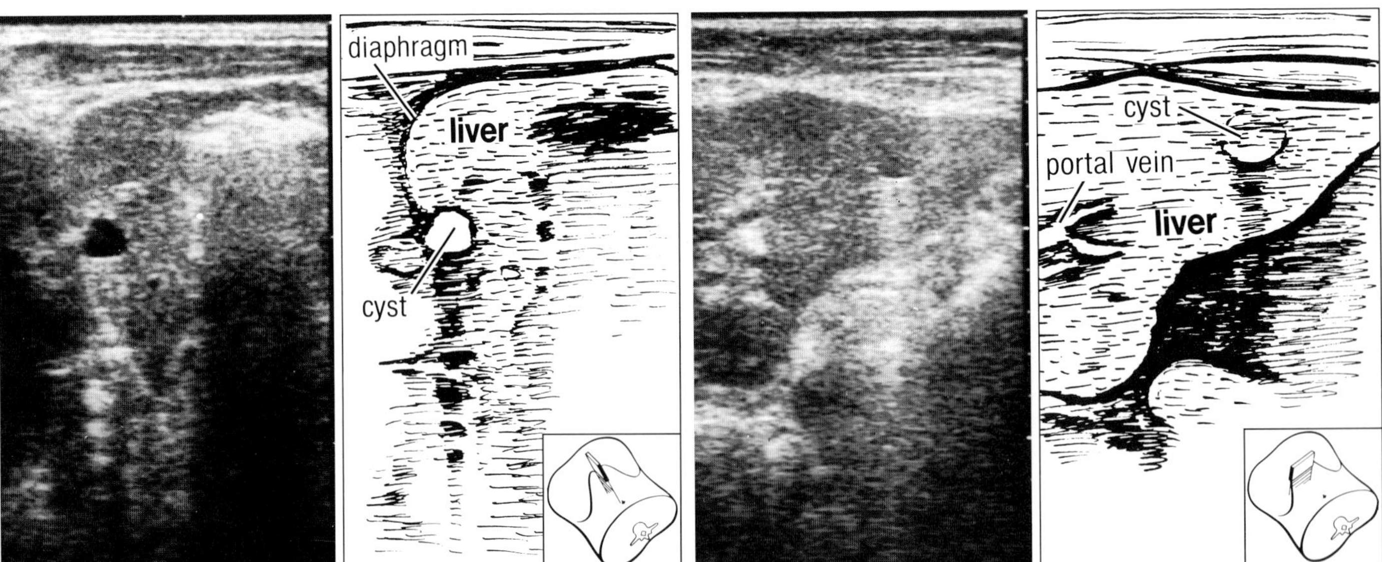

Fig. 3.70. *Case 1.* A 1-cm hepatic cyst with a typical cystic pattern

Fig. 3.71. *Case 2.* A 1.5-cm hepatic cyst with internal echoes and an ill-defined margin caused by reverberation echoes arising from the abdominal wall due to this lesion's superficial location. In this case, relatively thick subcutaneous fat increases the strength of the reverberation artifact

artifact, or they may appear solid. Most of the cysts are rounded with smooth walls, but rarely there is septation or a slight irregularity or spiculation of the wall. In these atypical cases, superimposed carcinoma should be considered, although it is quite rare in our experience.

How to Confirm a Cystic Lesion with Real-Time Scanning

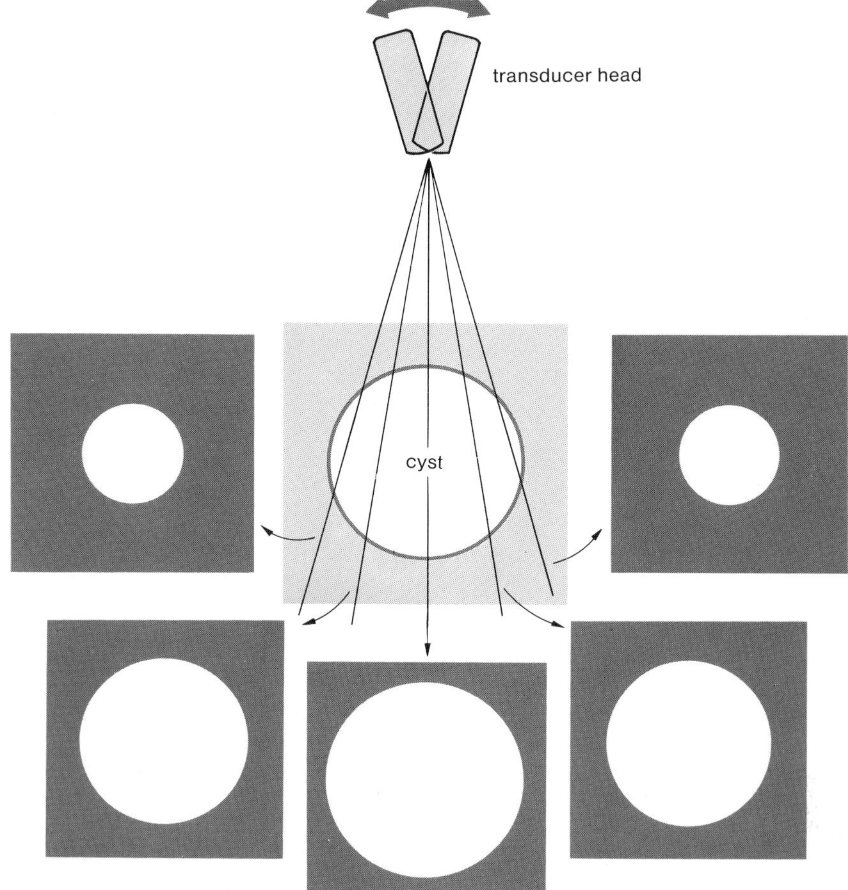

Fig. 3.72. Fan-shaped movement of the transducer head during examination of a hepatic cyst. When the ultrasound beam passes the center of the cyst, the cyst has its maximal diameter. As the ultrasound beam moves away from the center, the cyst appears smaller and finally disappears. In contrast to a tubular structure, a cyst is rounded irrespective of the direction of the beam

Cystic Diseases, Cystic Pattern

Simple hepatic cysts are the most common of the cystic diseases of the liver, but other liver diseases, such as liver abscesses, echinococcal disease, and solid tumors with central necrosis, also exhibit a cystic pattern. Not all structures with a cystic pattern are cysts, and not all cysts exhibit a typical cystic pattern. Examples of the former are the gallbladder, the urinary bladder, and sections of the great vessels. Examples of the latter are superficially located hepatic cysts and ovarian chocolate cysts.

Because of the wide range of detectable ultrasound intensities (dynamic range – comparable to window width on CT), recent advanced ultrasonographic equipment can detect weak echoes from crystals in the cyst fluid (most of these are cholesterol crystals) which could not be visualized on older equipment. Also, low-level noise from the equipment or a reverberation artifact may project within the cyst. As a consequence, not all cysts are anechoic.

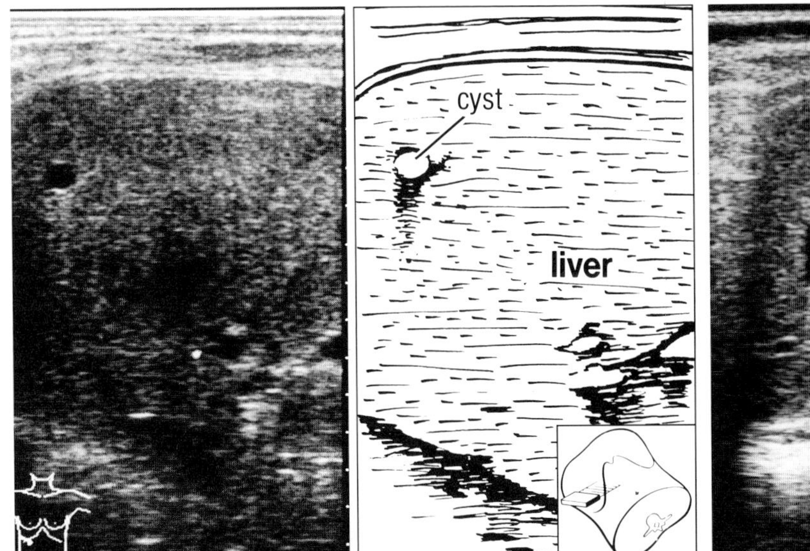

Fig. 3.73. *Case 1.* A hepatic cyst 6 mm in size. Although it is not possible to differentiate a cyst from a tubular structure on a single static image, we can probably safely say that, in this case, this is a hepatic cyst, as the lesion is in the peripheral portion of the liver where no normal tubular structure of this size exists

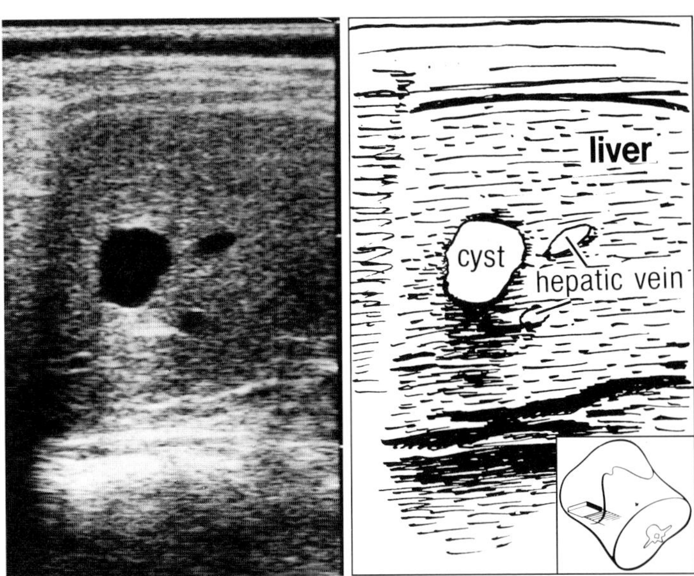

Fig. 3.74. *Case 2.* A 2-cm hepatic cyst. A section of the hepatic vein is visualized nearby

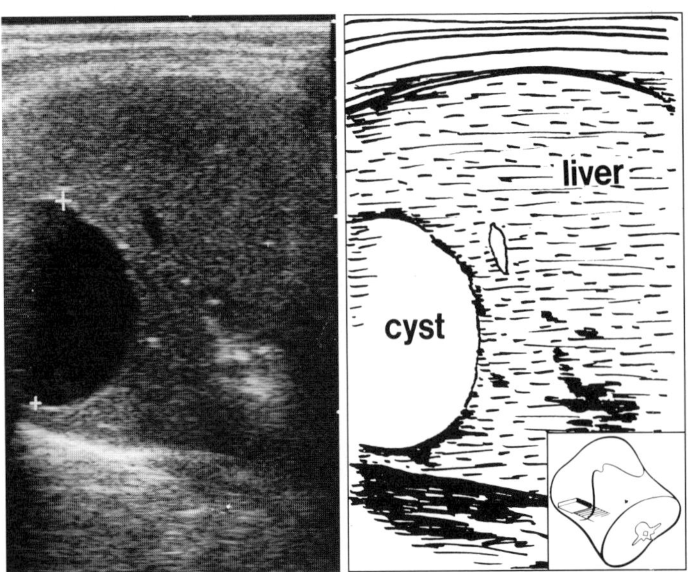

Fig. 3.75. *Case 3.* There is a 5-cm cyst in the superior portion of the right lobe of the liver. Half of the cyst is obscured by overlying lung. In this situation, images should be obtained in expiration when a smaller portion is covered by air in the lung

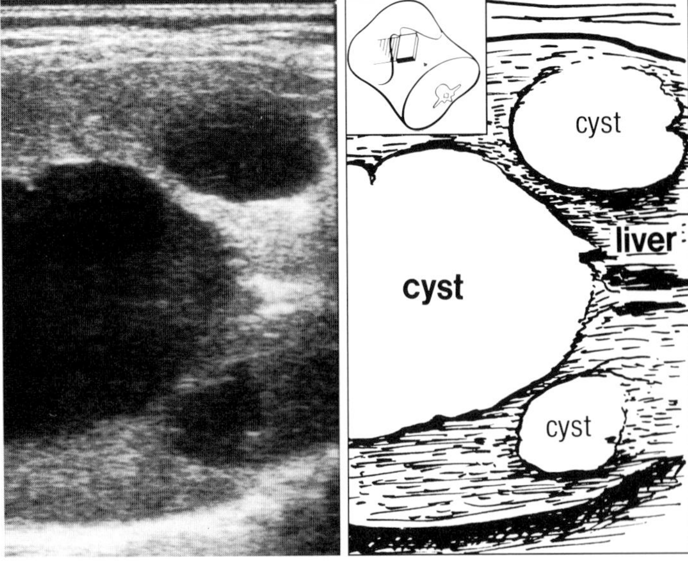

Fig. 3.76. *Case 4.* There are three cysts of various sizes in the superior portion of the right lobe. The walls of the cysts are slightly irregular, but irregularity of this extent is usually of no significance

Polycystic Disease

Polycystic disease is an autosomal dominant disease manifested by multiple cysts in the kidneys. Approximately two-thirds of the patients also have multiple hepatic cysts. Cysts can occur in the pancreas and spleen, but only rarely. Some patients may have multiple cysts only in the liver (polycystic liver) without any cysts in the kidneys. These entities are pathologically quite different from multiple simple cysts in the liver. Cysts in the kidneys or liver vary in size, and their shapes are not always round. In many cases there is severe enlargement of both kidneys and the liver. The border between the right kidney and the liver is often indistinct because of multiple cysts in these organs.

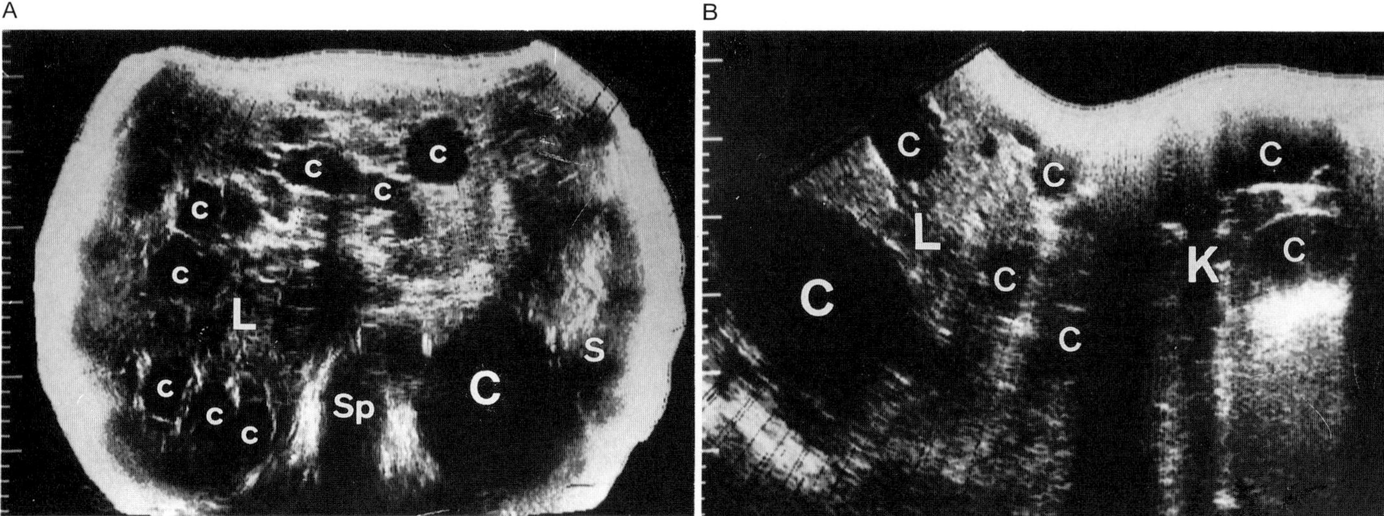

Fig. 3.77 A, B. *Case 1.* **A** Transverse section. The liver is enlarged with multiple cysts of various sizes. There are multiple cysts in the kidneys, but, on this image, the border between the right kidney and the liver is not clearly seen. **B** Longitudinal section through the right kidney.

Multiple cysts are seen in the liver and right kidney, but these organs cannot be distinctly delineated. *L,* liver; *S,* spleen; *Sp,* spine; *K,* right kidney; *C,* cysts

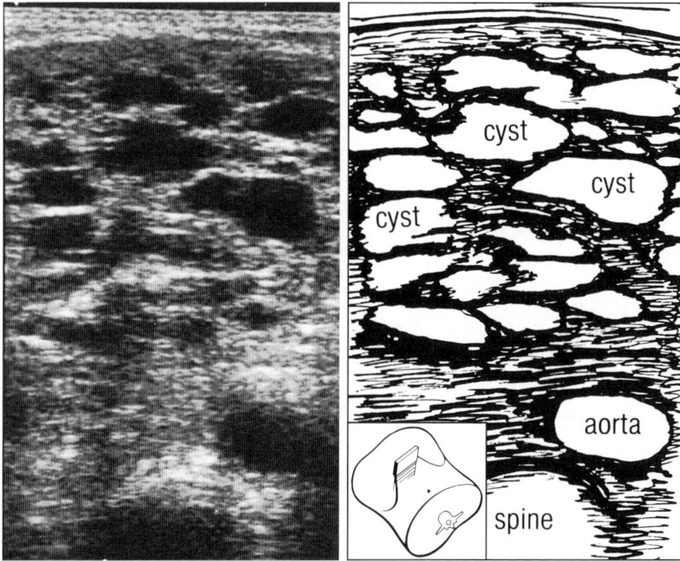

Fig. 3.78. *Case 2.* Polycystic disease. There are multiple cysts of various sizes in the liver, some with irregular shapes

Differential Diagnosis of Hepatic Cysts

There are ultrasonographic findings which may simulate hepatic cysts:

1. *Cysts in the right kidney:* cysts arising from the upper pole or middle portion of the right kidney may indent the surface of the liver as they grow. Most of the cystic lesions at the hepatorenal junction which appear to involve both organs are renal cysts. In order to determine the origins of a cyst, it is important to observe with which organ the cyst moves during deep inspiration or when changing the patient's position (erect position is especially useful).

2. *Intrahepatic vascular structures:* on static images, it is difficult to differentiate a cross-section of a hepatic or portal vein (especially the former) from a small hepatic cyst. Needless to say, it is easy to differentiate a cyst from a vascular structure during real-time scanning by tracing the course of the latter.

3. *Neck of the gallbladder:* when the neck of the gallbladder is tortuous, a portion of it may simulate a small hepatic cyst near the porta hepatis. Careful observation from different directions can distinguish this from a true hepatic cyst.

4. *Central necrosis of a solid tumor:* some of the metastatic liver tumors tend to have central necrosis with liquefaction. Even in these cases, the solid portion of the tumor is seen around the necrosis and therefore can usually be differentiated from a hepatic cyst.

5. *Hepatic abscess:* typically, hepatic abscesses appear anechoic, but on careful observation low-amplitude echoes are seen within the anechoic area. The contour of a hepatic abscess is more irregular than that of a cyst.

6. *Hepatic cystadenocarcinoma:* usually, there is a solid portion adjacent to the cyst wall, and it may be multiloculated.

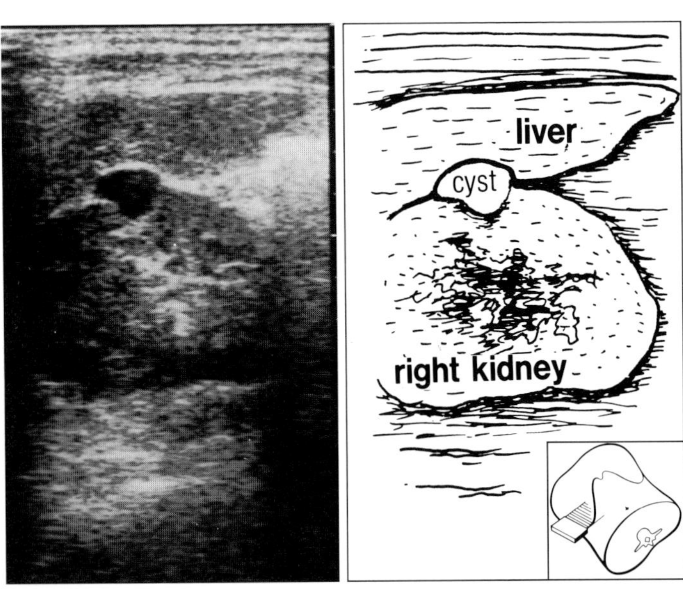

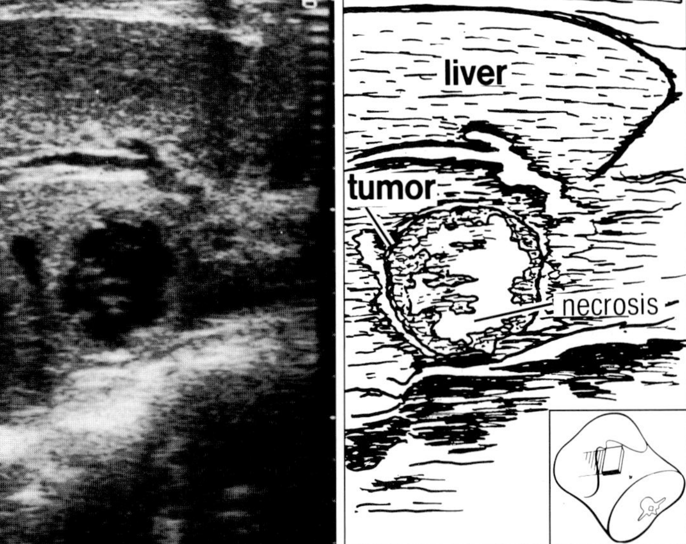

Fig. 3.79. *Right renal cyst.* There is a cyst at the junction of the liver and the right kidney. This cyst originates from the right kidney and is compressing the liver

Fig. 3.80. *Metastatic tumor with necrosis from gastric carcinoma.* Most of the tumor is liquefied. Irregularity of the wall and surrounding abnormal echoes help differentiate this lesion from a simple hepatic cyst

Hepatic Abscess

Hepatic abscess is one of the disease processes which has a cystic pattern on ultrasonographic examination. However, the purulent material within the abscess cavity is not entirely anechoic. An abscess wall is usually more irregular and indistinct compared with that of a cyst, and frequently there is adjacent liver tissue with decreased echogenicity suggesting parenchymal inflammation.

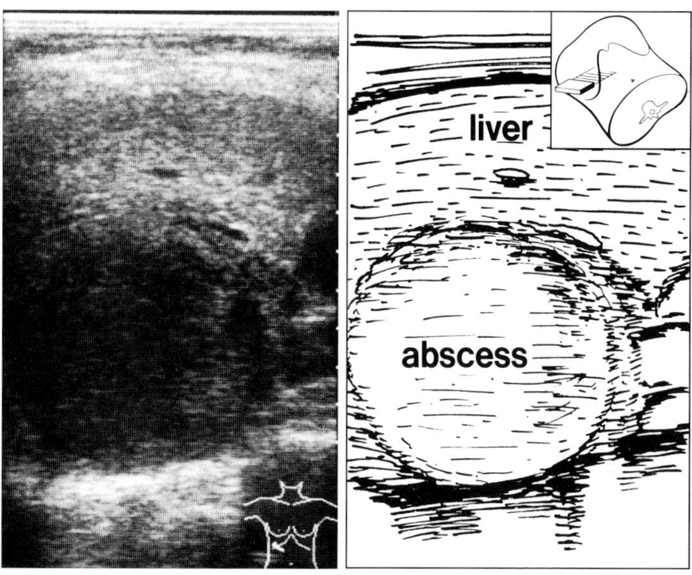

Fig. 3.81. *Case 1.* There is an 8-cm hypoechoic mass in the posterior portion of the right lobe of the liver. This patient had been treated for an abscess

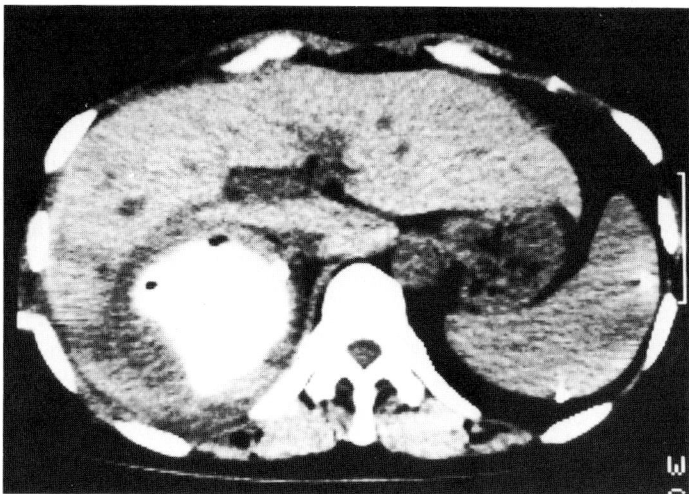

Fig. 3.82. *Case 1, CT scan, 4 days after the ultrasonographic examination.* Contrast material injected through the drainage tube is visualized in the central portion of the cystic space. The contrast material reveals the fluid nature of the lesion which appeared solid on ultrasonographic examination

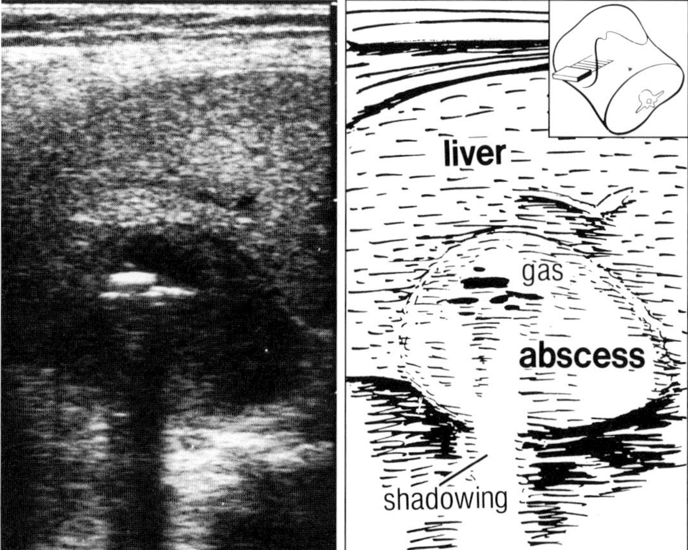

Fig. 3.83. *Case 1, ultrasonographic examination, 1 month after the initial ultrasonogram.* The abscess has decreased in size. There are strong echoes with posterior shadowing, indicating the presence of gas

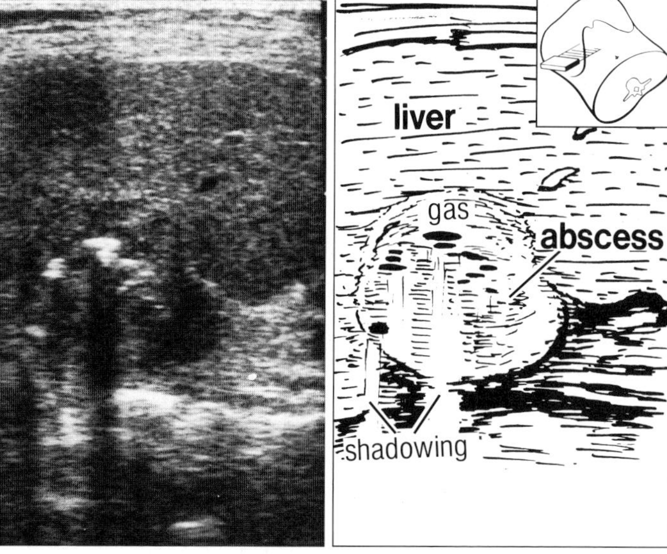

Fig. 3.84. *Case 1, ultrasonographic examination, 2½ months after the one in Fig. 3.83.* The abscess has further diminished in size and now measures 35 mm in diameter

Ultrasonographic Findings Which Suggest Hepatic Dysfunction

Deformity of the Liver Contour

The liver is enlarged in acute hepatitis; in chronic hepatitis the liver is normal in size. In hepatic cirrhosis, there is atrophy of the liver, especially around the gallbladder bed, while the lateral segment of the left lobe and the caudate lobe typically become enlarged.

Atrophy of the region of the gallbladder bed is clearly visualized on longitudinal sections of the liver through the gallbladder. As shown in Fig. 3.85, the normal liver covers the anterior surface of the gallbladder, and the gallbladder is oblong in shape. When there is atrophy of the liver in the region of the gallbladder bed, the gallbladder is pulled cephalad, and its shape is altered. Deformity of the gallbladder on oral cholecystography may be interpreted as an abnormality of the gallbladder itself, but deformity of the gallbladder is frequently secondary to deformity of the liver.

It is easy to identify the caudate lobe of the liver as it is clearly demarcated from the lateral segment of the left lobe by the fissure of the ligamentum venosum. The shape and size of the caudate lobe can be evaluated on the midline sagittal section or on transverse sections. When the caudate lobe is enlarged, the connective tissue in the fissure of ligamentum venosum becomes thickened.

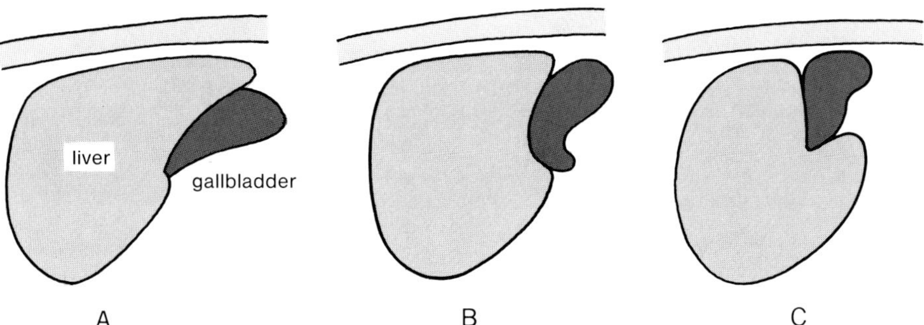

· **Fig. 3.85 A–C.** *Hepatic dysfunction and change of location and shape of the gallbladder.* When the liver is normal, the gallbladder is posterior to the right lobe of the liver (**A**). As hepatic dysfunction progresses, the liver decreases in size resulting in a deformity of the gallbladder bed. The fundus of the gallbladder becomes more cephalad in position (**B**). In hepatic cirrhosis with marked atrophy and deformity of the liver, the neck of the gallbladder becomes buried in the liver like a "wedge." The fundus of the gallbladder is in direct contact with abdominal wall (**C**)

Irregularity of the Liver Surface

In cases of severe hepatic dysfunction, the surface of the liver becomes irregular. This finding reflects formation of regenerative nodules associated with liver cirrhosis. With the accumulation of ascites, this finding becomes more apparent. The inferior edge of the liver becomes blunted, and the posterior surface of the liver becomes convex. (Fig. 3.88).

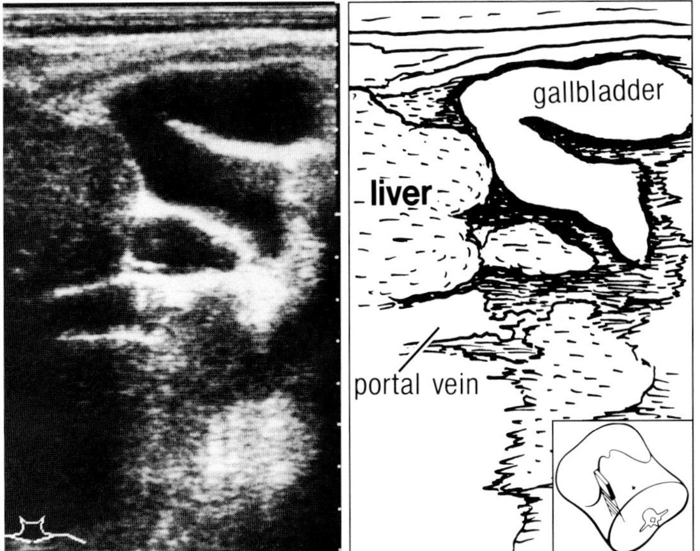

Fig. 3.86. *Case 1.* There is atrophy of the liver in the region of the gallbladder bed. As the liver becomes deformed, there is deformity of the gallbladder, and it appears S-shaped on the longitudinal section

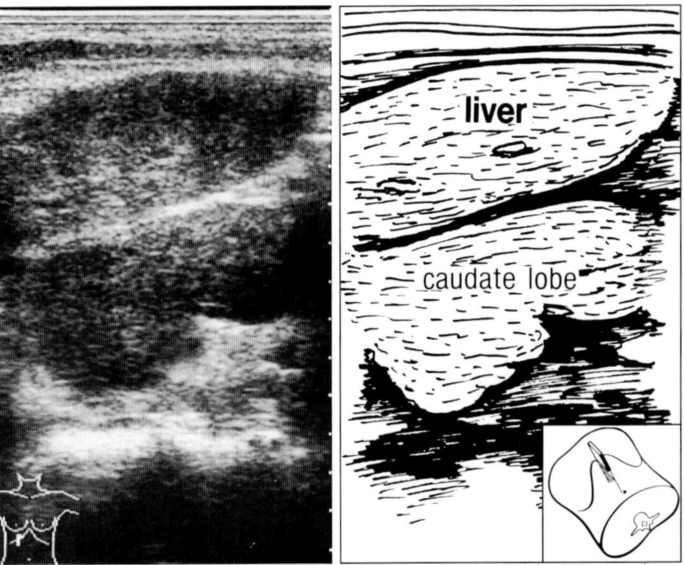

Fig. 3.87. *Case 2.* An enlarged caudate lobe is visualized posterior to the left hepatic lobe. There is thickening and prominence of the connective tissue between the caudate lobe and the left lobe (in the fissure of the ligamentum venosum). Because of its deep location, the caudate lobe appears hypoechoic and it can be mistaken for a hypoechoic hepatocellular carcinoma, particularly when it is enlarged

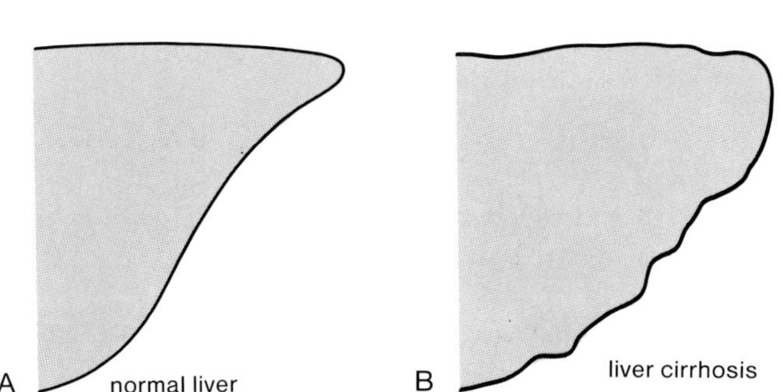

Fig. 3.88 A, B. The surface of the normal liver (**A**) is smooth and the inferior edge is acute. The posterior surface of the liver is concave. In case of liver cirrhosis (**B**), the inferior edge becomes blunted, and the surface becomes irregular. The posterior surface becomes convex

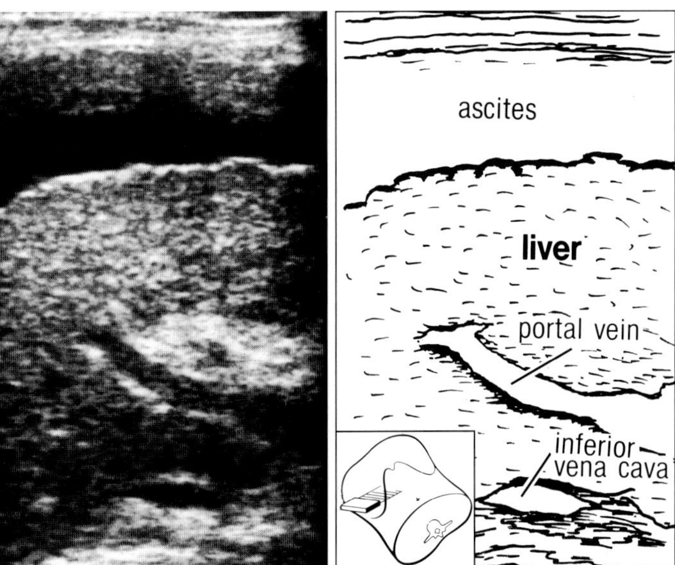

Fig. 3.89. *Case 1.* Cirrhosis with ascites. Irregularity (nodularity) of the surface of the liver is clearly visualized

Coarsening of the Internal Echo Texture of the Liver

The normal liver has a fine homogeneous echo pattern, but in cirrhosis the internal echo texture of the liver becomes coarse and heterogeneous. When there is severe regeneration, differentiation from diffuse infiltrating hepatocellular carcinoma becomes difficult. However, when there is tumor thrombus in the portal vein, it is a case of diffuse hepatocellular carcinoma.

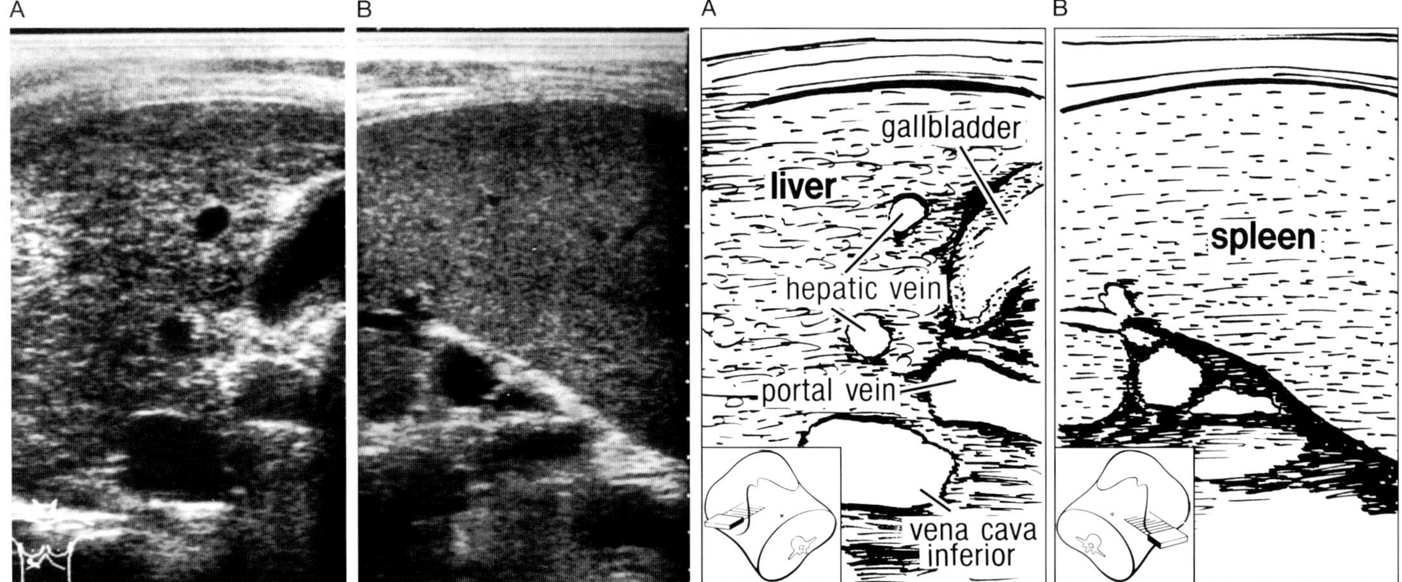

Fig. 3.90 A, B. *Case 1.* **A** Intercostal scan of the liver. **B** Intercostal scan of the spleen. There is marked splenomegaly. Normal liver has a fine homogeneous echo pattern, similar to that of the spleen. In this case, the internal echo pattern of the liver has become coarsened compared to that of the spleen. There is thickening of the wall of the gallbladder

Splenomegaly

The presence or absence, and, if present, the degree of splenomegaly, is a good indicator of hepatic dysfunction. Since splenomegaly is seen in many diseases (see p. 45), splenomegaly alone does not necessarily indicate hepatic dysfunction. However, in a case of known hepatic dysfunction, the degree of splenomegaly may indicate the extent of hepatic dysfunction.

Many methods have been reported to measure splenic volume by ultrasonography. However, it is impossible to accurately calculate the volume of the spleen using a linear scanner since the portion of the spleen adjacent to the lung cannot be adequately visualized. One generally accepted method of estimating splenic volume is to measure the spleen on the image in which the largest portion of the spleen is visualized. With this method, the closer the splenic size is to normal, the larger the degree of error can be.

We divide splenomegaly into four groups, using the standard linear scanner with an effective visual field of 8 cm (Fig. 3.91). A normal-sized spleen is in contact with the abdominal wall for 4 cm or less. Minimal splenomegaly is present when the spleen is in contact with the abdominal wall for 5–7 cm, mild splenomegaly 7–9 cm, and moderate enlargement more than 9 cm. The massive spleen, as seen in cases of leukemia, is designated as marked splenomegaly. It should be noted that the spleens of children are relative large considering their body size. (See pp. 142–145, "Splenomegaly.")

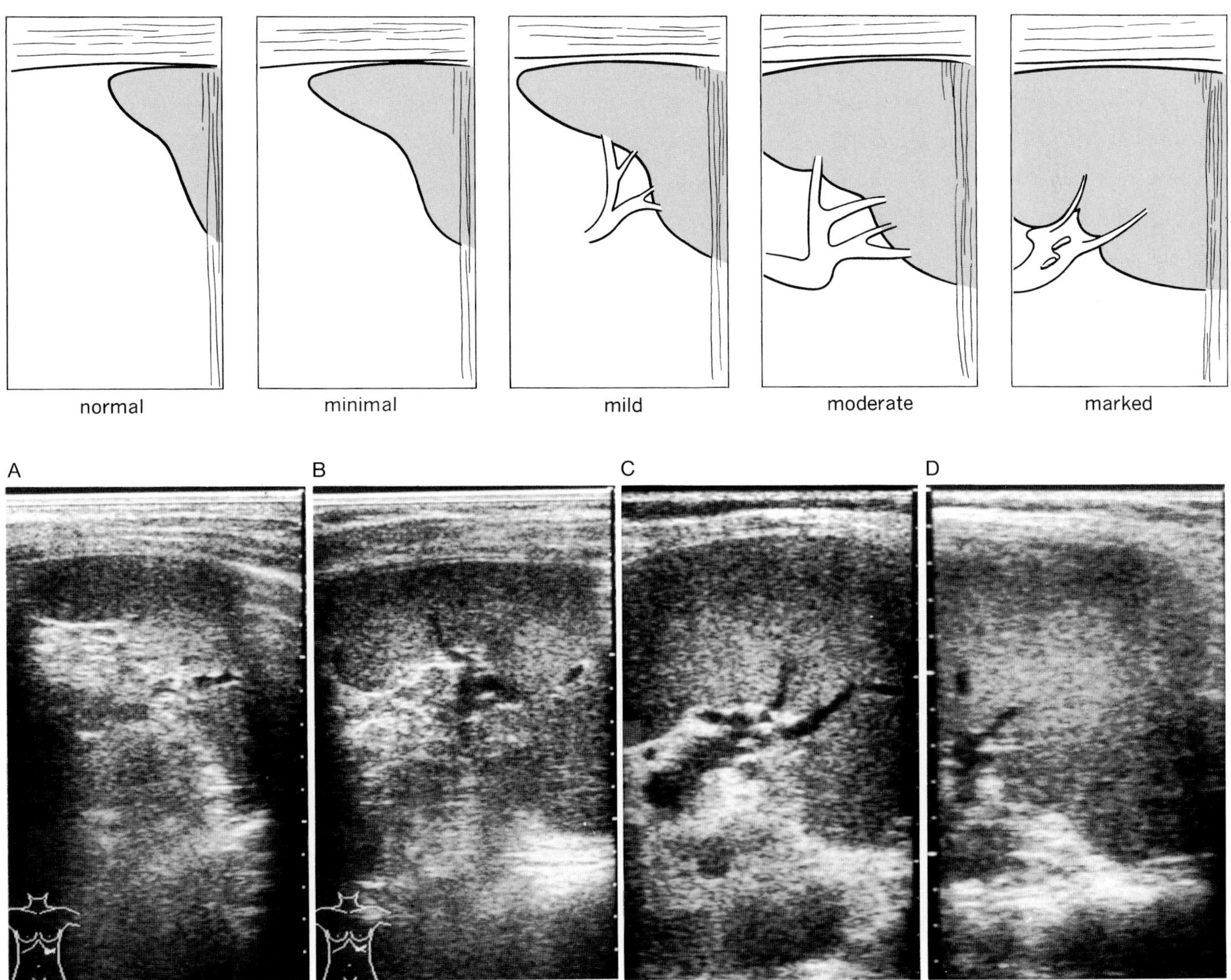

Fig. 3.91 A–D. *Evolution of splenomegaly*. Using a linear scanner with an effective field of 8 cm, splenomegaly can be divided into four groups: **A** minimal; **B** mild; **C** moderate; **D** marked (see text)

**Development
of Collateral Pathways**

Portal venous pressure is elevated in hepatic cirrhosis; and the portal, splenic, and superior mesenteric veins become enlarged. Part of the portal flow drains into the systemic venous system via collateral pathways. There are several collateral pathways which develop in portal hypertension, as shown in Fig. 3.92. Dilatation of the left gastric vein and the paraumbilical vein can be visualized on ultrasonography. Normally, the left gastric vein cannot be visualized, but, when dilated, it is visualized as a serpiginous structure posterior to the left lobe of the liver. As the portal pressure rises, the paraumbilical vein becomes dilated and anechoic centrally.

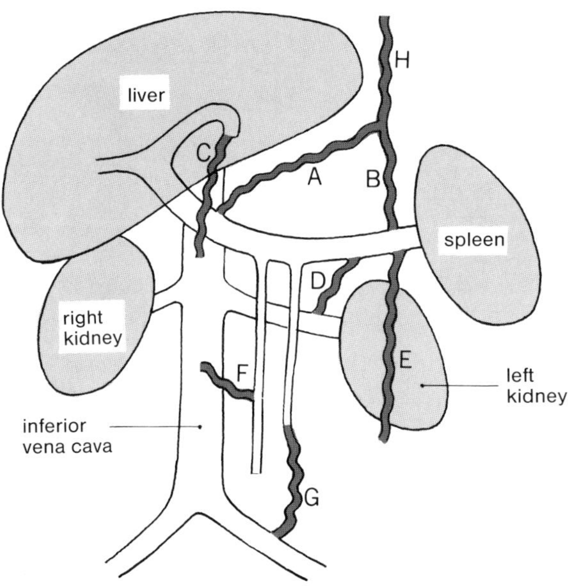

Fig. 3.92. *Portal collateral pathways. A*, left gastric vein; *B*, short gastric vein; *C*, paraumbilical vein; *D*, splenorenal shunt; *E*, splenoretroperitoneal shunt; *F*, superior mesenteric vein–inferior vena cava shunt; *G*, hemorrhoidal vein; *H*, esophageal vein

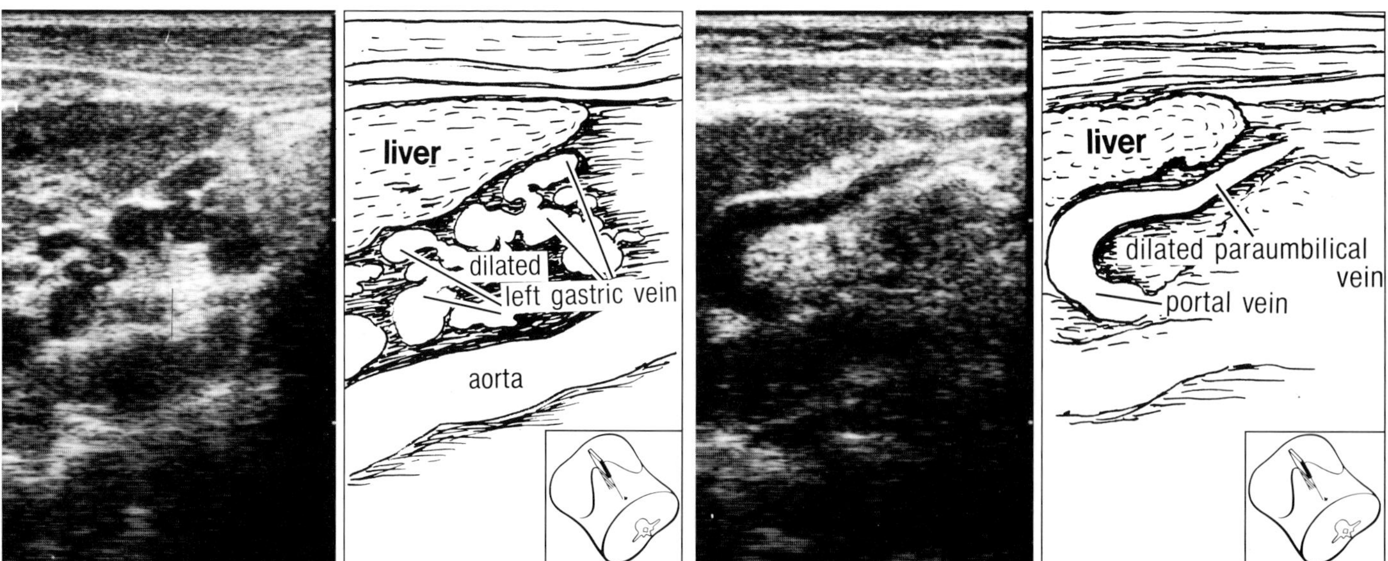

Fig. 3.93. *Case 1.* A dilated left gastric vein is visualized between the left lobe of the liver and the aorta

Fig. 3.94. *Case 2.* Dilated paraumbilical vein penetrates the liver and is subjacent to the anterior abdominal wall

**Thickening
of the Gallbladder Wall**

The normal thickness of the gallbladder wall is only 2 mm. In hepatic cirrhosis, it can be as thick as 5 mm. The internal echo texture of the thickened gallbladder wall is frequently hypoechoic.

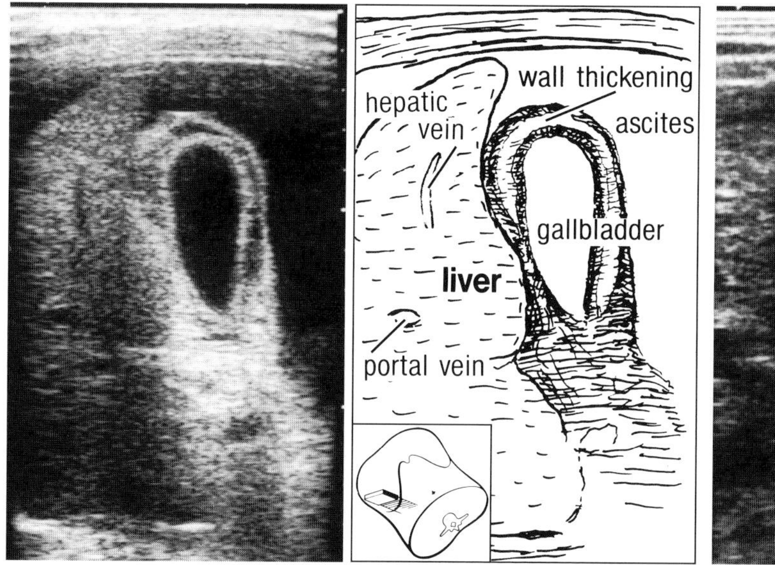

Fig. 3.95. *Case 1*. There is marked thickening of the gallbladder wall and a hypoechoic central layer; hence, three distinct wall layers are visualized. Abundant ascites is present

Fig. 3.96. *Case 2*. The entire gallbladder wall is thickened and hyperechoic. The liver parenchyma around the gallbladder has a coarse echo texture

Ascites

When ascites is present, anechoic spaces between the liver and right kidney (Morison's pouch), or between the liver and the abdominal wall are identified. With a large amount of ascites, the intestine will be seen floating within the peritoneal cavity.

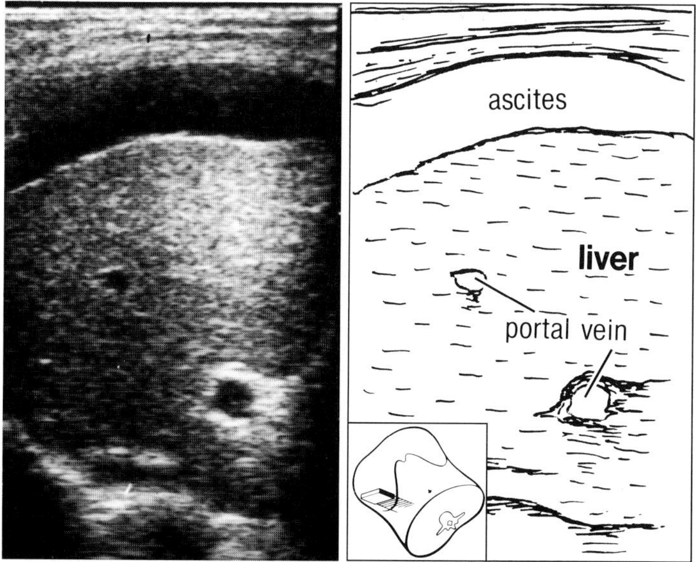

Fig. 3.97. *Case 1*. There is a 2-cm anechoic space between the liver and abdominal wall

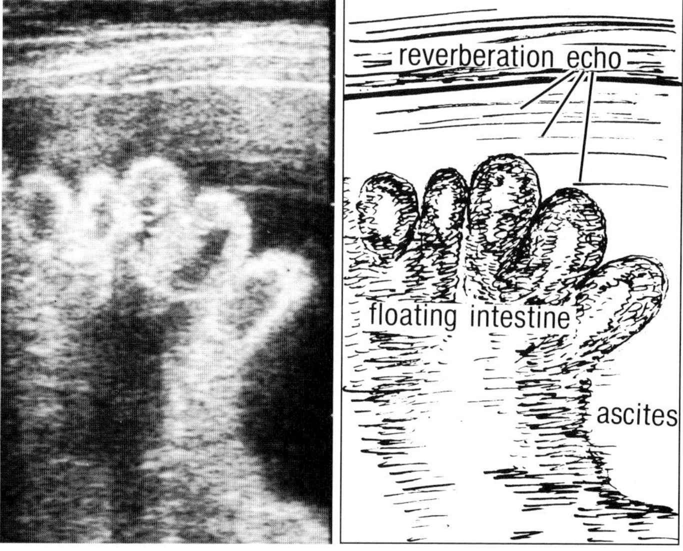

Fig. 3.98. *Case 2*. Small intestinal loops float within the ascites to give a characteristic appearance

Acute Hepatitis

In acute hepatitis, the liver becomes enlarged. The gallbladder appears small with a thick wall secondary to decreased biliary excretion from the liver. There may be echoes within the lumen of the gallbladder representing sludge. With improvement of hepatic function, the gallbladder becomes normal in appearance.

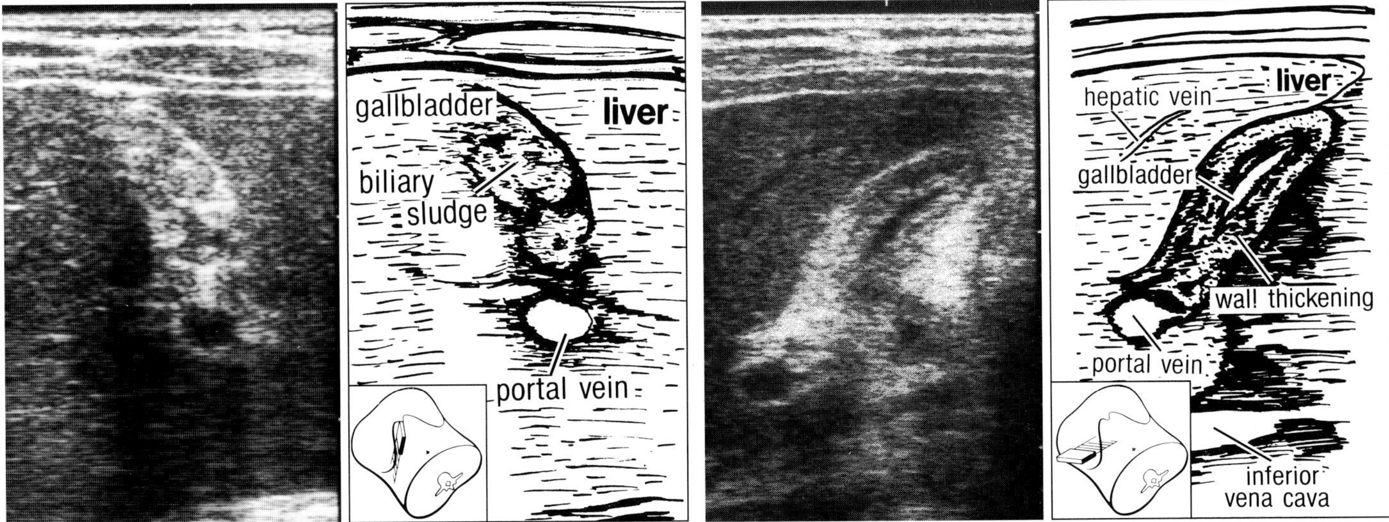

Fig. 3.99. *Case 1*. Acute viral hepatitis. Laboratory findings: SGOT 1190 IU/l, SGPT 1105 IU/l, LDH 1921 IU/l (IU: International Unit)

Fig. 3.100. *Case 2*. There is diffuse thickening of the gallbladder wall with a central hypoechoic layer. The lumen of the gallbladder is abnormally small. The liver is unremarkable

Chronic Hepatitis

Findings clearly visualized on ultrasonography are minimal-to-mild splenomegaly and a blunting of the inferior edge of the liver. Presence of a coarsened internal echo texture, deformity of the liver, collateral pathways, or ascites suggests hepatic cirrhosis.

Can Liver Size Be Measured by Ultrasonography?

Using a linear scanner, the size of the liver may be estimated by measuring several craniocaudal sections of the liver at certain representative sites. However, there are many problems with this method. First of all, it is difficult to visualize the dome of the right lobe using a linear scanner because of adjacent air in the lungs. In order to measure the size of the right lobe, it is necessary to utilize two images as the length of the right lobe exceeds the size of the transducer head, and there are no guarantees that this composition has been done accurately. Even if the craniocaudal dimension of the liver could be accurately measured, it is difficult to decide where the measurement should be taken because of large variations in hepatic shape as seen, for example, on hepatic scintigraphy. It is possible to calculate the volume of the spleen by measuring several axes (such as long and short axes) as the spleen enlarges relatively symmetrically. The liver, on the other hand, enlarges or shrinks with its shape changing in a complex rather than a symmetric fashion; therefore, it is not possible to accurately calculate (or even estimate) the volume of the liver.

Cirrhosis of the Liver

In cirrhosis of the liver, various combinations of the previously mentioned findings that suggest hepatic dysfunction are present. Atrophy of hepatic parenchyma in the area of the gallbladder fossa is characteristic and is frequently observed. If collateral pathways or ascites are present, advanced cirrhosis is suggested. Rarely, there is only minimal splenomegaly in the presence of liver cirrhosis.

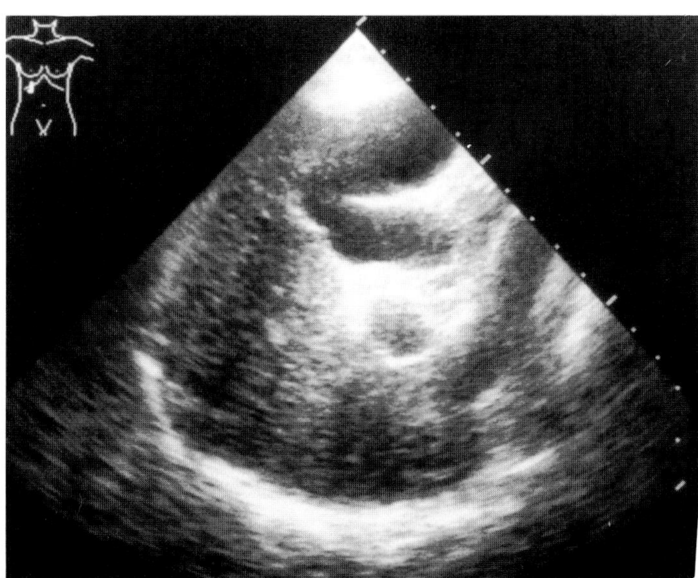

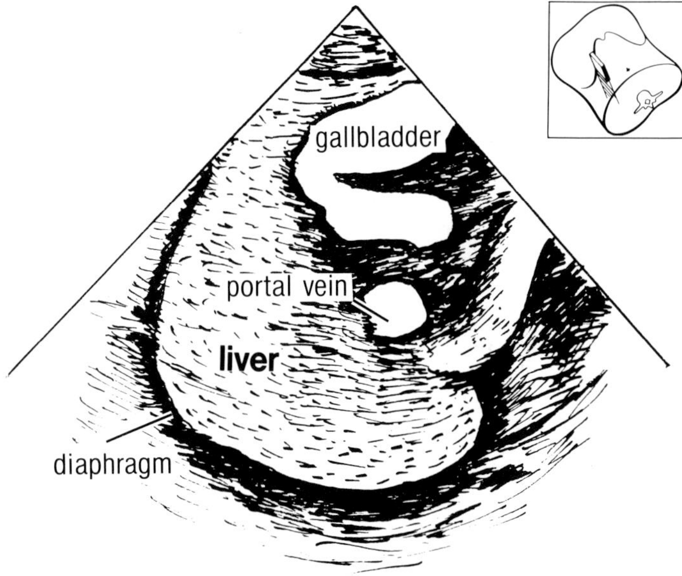

Fig. 3.101. *Case 1.* A longitudinal section of the right lobe of the liver through the gallbladder. There is severe deformity of the liver. The gallbladder is more cephalad than normal secondary to atrophy of liver in the area of gallbladder fossa and appears C-shaped

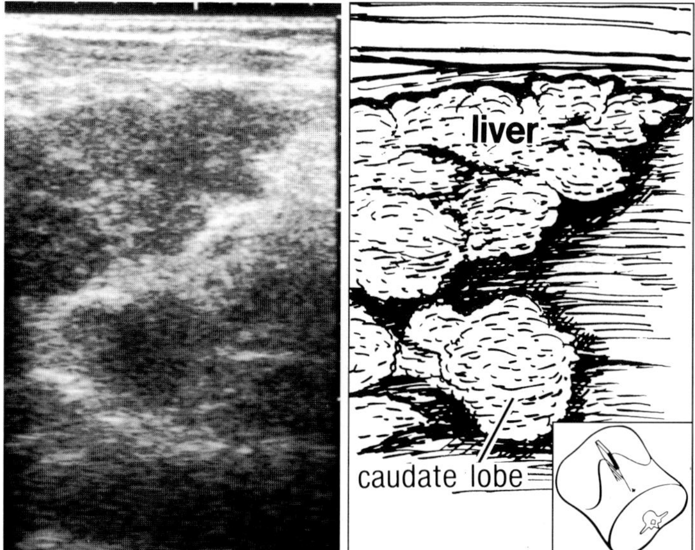

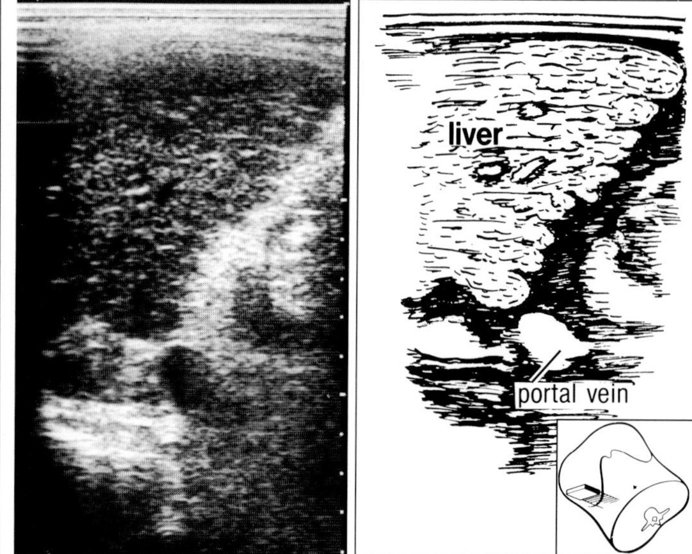

Fig. 3.102. *Case 2.* Midline sagittal image. There is marked irregularity of the liver surface and coarsening of the internal echo texture

Fig. 3.103. *Case 3.* Irregularity of the liver surface, particularly on the posterior surface, is well visualized. There is a coarse internal echo texture throughout the liver

Fatty Infiltration of the Liver

The clinical diagnosis of fatty infiltration of the liver is difficult because there are few characteristic biochemical abnormalities on analysis of the serum, but ultrasonographic diagnosis is relatively easy due to several characteristic findings. This disease can be also diagnosed on CT, but ultrasonography is more sensitive. The ultrasonographic findings of fatty infiltration of the liver are as follows:

1. Increased echogenicity throughout the liver (bright liver)
2. Hepatomegaly
3. Poor visualization of the intrahepatic tubular structures

Increased echogenicity of the liver is caused by an increased number of interfaces between hepatic parenchyma and fatty droplets which reflect the ultrasound beam. Because of increased attenuation of the ultrasound beam in the liver, there is a decrease in the echo level in the deep portions of the liver. In order to determine the echogenicity of the liver objectively, it should be compared with that of the right kidney or the spleen. In obese patients, the echo level of the liver may appear increased, simulating fatty infiltration of the liver because of reverberation artifacts produced by an increased thickness of the abdominal wall.

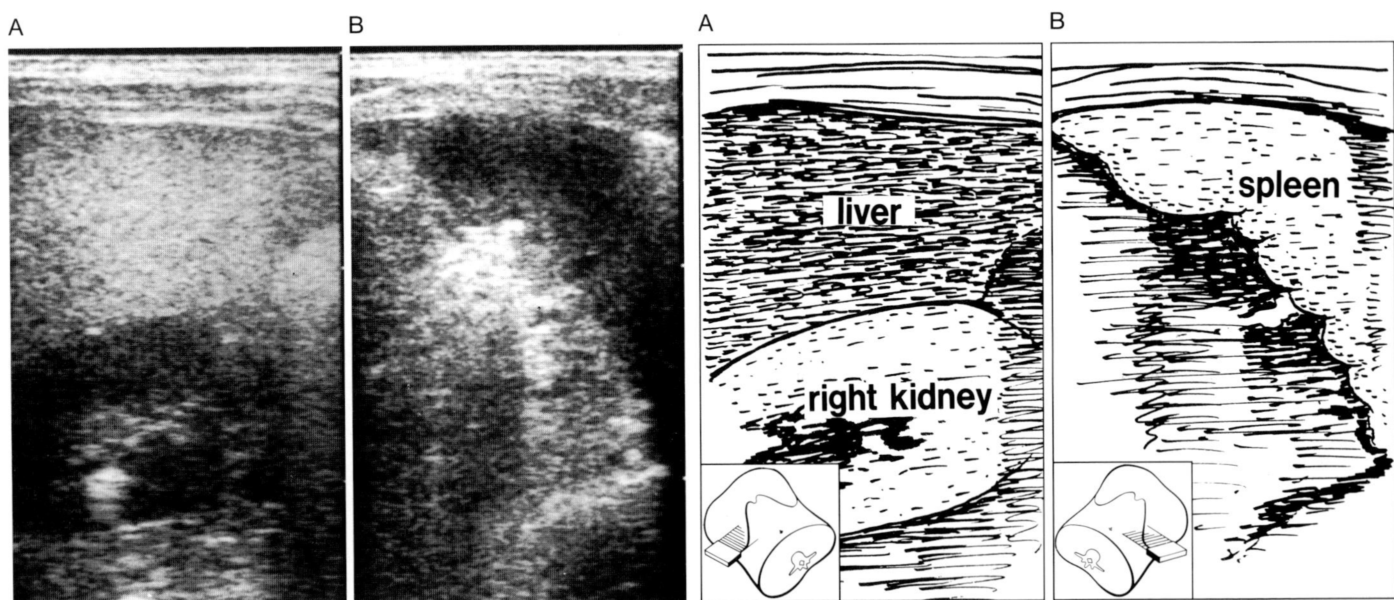

Fig. 3.104 A, B. *Case 1.* **A** Liver with increased echogenicity (bright liver). Note the large differences in echogenicity relative to the right kidney. **B** Images of the spleen using the same technique; this indicates that only the echo level of the liver is increased

Focal Fatty Infiltration of the Liver

Fatty infiltration of the liver has become a relatively common ultrasonographic diagnosis, and some of these cases are associated with what appears to be a small solid tumor in the liver. This finding is most frequently seen adjacent to the gallbladder (area of the gallbladder fossa) or adjacent to the horizontal portion of the portal vein. The abnormal area is hypoechoic relative to the surrounding hepatic parenchyma. These lesions are most often oblong or irregular rather than rounded in shape. On the basis of CT, biopsy, and the clinical course, this finding is believed by many to be spared normal liver tissue; i.e., the relatively hypoechoic area is residual normal liver tissue surrounded by fatty liver which is hyperechoic. A variation of this phenomenon is seen when two segments separated by a hepatic vein have different degrees of fatty infiltration.

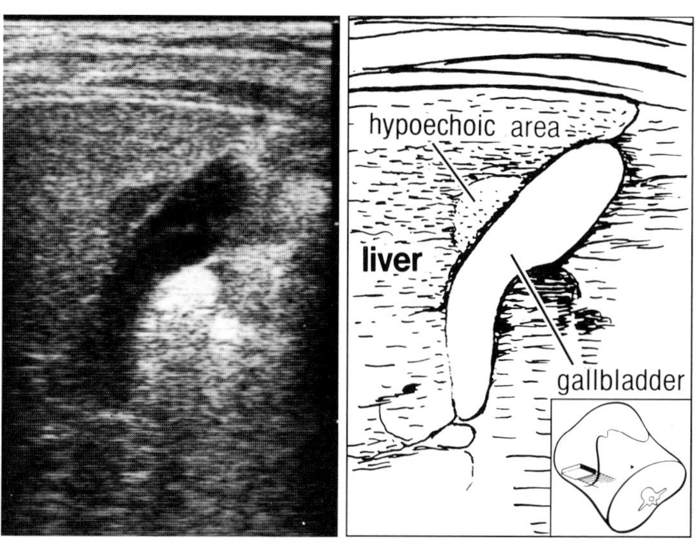

Fig. 3.105. *Case 1.* A triangularly shaped hypoechoic area adjacent to the gallbladder resembles a tumor, but this area is normal liver tissue surrounded by hyperechoic fatty liver

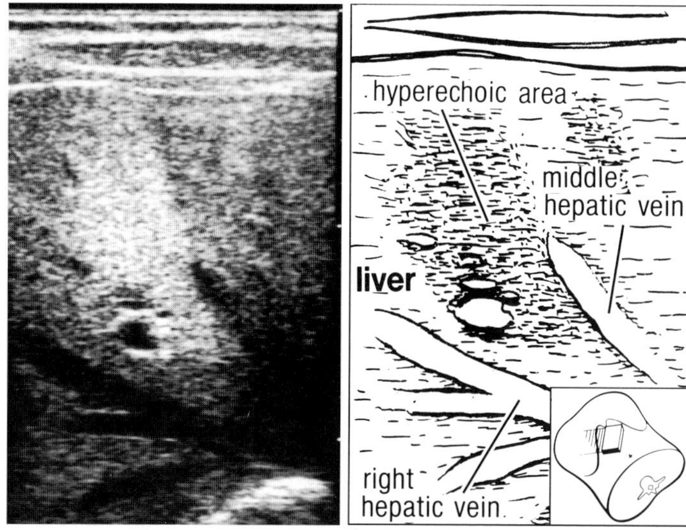

Fig. 3.106. *Case 2.* Focal fatty infiltration of the liver. The echo level is particularly elevated posterior to the middle hepatic vein (anterior segment of the right lobe)

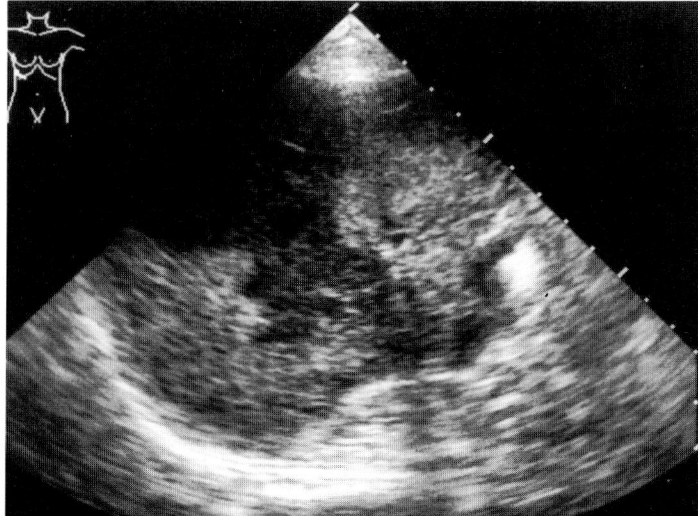

Fig. 3.107. *Case 3.* Patient with diabetes. There is a map-like hypoechoic area in the anterosuperior portion of the right lobe. This geographic area appears abnormal, but it actually represents normal liver

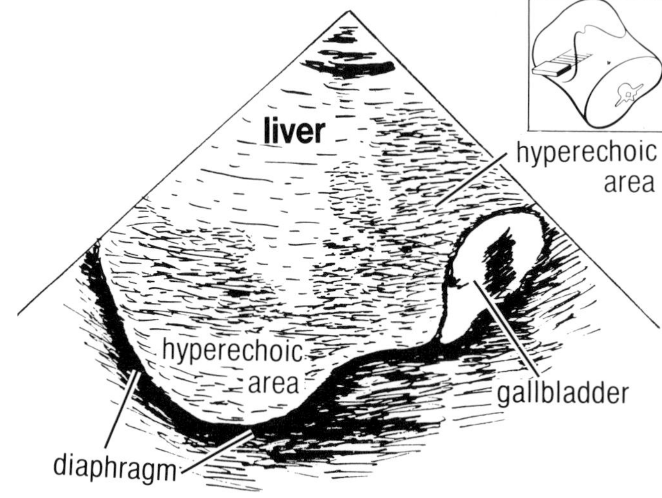

tissue, whereas other portions have increased echogenicity secondary to focal fatty infiltration

Intrahepatic Biliary Dilatation

Tertiary branches of the intrahepatic portal vein can be visualized ultrasonographically, but only primary branches of the intrahepatic bile duct (hepatic duct) can normally be visualized. However, using high-resolution equipment, careful examination of the lateral segment of the left lobe in a thin patient can at times reveal the secondary branches of the hepatic duct.

When dilated, the intrahepatic bile duct is visualized parallel to the portal vein. This is called the parallel channel sign. When there is severe biliary dilatation, the biliary ducts become quite prominent in the liver, and it becomes rather difficult to identify the portal vein and its radicles. Since ultrasonography is very sensitive for biliary tract dilatation, ultrasonographic examination of a jaundiced patient can differentiate surgical (obstructive) from medical (hepatocellular) etiologies with ease.

When there is relatively acute biliary tract obstruction, such as with cancer of the pancreatic head, cancer of the common bile duct, or an incarcerated gallstone in the distal common bile duct, the intra- and extrahepatic bile ducts and the gallbladder become markedly dilated. In contrast, when there is long-standing subtotal obstruction by chronic pancreatitis or cholangitis, only the extrahepatic biliary duct becomes dilated and the intrahepatic ducts and the gallbladder remain normal in size. Dilatation of the extrahepatic bile duct alone is also seen after cholecystectomy, and in elderly patients.

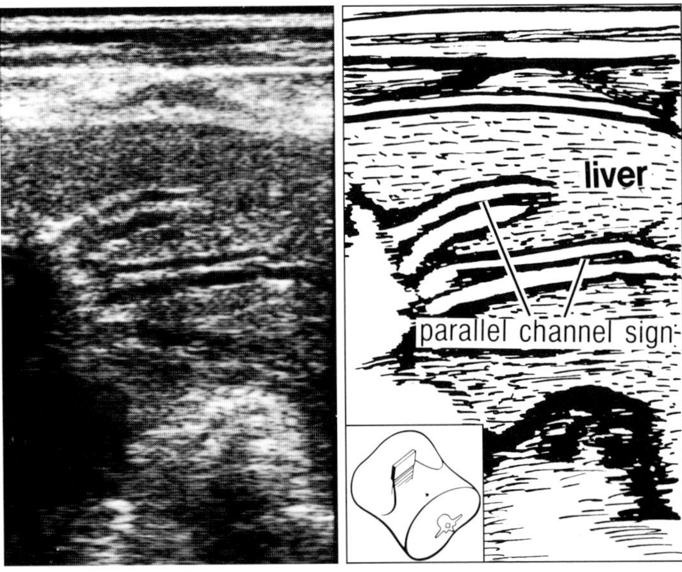

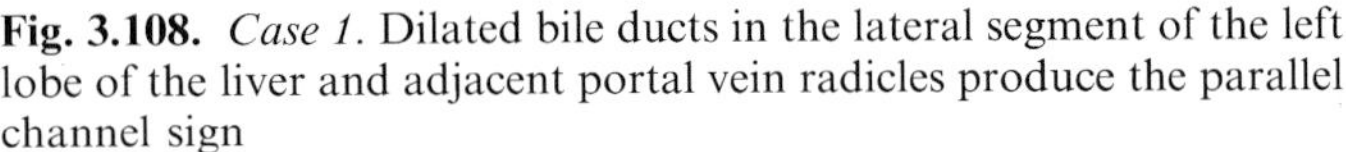

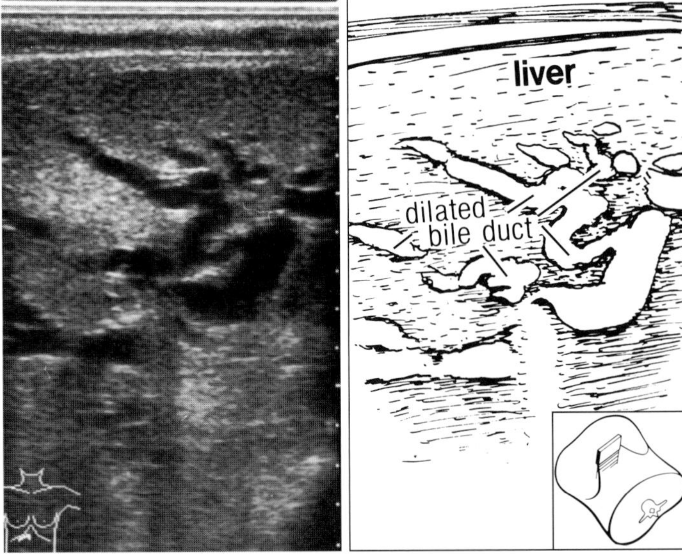

Fig. 3.108. *Case 1.* Dilated bile ducts in the lateral segment of the left lobe of the liver and adjacent portal vein radicles produce the parallel channel sign

Fig. 3.109. *Case 2.* There is dilatation of the bile ducts in the left lobe of the liver. With dilatation of this extent, it is difficult to differentiate bile ducts from portal veins

Intrahepatic Biliary Stones

Intrahepatic biliary stones usually do not produce echoes as strong as those from gallstones in the gallbladder because of the absence of fluid anterior to the stones. With intrahepatic biliary stones, the bile ducts may be filled with stones, and therefore these stones will appear buried within the liver parenchyma. This situation is similar to that of gallstones within a contracted gallbladder.

Recall that the reflection of ultrasound is proportional to the differences in acoustic impedances of two tissues that constitute an interface. While there is a large difference in acoustic impedances between bile and gallstones, there is a smaller difference between the acoustic impedances of liver tissue and intrahepatic biliary stones. This small difference accounts for the weaker echoes produced by intrahepatic biliary stones compared to gallstones in the gallbladder.

The combinations of weaker echoes and the absence of adjacent hypoechoic bile creates an image with less contrast, and therefore the intrahepatic biliary stones are not visualized as clearly as stones in the gallbladder. Dilatation of the bile ducts peripheral to the stones may or may not be present.

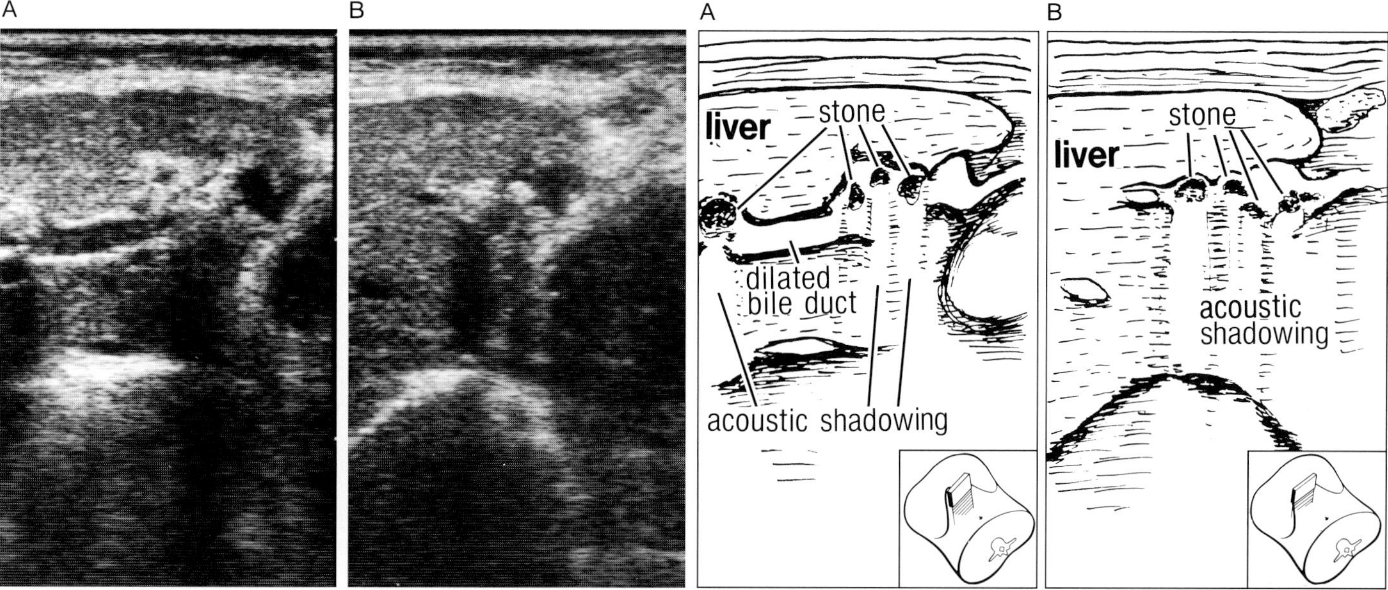

Fig. 3.110 A, B. *Case 1.* There are multiple hyperechoic areas with associated acoustic shadowing in the lateral segment of the left lobe of the liver. There is also dilatation of a peripheral bile duct and a 2-cm hyperechoic focus in a bile duct located in the hepatic hilum

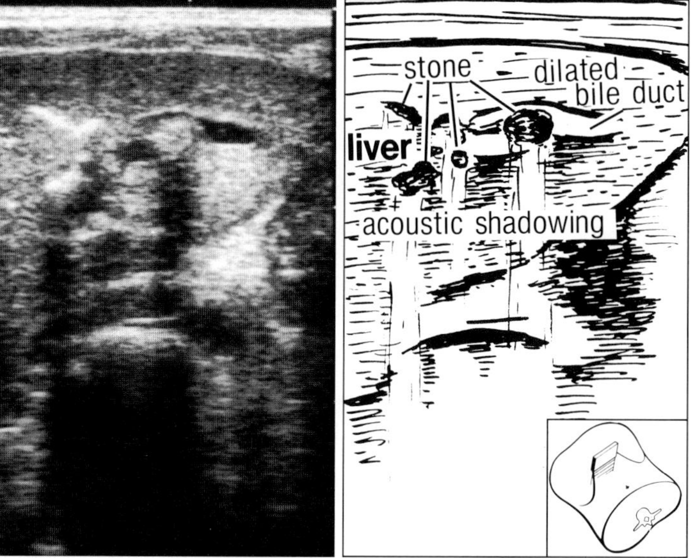

Fig. 3.111. *Case 2.* A bile duct is dilated in the left lobe of the liver, and there are several hyperechoic areas ranging in size from 5 to 12 mm. The patient also had three stones within the extrahepatic bile duct

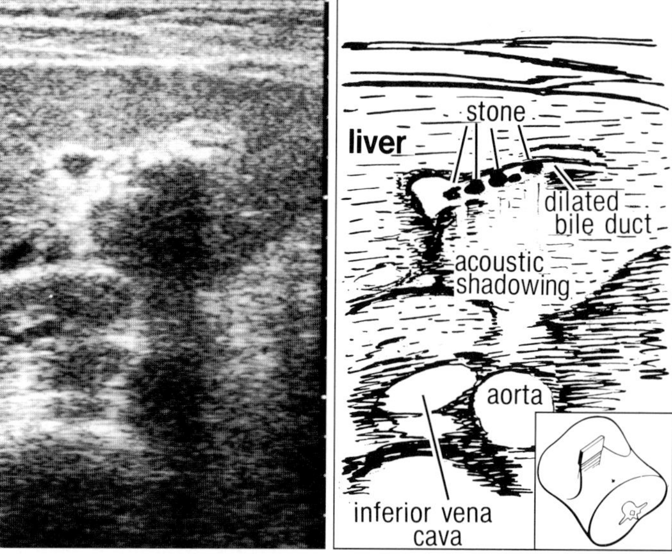

Fig. 3.112. *Case 3.* There are several stones in a bile duct in the lateral segment of the left lobe

Biliary Emphysema

Air normally refluxes into the biliary tract following certain types of surgery such as choledochojejunostomy for cancers of the pancreatic head, gallbladder, or duodenal papilla; after papillotomy for stones in the common bile duct; or, rarely, when the gallbladder ruptures into the duodenum. Since the interface between air and soft tissue strongly reflects ultrasound, even small air bubbles in the bile duct appear hyperechoic.

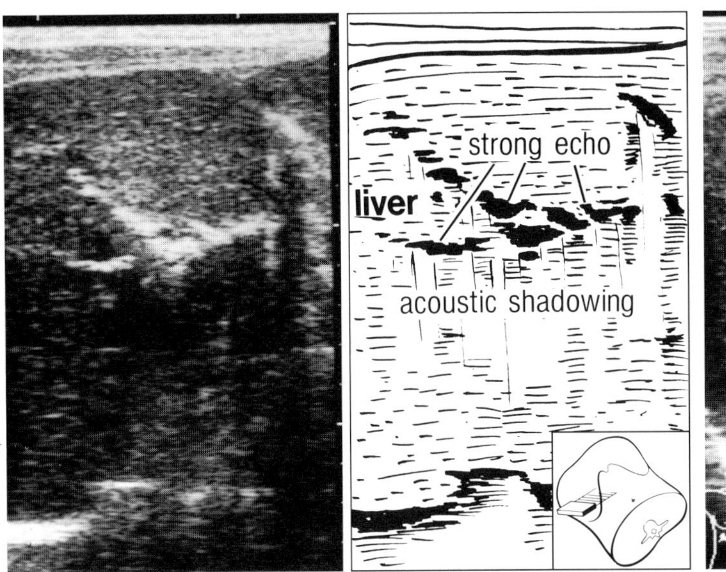

Fig. 3.113. *Case 1.* There are hyperechoic areas along the course of the portal vein. This patient had had cholecystectomy 23 years earlier. Radiography of the abdomen demonstrated gas along the course of the intrahepatic bile ducts

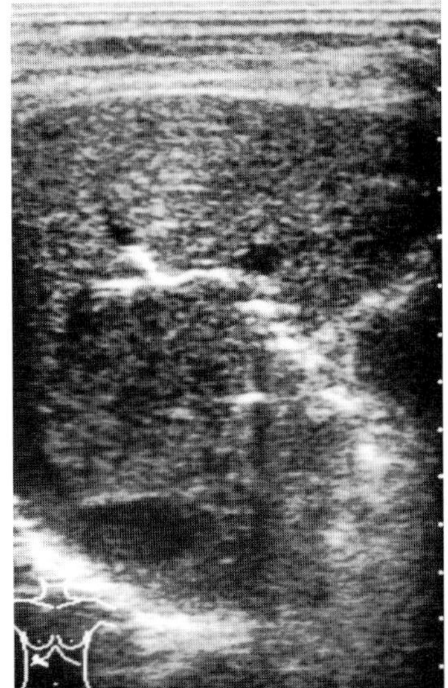

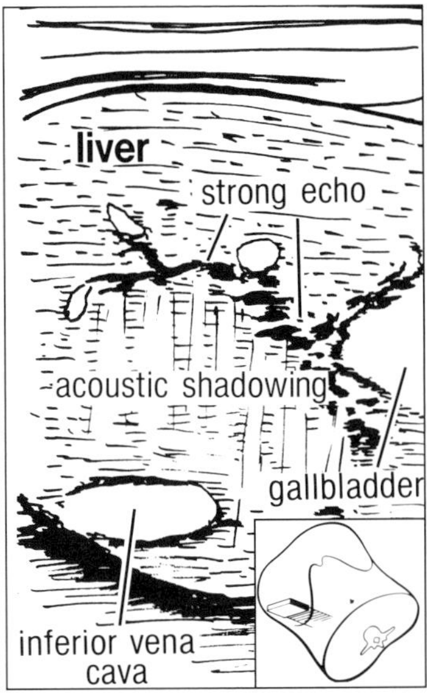

Fig. 3.114. *Case 2.* Multiple hyperechoic areas in the distribution of the intrahepatic bile ducts. This patient had had cholecystectomy for cholelithiasis 11 years earlier, and 8 years earlier, had had anastomosis of the left hepatic duct and jejunum with papillotomy for choledocholithiasis

Intrahepatic Calcification

During ultrasonographic examination of the liver, hyperechoic areas of 3–5 mm in size associated with posterior shadowing are occasionally observed. This finding indicates either small stones in the peripheral biliary radicles or calcifications within the liver parenchyma.

As stated before (p. 86), stones within the intrahepatic bile ducts do not usually produce strong echoes with clear posterior shadowing. They are usually multiple and distributed along the course of bile ducts. In contrast, parenchymal calcifications are usually solitary, or two or three in number and they do not follow the course of the bile ducts.

Parenchymal calcifications show high attenuation on CT owing to a high calcium content. These calcifications are thought to be secondary to abscess, hemorrhage, tuberculous granuloma, parasitic granuloma, etc. In individual cases, the cause for the calcification is rarely determined.

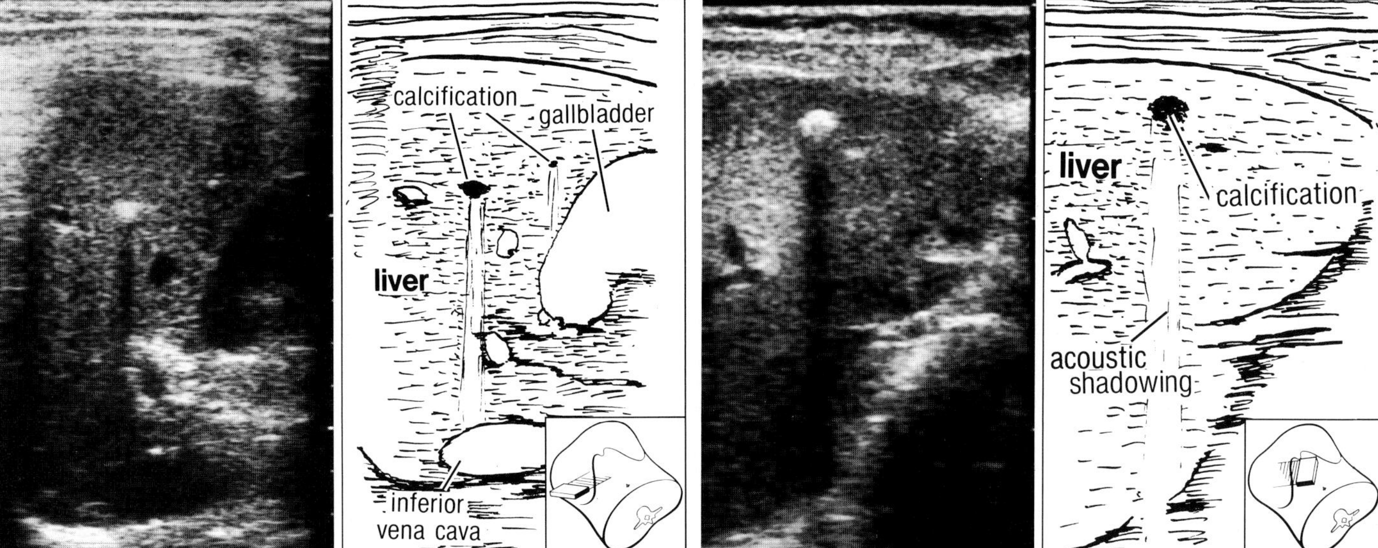

Fig. 3.115. *Case 1.* There is a hyperechoic area, 6 mm in size, in the right lobe of the liver and distinct posterior acoustic shadowing. This is a solitary lesion having no association with the biliary tract

Fig. 3.116. *Case 2.* There is a 1-cm hyperechoic area with posterior acoustic shadowing in the right lobe of the liver

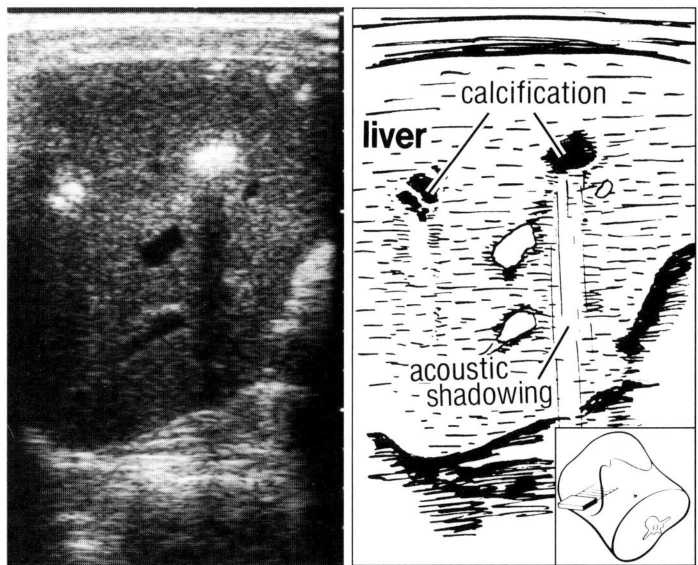

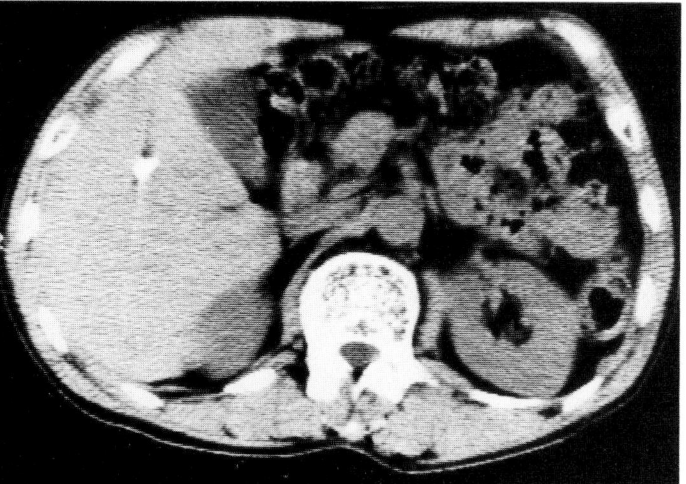

Fig. 3.117. *Case 3.* There are two hyperechoic areas in the right lobe. The larger one is associated with distinct acoustic shadowing

Fig. 3.118. *Case 3, CT scan.* There is a high-density focus indicating calcification

Schistosomiasis Japonica

Schistosomiasis japonica is a parasitic disease which affects the rural population in Japan, China, and some other Asian countries. Liver lesions in this disease show characteristic findings on ultrasonography. The liver lesion is referred to as a "tortoise shell" or network pattern and is characterized by hyperechoic septations. The septated appearance is produced by linear fibrosis. The larvae, with or without calcifications, may be found within the fibrosis.

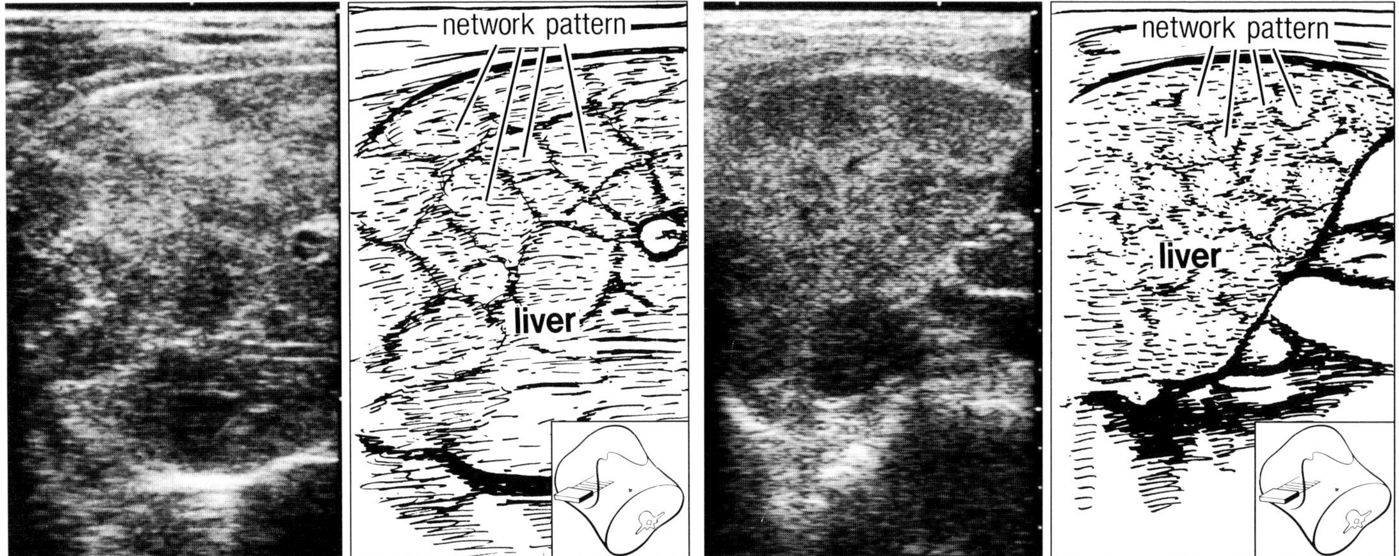

Fig. 3.119. *Case 1.* Typical appearance of schistosomiasis japonica. Diffuse network pattern of the liver

Fig. 3.120. *Case 2.* Findings similar to case 1 (Fig. 3.119)

Liver Congestion

Liver congestion is seen in patients who have increased right-sided heart pressures secondary to cardiac disease. Ultrasonographic findings include dilatation of the inferior vena cava and the hepatic vein, and hepatomegaly. The inferior vena cava not only dilates, but also loses its normal pulsation. The size of the inferior vena cava normally changes secondary to pressure changes which vary according to cardiac and respiratory cycles (e.g., the inferior vena cava dilates on expiration). However, in a patient with increased right-sided heart pressures, the inferior vena cava remains dilated even on inspiration.

Whereas a cross-section of the inferior vena cava is either oval or almost flat at the level of the pancreas in normal subjects, in patients with right-sided cardiac failure, it is a round structure which is larger than the aorta. Dilatation of the inferior vena cava and the hepatic veins is seen first; hepatomegaly is present only in advanced cases.

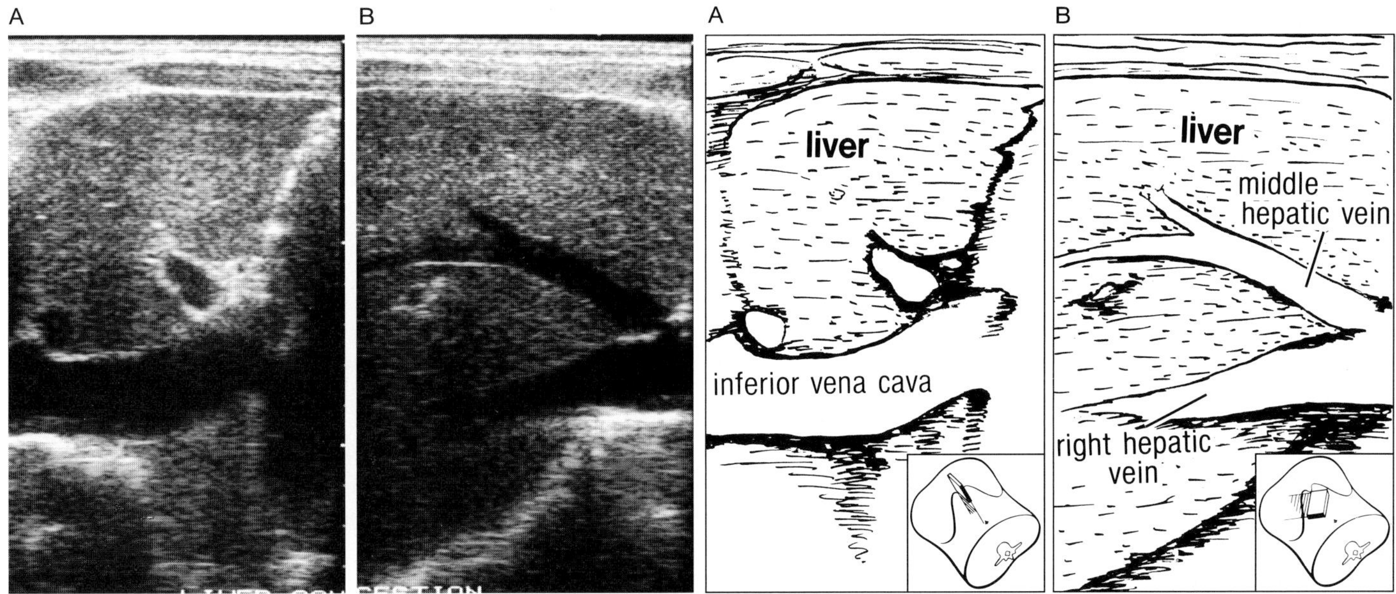

Fig. 3.121 A, B. *Case 1.* Dilatation of the inferior vena cava with loss of pulsation (**A**). Mild dilatation of the right and middle hepatic veins (**B**). This is a case of mitral stenosis

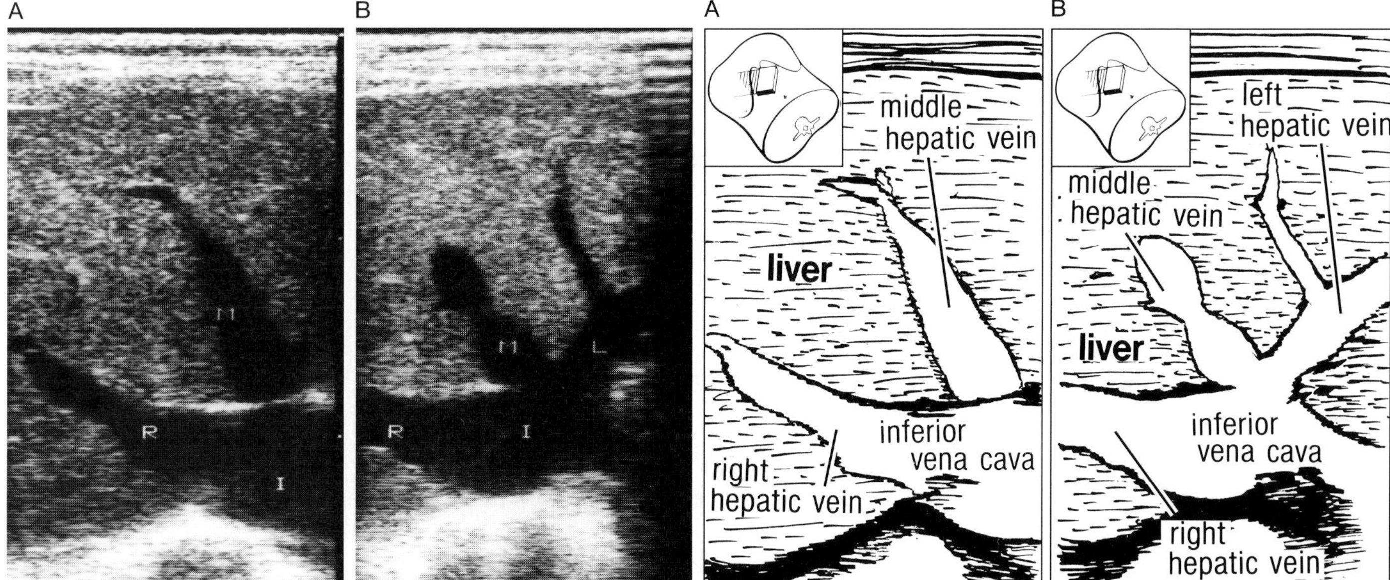

Fig. 3.122 A, B. *Case 2.* There is marked dilatation of the inferior vena cava and the right, middle, and left hepatic veins. There is mild hepatomegaly. This patient's status is post mitral valve replacement for mitral stenosis and mitral insufficiency. Aortic stenosis was present as well

4 Gallbladder and Bile Ducts

**Anatomy
of the Intrahepatic
Bile Ducts**

The intrahepatic bile ducts course through the liver along the portal venous system. The right hepatic duct, a portion of the right anterior segmental branch, the left hepatic duct, and a portion of the lateral segmental branch in the left lobe can be visualized ultrasonographically. The left hepatic duct runs anterior to the transverse segment of the left portal vein, passes cephalad to the umbilical portion of the portal vein, and then connects to the lateral segmental branch in the left lobe. The lateral segmental branch runs parallel to and superoposterior to its accompanying portal vein radicle.

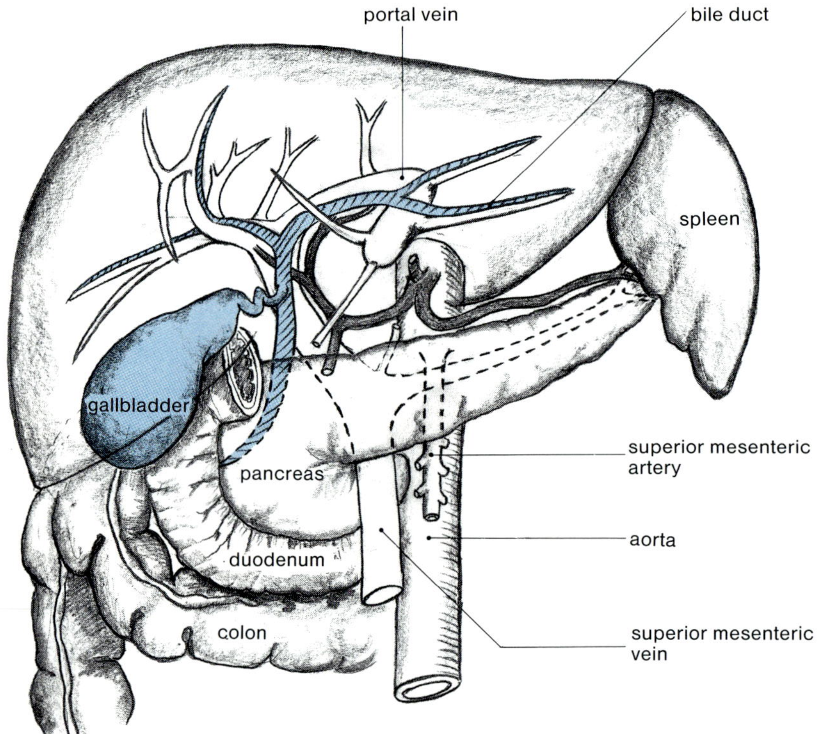

Fig. 4.1. Anatomy of the intrahepatic bile ducts

Anatomy of the Extrahepatic Bile Ducts

The right and left hepatic ducts join at the porta hepatis to form the common hepatic duct. The common hepatic duct courses inferiorly anterior to the main trunk of the portal vein, joins with the cystic duct becoming the common bile duct. It is difficult to visualize the confluence of the cystic duct and the common hepatic duct on ultrasonography so it is impossible to precisely differentiate the common hepatic from the common bile duct. It is generally acceptable to refer to the superior segment (close to the liver) as the common hepatic duct and the inferior segment (close to the pancreas) as the common bile duct.

The common bile duct is initially in contact with the main portal vein and descends anterior and to the right of it, then it becomes separated from the portal vein as it passes posterior to the head of the pancreas, curving to the right to reach the medial surface of the duodenum. The inner diameter of the extrahepatic bile duct measured ultrasonographically is usually 2–3 mm smaller than that measured by percutaneous transhepatic cholangiography or endoscopic retrograde cholangiopancreatographic examination. Using ultrasonography, the upper limit of normal is 6 mm; 8 mm is acceptable in a patient with a previous cholecystectomy.

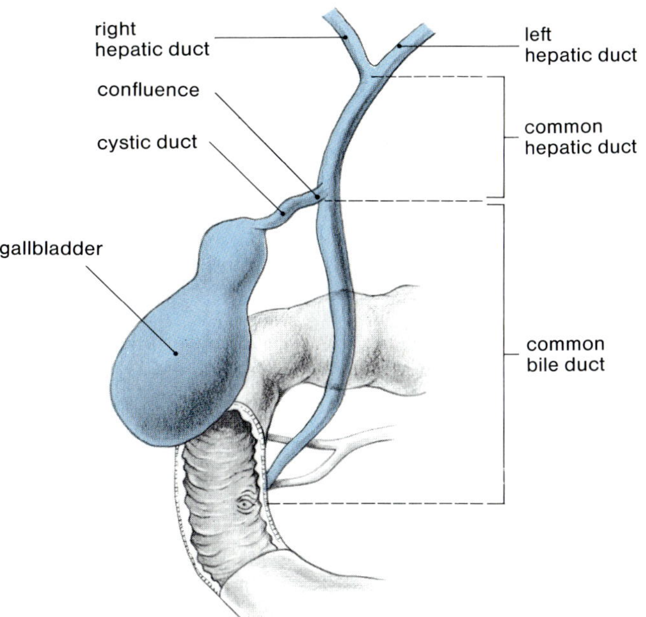

Fig. 4.2. Anatomy of the extrahepatic bile duct system

Anatomy of the Gallbladder

The gallbladder is on the inferior surface of the liver and is fixed to the serosa of the liver between the right and left hepatic lobes (Fig. 4.3). The fundus of gallbladder is near the anterior edge of the liver, and its neck points toward the porta hepatis. Its body and neck are often marginated by mucosal folds, forming Hartman's pouch. These folds are visualized as septae within the lumen of gallbladder on ultrasonography.

Ultrasonographic examination of the gallbladder may be adversely affected by intestinal gas artifacts from the duodenal bulb, hepatic flexure, and transverse colon. The duodenal bulb is located on the medial-caudal aspect of the gallbladder. The colon is located lateral and anteroinferior to the neck of the gallbladder. Ultrasonographic visualization of the gallbladder is difficult in patients who have a thick thorax, obese abdomen, or liver atrophy, because the liver retracts up under the rib cage bringing the colon near the costal angle. Normal ultrasonographic measurements of the gallbladder include a long axis length of 7–8 cm and a short axis length of 2–3 cm.

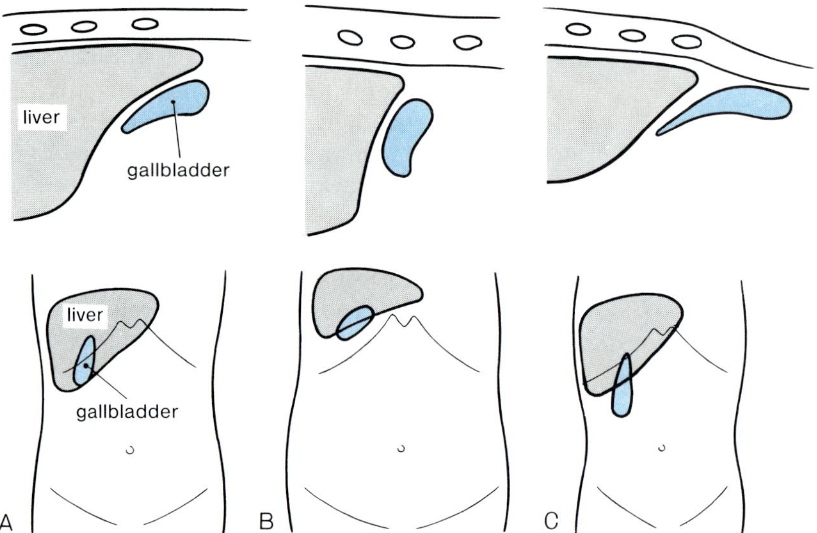

Fig. 4.3 A–C. *Positional relationship of the liver and gallbladder.* In a patient with a standard body habitus (**A**), the gallbladder resides on the posterior surface of the liver and is visualized posterior to the liver on a scan obtained from the anterior abdominal wall. In an obese patient (**B**), the posterior surface of the liver and long axis of the gallbladder are often nearly perpendicular to the anterior abdominal wall. In this situation, visualization of the gallbladder can be difficult due to intestinal gas. In a thin patient (**C**), the gallbladder is usually elongated in shape and is in contact with the anterior abdominal wall. In this situation, owing to its superficial location, the lumen of the gallbladder may not appear anechoic because of reverberation artifacts from the abdominal wall

Ultrasonographic Appearance of a Normal Gallbladder

Subcostal Scanning

After visualizing the portal bifurcation on a subcostal scan, the neck of the gallbladder can be located by slightly tilting the transducer head toward the feet. The lumen of the gallbladder can be well visualized by a fan-shaped movement of the transducer head in this location. Images should be recorded during the real-time examination documenting the largest lumen of the gallbladder. Images of the gallbladder neck should be included. Note, however, that on subcostal scanning, even large stones can be missed when they are located in the gallbladder fundus which may not be well visualized due to colonic gas.

With the patient in the left decubitus position, gallstones roll to the gallbladder neck. Therefore, to fully evaluate the gallbladder, it is necessary to obtain intercostal and subcostal scans with changes in the patient's position. When the anterior edge of the liver is retracted high above the costal margin, maneuvers such as deep inspiration or the erect position will move the liver caudally, making examination of the gallbladder possible. If there is inadequate descent of the liver by these methods, intercostal scanning should be performed.

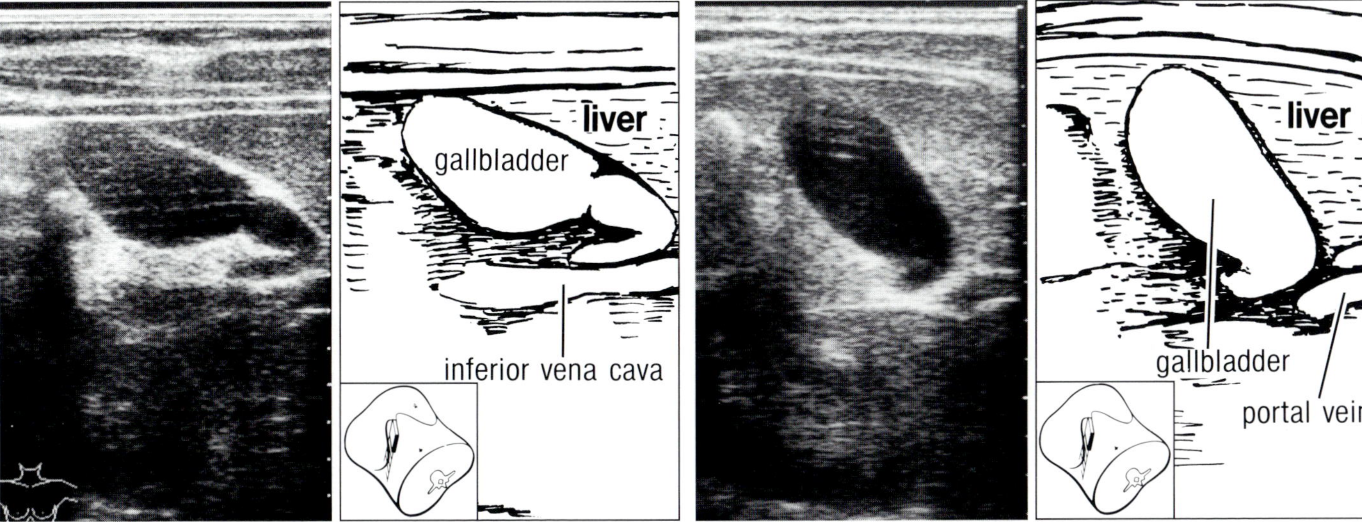

Fig. 4.4. *Case 1*. Subcostal image of a normal gallbladder

Fig. 4.5. *Case 2*. Subcostal image of a normal gallbladder (another patient to Fig. 4.4)

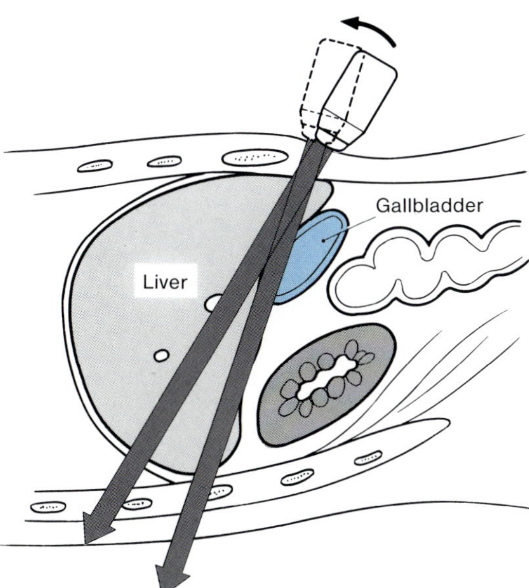

Fig. 4.6. *How to image the gallbladder from a subcostal approach*. It is important to direct the transducer head so that the beam encounters the gallbladder after traversing the liver when scanning from a subcostal approach. Because the liver transmits the ultrasound beam well, the gallbladder is well visualized by this method. When the position of the transducer head is too low on the abdominal wall, the gallbladder cannot be visualized because of interposed intestinal gas which will not transmit the ultrasound beam. On subcostal scanning, the transducer head is gently pushed against the abdominal wall at the costal margin. The liver should be visualized first. Then by rocking the transducer head (as shown in this figure) or by moving the transducer head downward, the gallbladder can be observed using the liver as an acoustic window

Longitudinal Scanning   On a longitudinal scan, the gallbladder is visualized as a cystic structure on the inferior surface of the liver. Only in a thin patient, in whom the long axis of the gallbladder parallels the abdominal wall, is the entire length of the gallbladder visualized on longitudinal scans. The fundus of the gallbladder is difficult to visualize from a subcostal approach.

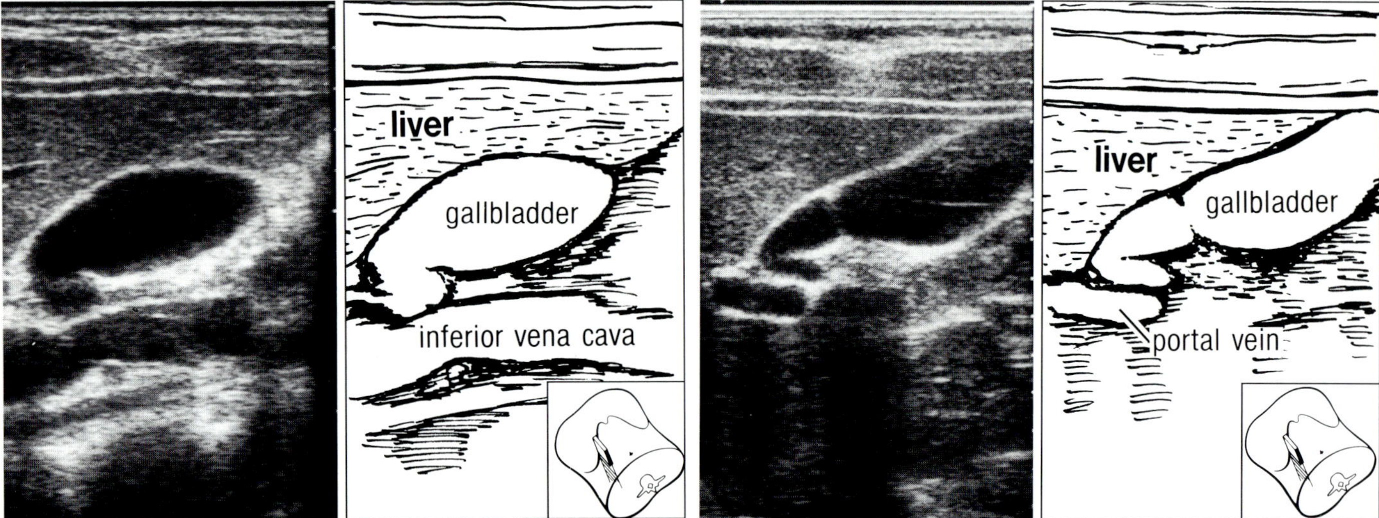

Fig. 4.7. *Case 1.* Longitudinal image of a normal gallbladder

Fig. 4.8. *Case 2.* Longitudinal image of a normal gallbladder (another patient to Fig. 4.7)

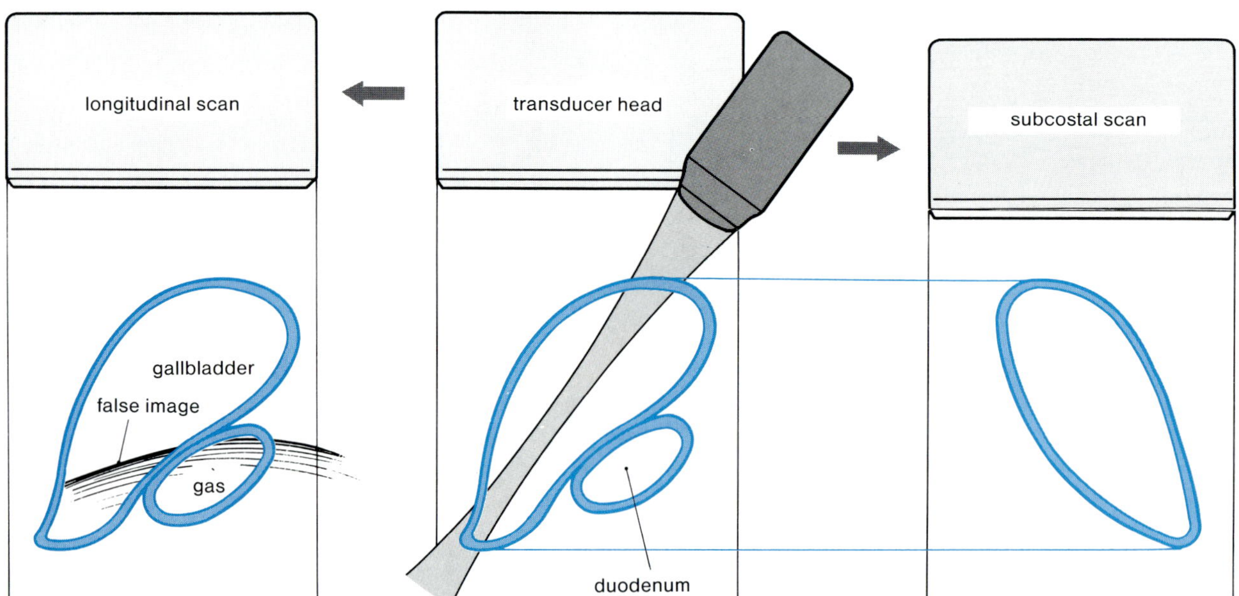

Fig. 4.9. *How to Recognize a False Image Due to Side Lobe Artifacts.* When obtaining longitudinal scans of the gallbladder, intestinal gas posterior to the gallbladder may be detected by a side lobe of the beam, and this may produce sludge-like echoes within the gallbladder lumen. By changing the direction of the transducer head in the subcostal position, this artifact disappears, whereas real sludge will be visualized as a collection of fine echoes from all scanning directions

Intercostal Scanning

The position of the gallbladder varies according to the patient's position, body habitus, and respiration. The intercostal space allowing optimal access to the gallbladder should be determined. On intercostal scanning, the main portal vein is well visualized. The common hepatic duct and the common bile duct are visualized coursing along the main portal vein. The gallbladder is visualized as a cystic structure with its neck close to the right hepatic duct or the right branch of the portal vein. The neck of the gallbladder is well visualized by moving the transducer head in a fan-shaped fashion. The fundus of the gallbladder may not be visualized well because of intestinal gas, and therefore an intercostal scan cannot necessarily visualize the entire length of the gallbladder. Care must be taken not to confuse the false image created by the partial volume effect of the gallbladder and intestinal gas with gallstones (Fig. 4.10).

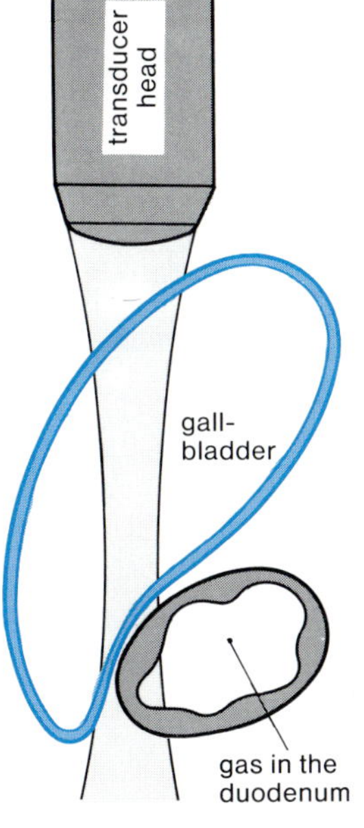

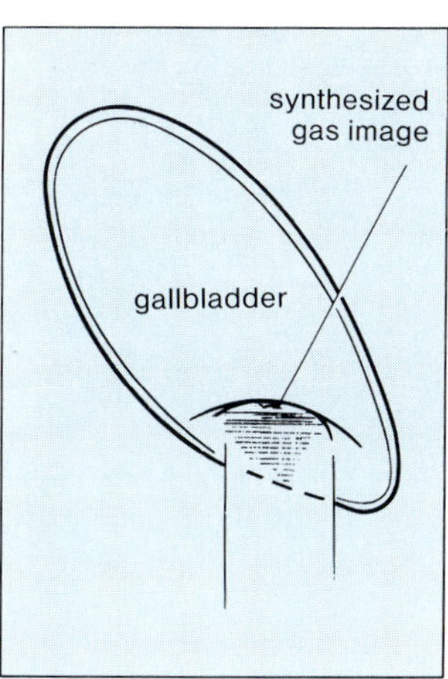

Fig. 4.10. *False image created by the partial volume effect.* A phenomenon similar to partial volume averaging in CT can occur in ultrasonography. Data (echoes) from tissue slices of 3–8 mm in thickness are projected into a single two-dimensional image. On examination of the gallbladder, intestinal gas outside the gallbladder can appear to be within the gallbladder lumen, simulating gallstones. By altering the angle of the transducer head, this false finding can be recognized as such. It is important that the questionable or misleading findings viewed on the real-time examination are not recorded on the static images. Note that there is a great deal of difference in the quality and quantity of information obtained between the static images and the dynamic images as viewed on the monitor during a real-time examination. Accurate diagnosis can only be made on the basis of information obtained at real time

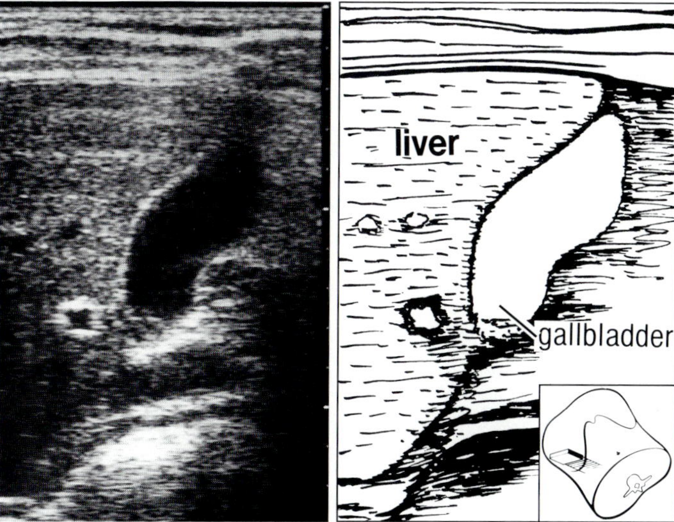

Fig. 4.11. *Case 1.* Intercostal image of a normal gallbladder

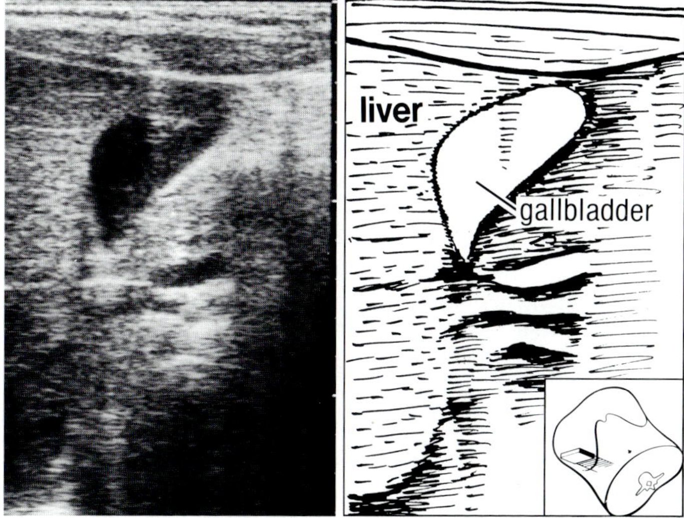

Fig. 4.12. *Case 2.* Intercostal image of a normal gallbladder (another patient to Fig. 4.11)

Comet-Like Echo

Comet-like echoes with long tails (synonyms: comet-tail sign, comet sign) can occasionally be seen arising from the wall of the gallbladder. This is an artifact secondary to reverberation (Fig. 4.13) and is caused by cholesterol polyps, intramural stones, or Rokitansky-Aschoff sinuses in the anterior wall of the gallbladder.

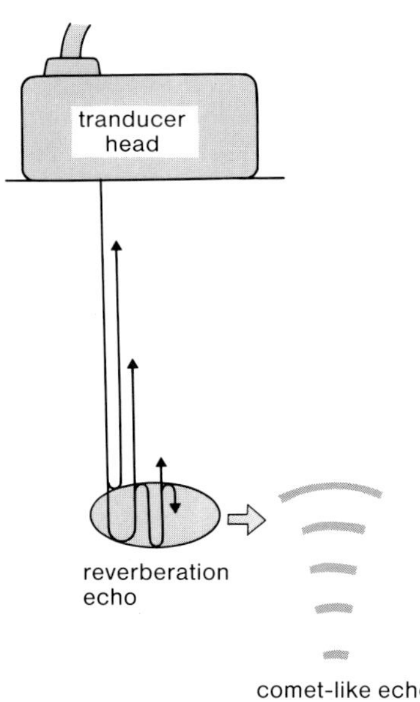

Fig. 4.13. *Principle of the comet-like echo.* The comet-like echo represents a reverberation artifact which occurs in a small structure with closely spaced anterior and posterior reflecting surfaces

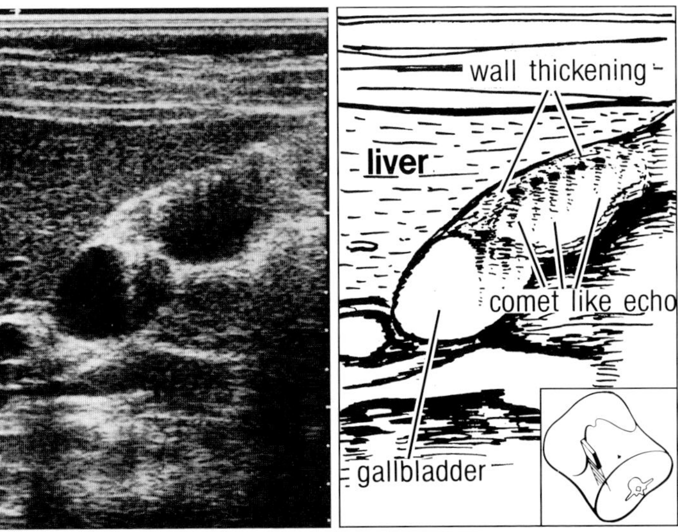

Fig. 4.14. *Case 1.* There are multiple comet-like echoes on the anterior wall of the fundus of the gallbladder. This is an example of the comet-like echo seen in adenomyomatosis

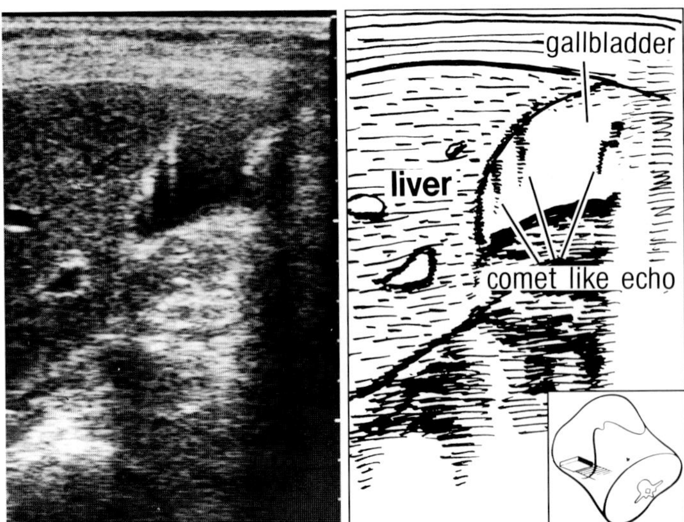

Fig. 4.15. *Case 2.* There are two comet-like echoes with long tails arising from the anterior wall of the gallbladder

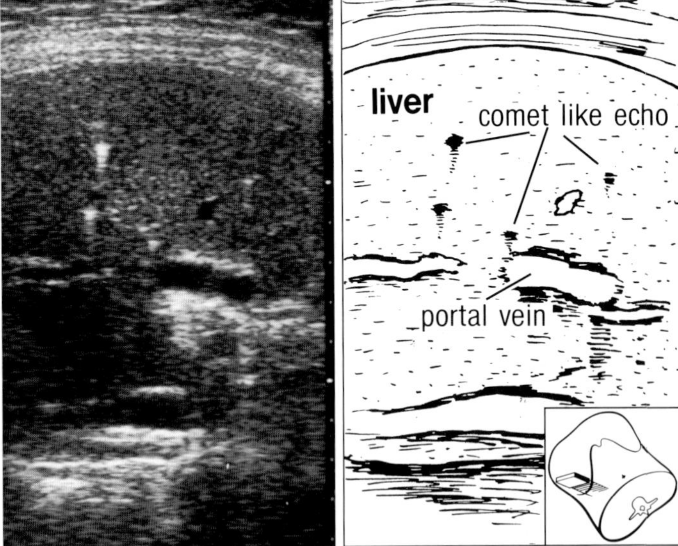

Fig. 4.16. *Case 3.* Comet-like echo seen in the liver. This finding is often seen in a patient with biliary stones. In this case, the comet-like echo is seen adjacent to the portal vein and is thought to represent small stones within the intrahepatic biliary ducts

Pitfalls in the Ultrasonographic Examination of the Gallbladder

During ultrasonographic examination of the gallbladder, care should be taken to visualize the entire gallbladder. One plane cannot visualize the entire gallbladder which is variable in shape. The fundus of the gallbladder may not be well visualized because of intestinal gas. Observation should be performed from different directions by altering the patient's respiratory phase or position.

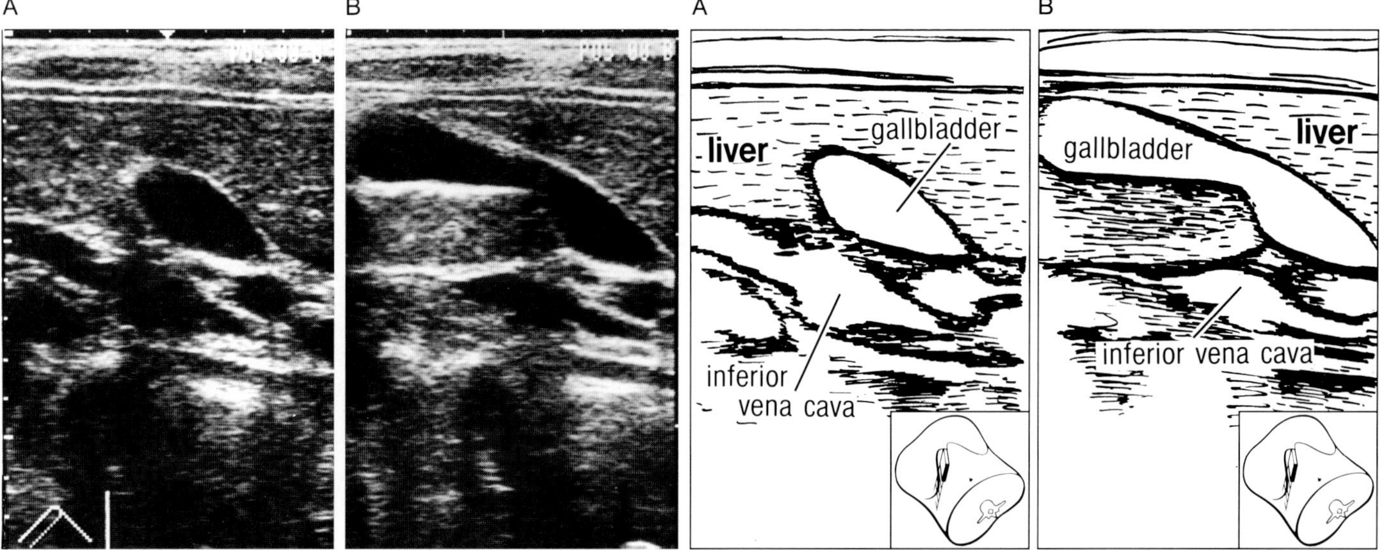

Fig. 4.17 A, B. *Case 1.* The subcostal image (**A**) shows a normally shaped gallbladder. However, **B** shows that, in this case, the gallbladder is elongated, nearly twice as long as seen in **A**; i.e., only half of the gallbladder is visualized in **A**

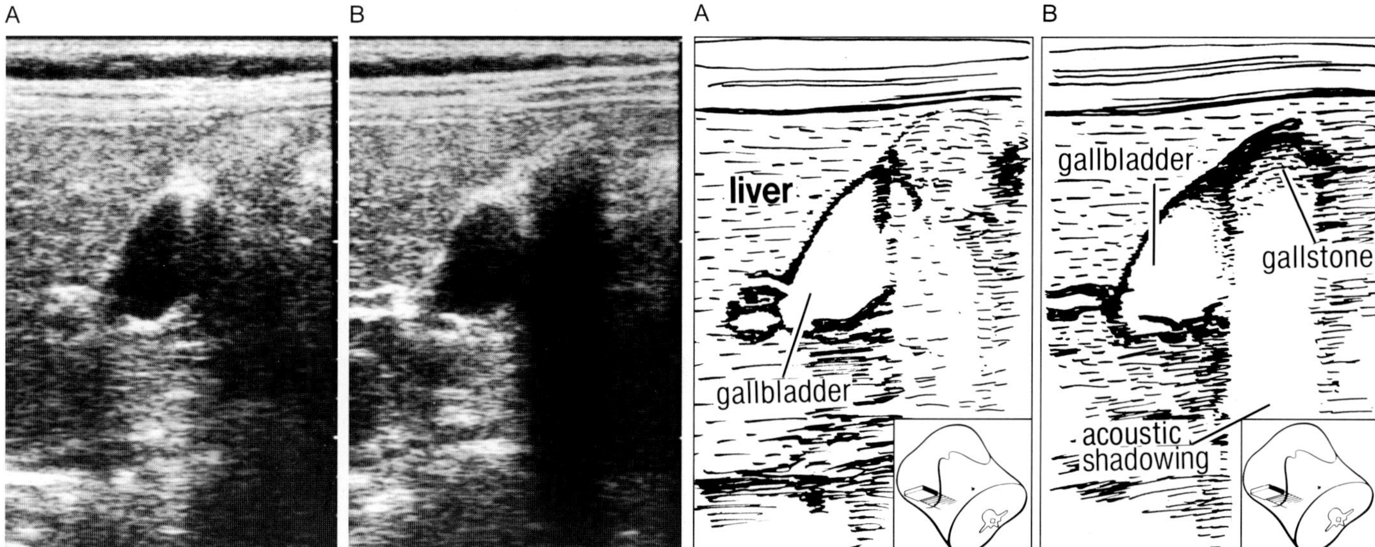

Fig. 4.18 A, B. *Case 2.* The inferior portion of the gallbladder is not visualized on the intercostal image (**A**) because of intestinal gas. The visualized portions of the gallbladder show no definite abnormalities. With a slight change in the direction of the transducer head (**B**), definite acoustic shadowing is seen arising from the region of the fundus of the gallbladder, suggesting a large stone. Usually, the gallstone moves toward the neck of the gallbladder in the supine position, but a large stone may not move at all when incarcerated in the fundus

Ultrasonographic Appearance of a Normal Extrahepatic Bile Duct

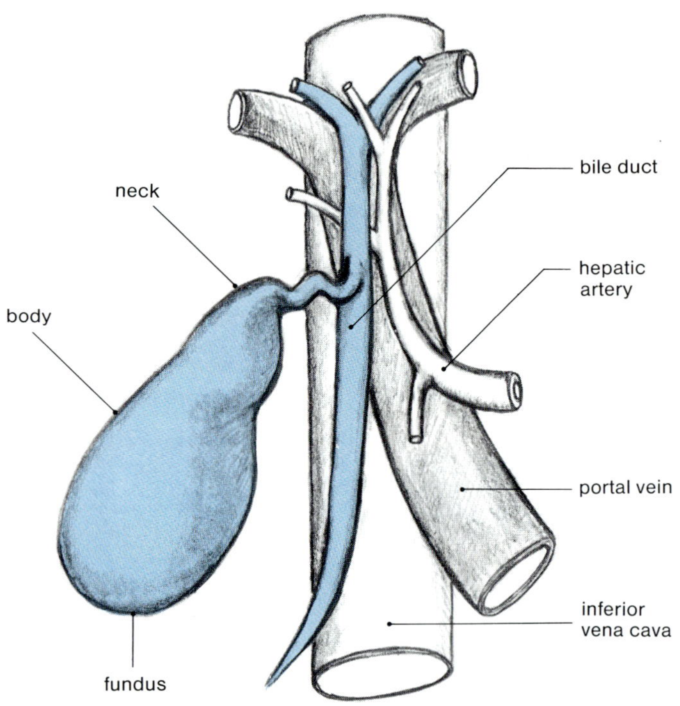

Fig. 4.19. Anatomy of the extrahepatic bile duct

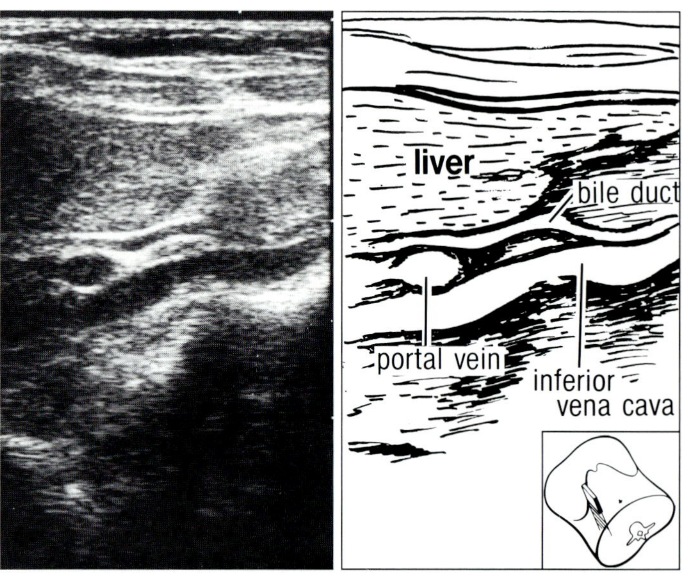

Fig. 4.20. *Case 1.* On the longitudinal scan of the porta hepatis, the common hepatic duct, the main trunk of the portal vein, and the inferior vena cava are visualized from anterior to posterior, in this order. The normal common hepatic duct lumen is 6 mm or less in diameter on ultrasonography

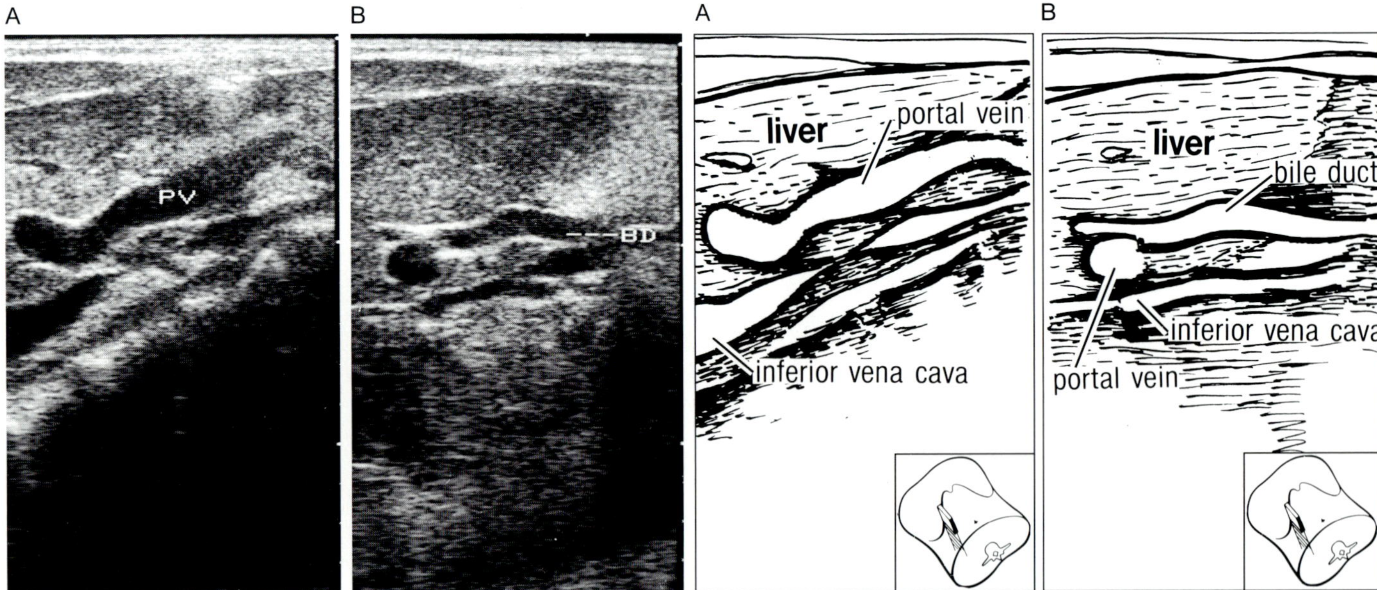

Fig. 4.21 A, B. *Case 2.* The bile duct and the portal vein are in the same sagittal plane near the porta hepatis; but, as they descend, the portal vein deviates toward the left, and it becomes difficult to visualize these two structures in a single plane. **A** was obtained with the transducer head positioned parallel to the portal vein; **B** was obtained with the transducer head parallel to the bile duct. In this case, the extrahepatic bile duct is 6 mm in diameter, which is at the upper limits of normal

Cholelithiasis

Typical cholelithiasis demonstrates a strong echo in the gallbladder with posterior acoustic shadowing, the width of which corresponds to the diameter of the stone (Fig. 4.22). When there is only one small stone, there may be only a strong echo without acoustic shadowing (Fig. 4.23). In this situation, if the stone is observed to move to the dependent portion when the patient's position is changed (Fig. 4.25), the diagnosis of cholelithiasis can be made.

When there are multiple small stones, the posterior shadowing may be weak because much of the ultrasound beam passes between the stones (Fig. 4.22). When there is a large stone with a smooth surface, often only the anterior surface of the stone is visualized as a crescent-shaped strong echo because most of the beam is reflected at the stone surface (Fig. 4.22).

When gallstones cannot be visualized in the supine position, the patient should be placed in the left lateral decubitus or erect position. This may facilitate visualization as the stones may move to a location which is more accessible to the ultrasound beam or overlying intestinal gas may shift away from the gallbladder.

The Ultrasonographic Pattern of Gallstones

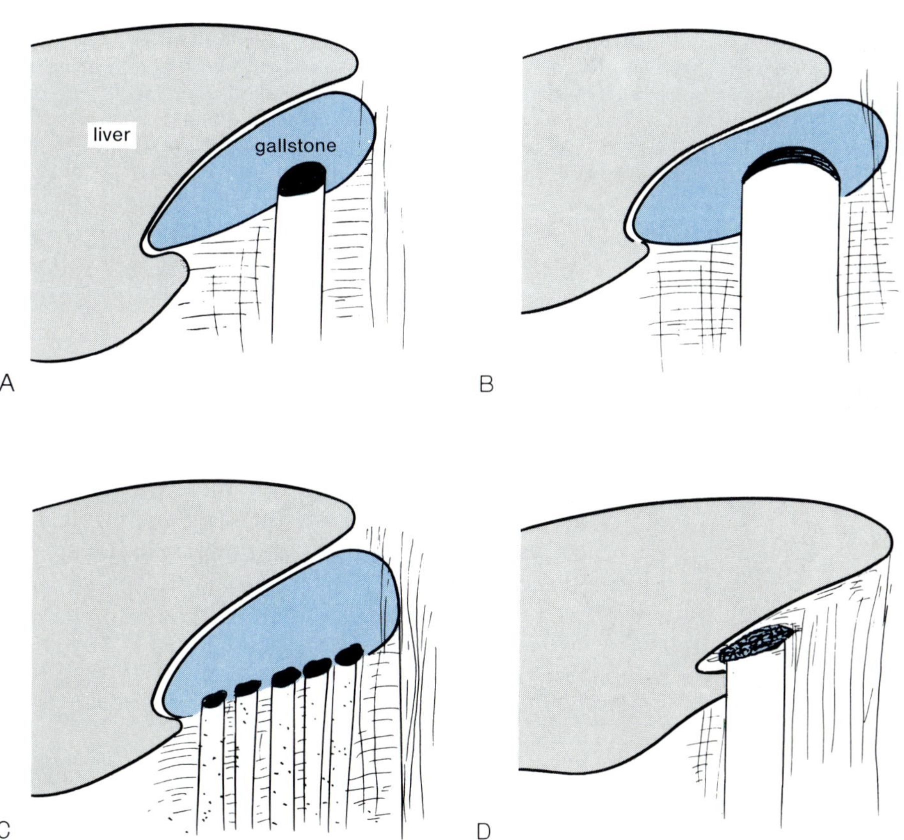

Fig. 4.22. A *Typical appearance:* There is a strong echo in the lumen of the gallbladder associated with posterior acoustic shadowing. **B** *Crescent shape:* When the stone is large, only the surface closest to the transducer head is visualized, appearing as a crescent-shaped strong echo within the gallbladder and associated with acoustic shadowing. **C** *Multiple small stones:* There are multiple hyperechoic foci, but no distinct acoustic shadowing. **D** *Contracted gallbladder:* In the gallbladder fossa, there is a hyperechoic focus with acoustic shadowing, but the lumen of the gallbladder cannot be identified. Differentiation from intestinal gas may be difficult

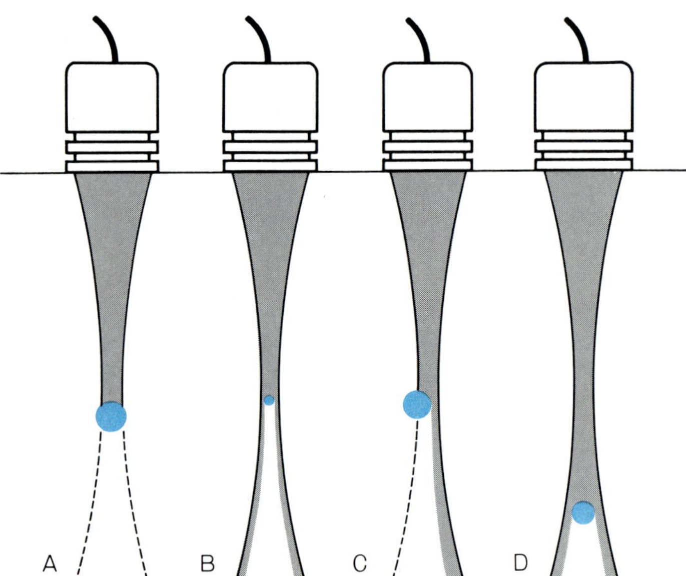

Fig. 4.23 A–D. *Gallstones and posterior acoustic shadowing.* Not all gallstones produce acoustic shadowing (**A**). For example, some stones are not large enough to completely block the ultrasound beam (**B**). Also, when the ultrasound beam encounters only a small portion of the stone (**C**), or when the stone is a distance beyond the focal zone of the beam (**D**), there will be no distinct acoustic shadowing

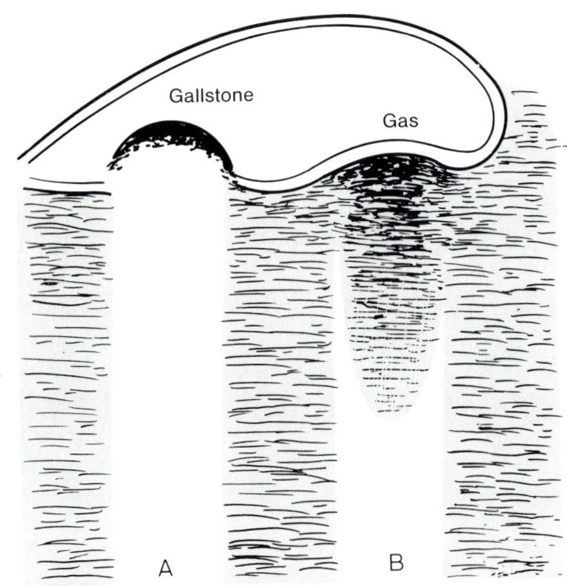

Fig. 4.24 A, B. *Clean shadow and dirty shadow.* The acoustic shadowing which is seen in association with a gallstone is clear immediately posterior to the stone; this is called a clean shadow (**A**). In contrast, the shadow from gas demonstrates a snowflake-like appearance beyond the gas, which becomes progressively clear as it continues posteriorly. This type of shadow is called a dirty shadow (**B**)

A stone incarcerated in the neck of the gallbladder or in the cystic duct may be difficult to visualize. When the gallbladder is contracted and there is no bile around the stone, the characteristic strong echo is not usually seen (Fig. 4.22). When there is a collection of relatively strong echoes with acoustic shadowing located on the posterior surface of the liver, in the expected location of the gallbladder (gallbladder fossa), cholelithiasis in a contracted gallbladder is highly probable. In this situation, differentiating acoustic shadowing due to gallstones from intestinal gas shadowing is important. With acoustic shadowing caused by stones, there will be no echoes immediately below the strong echoes, whereas with intestinal gas shadowing, there will be snowflake-like fine echoes immediately under the strong echoes, and there will be a gradual loss of echoes distally (Fig. 4.24).

Movement of Gallstones when the Patient's Position Is Changed

When there are small hyperechoic foci (< 5 mm) without definite acoustic shadowing within the gallbladder, or when it is uncertain whether echoes arise from gallstones or from intestinal gas, it is important to change the patient's position to determine whether the hyperechoic foci move within the gallbladder lumen. Strong echoes moving to the dependent portion of the gallbladder indicate the presence of stones.

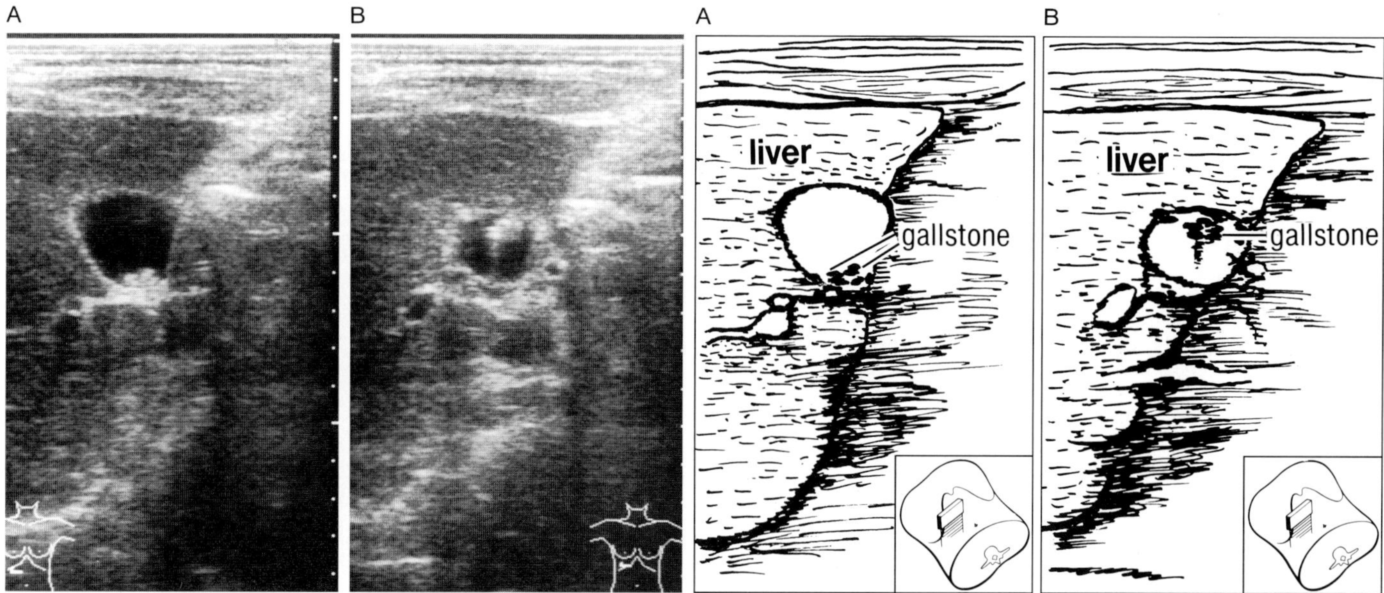

Fig. 4.25 A, B. *Case 1*. There are gallstones near the neck of the gall-bladder. The patient was instructed to assume a prone position, and subsequently the examination was performed with the patient in the left lateral decubitus position; the stones were observed to move toward the anterior wall of the gallbladder (**B**)

Typical Ultrasonographic Findings

There will be strong reflection of ultrasound at the surface of a gallstone due to the large differences in acoustic impedances between a stone and bile. Acoustic shadowing manifests as the absense of the ultrasound beam posterior to the stone. The hyperechoic gallstone will move to the dependent portion of the gallbladder when the patient's position is changed.

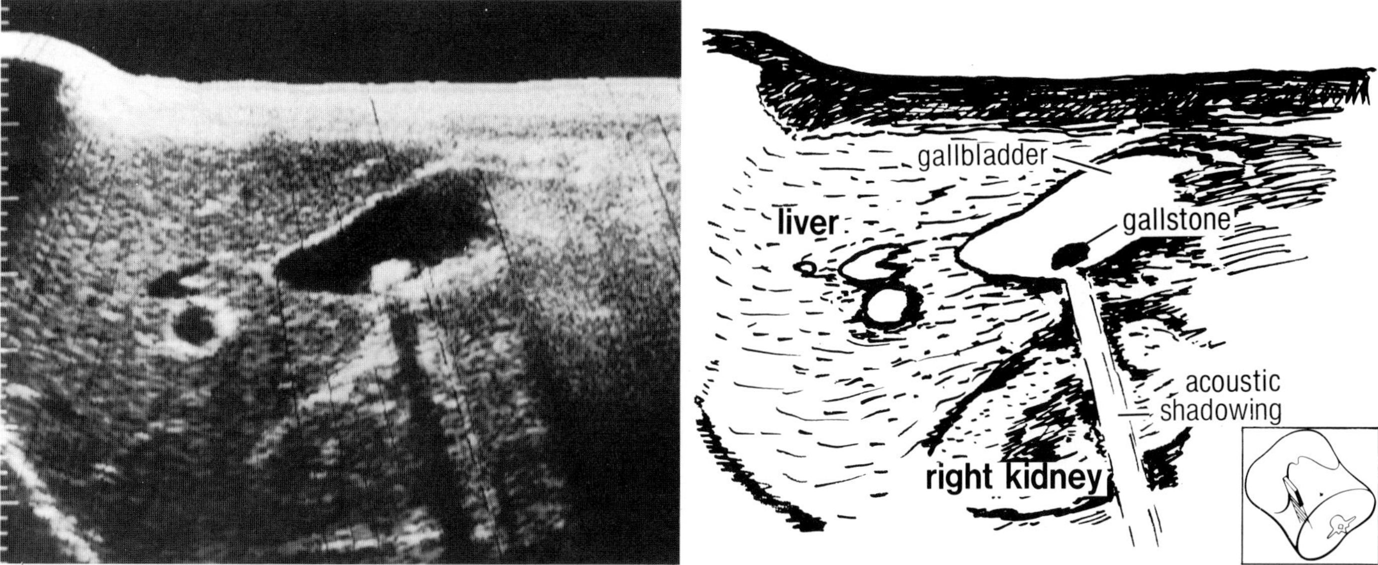

Fig. 4.26. *Case 1*. Image obtained with a contact compound scanner. There is a 2-cm strong echo on the dependent surface of the gallbladder, associated with clear posterior acoustic shadowing

Small Gallstones

Small stones may manifest as hyperechoic foci, but posterior shadowing may not be clear. A small stone may not block all of the ultrasound in a beam which has a finite width. A small stone which does not cause shadowing may be differentiated from a polyp by the mobility which occurs when the patient's position is changed.

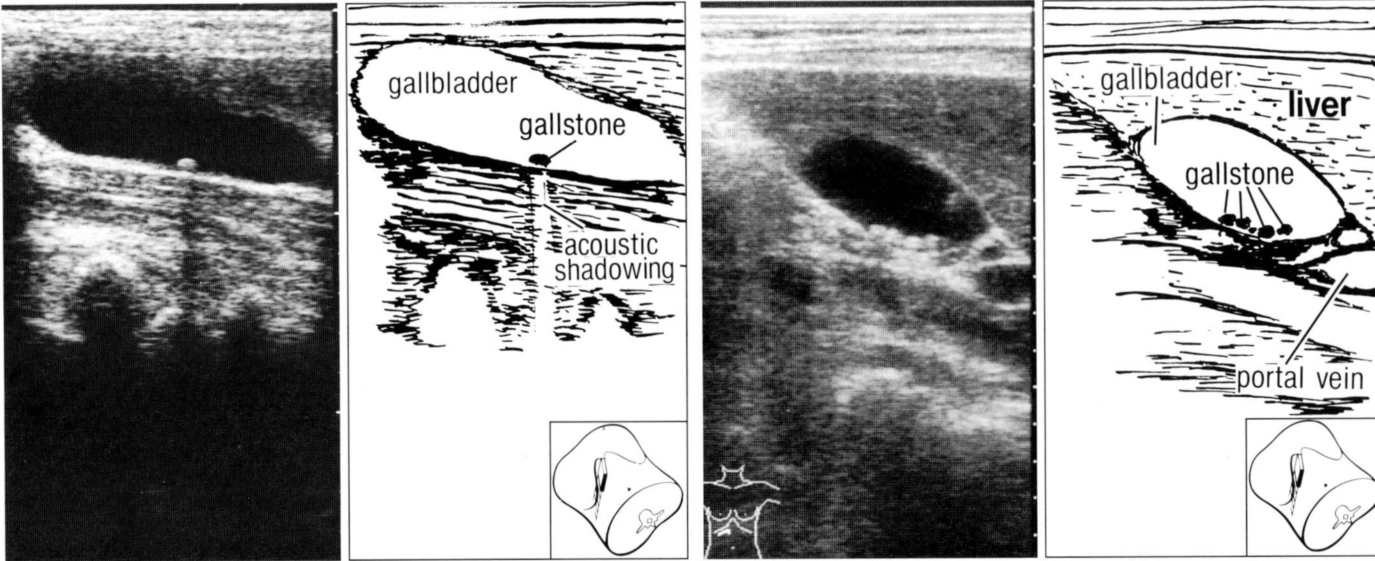

Fig. 4.27. *Case 1.* There is a 3-mm hyperechoic focus on the dependent surface of the gallbladder. In this case, acoustic shadowing is present

Fig. 4.28. *Case 2.* There are at least four small strong echoes. No definite acoustic shadowing is seen

Large Gallstones (Crescent-Shaped Appearance)

When a gallstone is large and its surface comprises a hard and compact substance, most of the ultrasound beam is reflected at its surface, and little of the beam reaches the interior of the stone. Consequently, there is a strong crescent-shaped echo reflected by the anterior surface. This is, of course, associated with posterior acoustic shadowing. These findings are often seen with cholesterol stones.

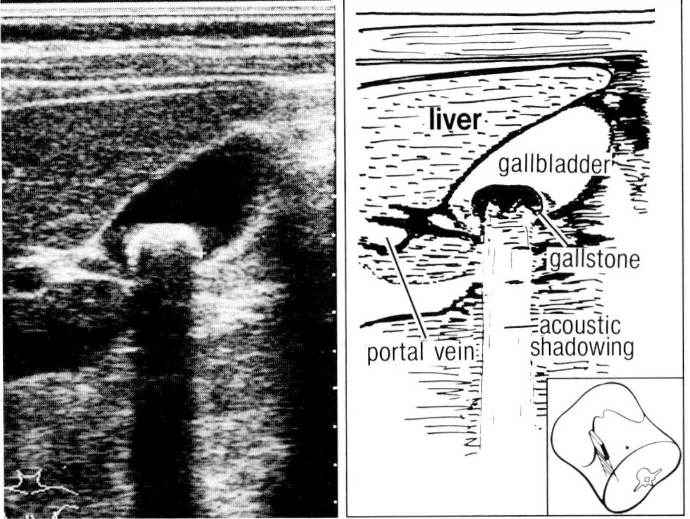

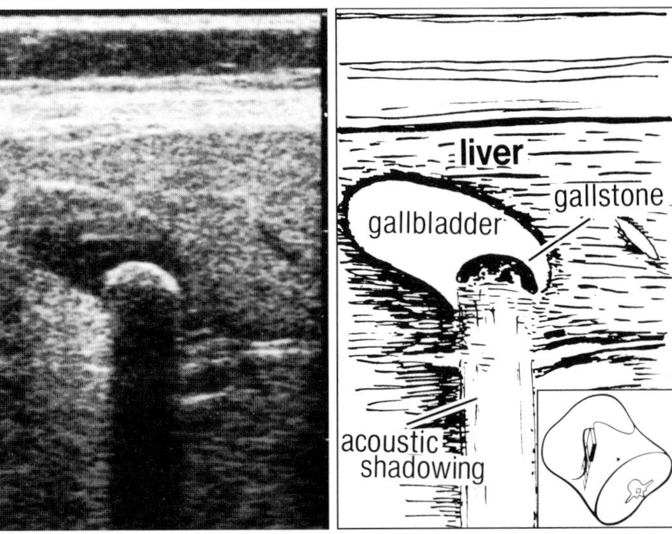

Fig. 4.29. *Case 1.* There is a crescent-shaped strong echo near the neck of the gallbladder

Fig. 4.30. *Case 2.* Crescent-shaped hyperechoic area near the neck of the gallbladder

Cholelithiasis in a Contracted Gallbladder

When the lumen of a contracted gallbladder is filled with stones, echoes from the stones are not distinct, but there is prominent acoustic shadowing. Differentiating this combination of findings from intestinal gas is possible by observing the gallbladder from various angles.

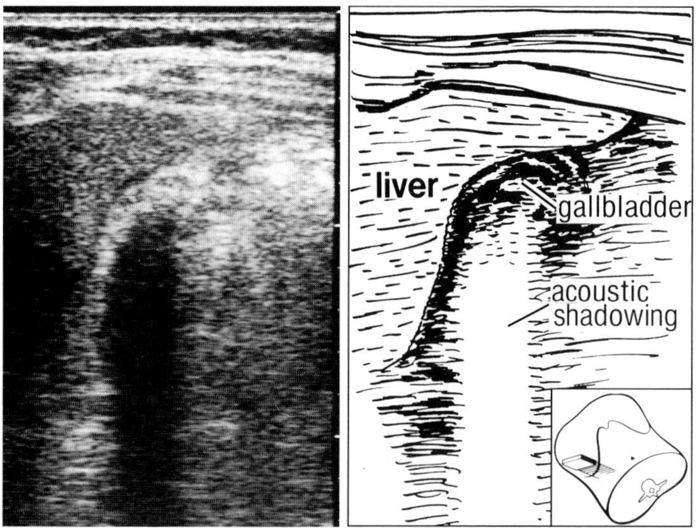

Fig. 4.31. *Case 1.* No cystic structure is identified in the expected location of the gallbladder. However, there is hyperechoic collection with acoustic shadowing on the inferior surface of the liver, representing a contracted, stone-filled gallbladder

Fig. 4.32. *Case 2.* There is an abnormal echo collection with clear posterior acoustic shadowing in the gallbladder bed

Incarcerated Stone in the Neck of the Gallbladder

The gallbladder dilates when a stone becomes incarcerated in the neck of the gallbladder. The bile in the enlarged gallbladder remains anechoic for a short period of time, but subsequently the combination of infected bile and desquamated cells from the gallbladder wall produce a mixed pattern of strong and weak echoes. This condition is referred to as empyema of the gallbladder.

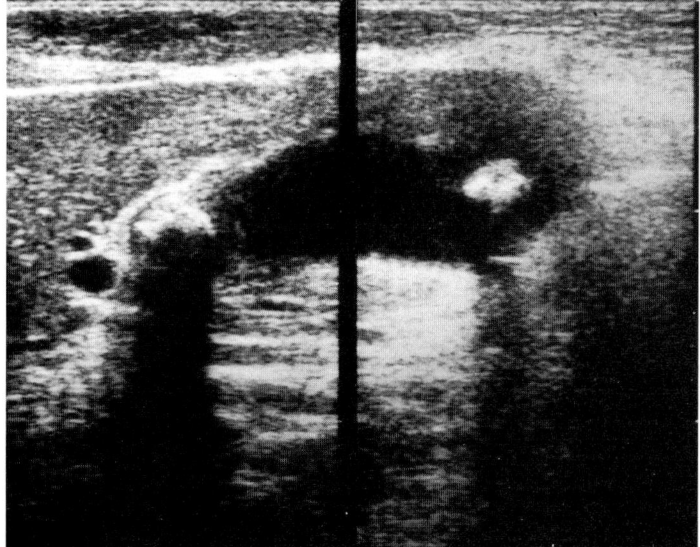

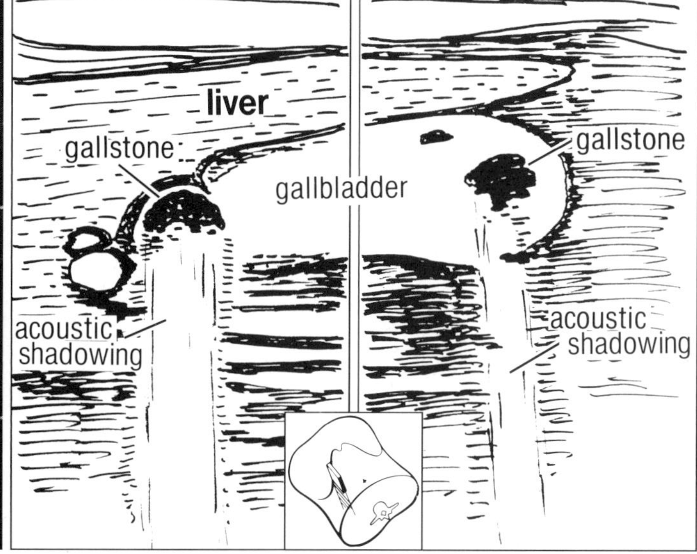

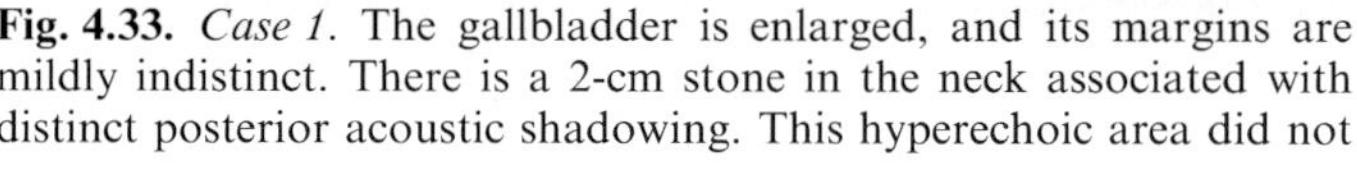

Fig. 4.33. *Case 1.* The gallbladder is enlarged, and its margins are mildly indistinct. There is a 2-cm stone in the neck associated with distinct posterior acoustic shadowing. This hyperechoic area did not move despite changing the patient's position and rocking the patient's body. The hyperechoic area in the fundus of the gallbladder did move

Small Floating Gallstones

When gallstones are small, they may float within the lumen of the gallbladder. This occurs because there is little difference in specific gravity between small gallstones and bile. This finding is frequently seen immediately after the patient's position is changed. Then, in time, these floating gallstones may descend to the dependent portion of the gallbladder.

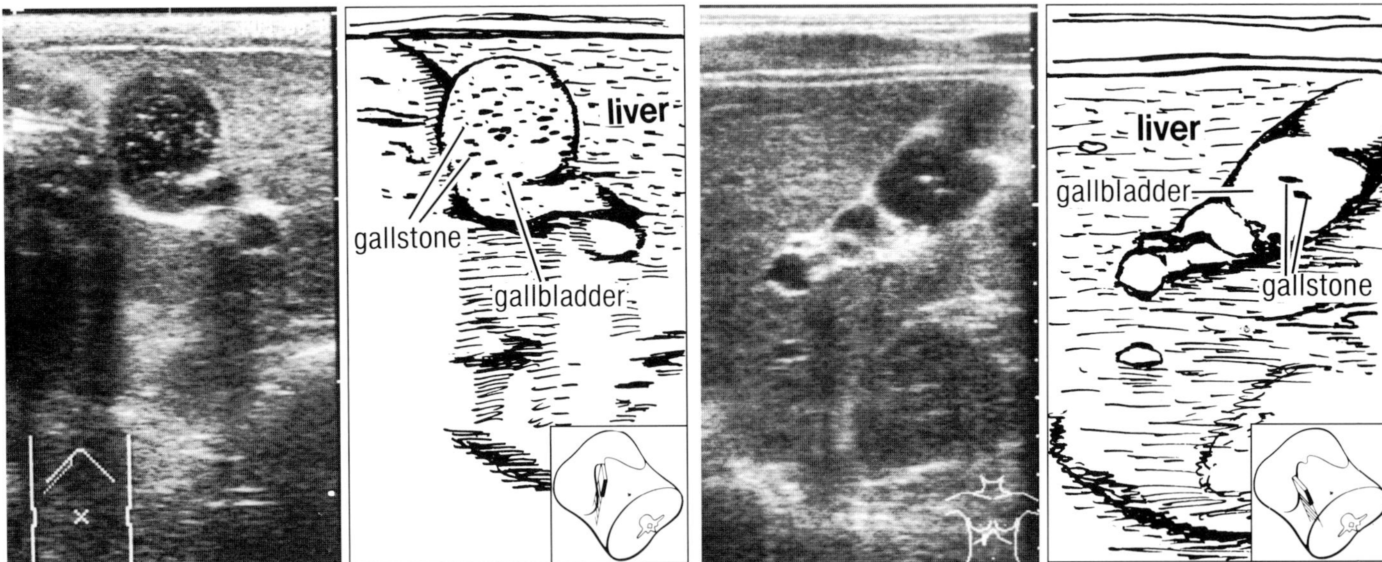

Fig. 4.34. *Case 1.* There are multiple punctate hyperechoic foci within the gallbladder lumen, which persisted throughout the ultrasonographic examination

Fig. 4.35. *Case 2.* There are two hyperechoic foci floating within the lumen of the gallbladder

Various Conditions Which Mimic Gallstones

During examination of the gallbladder, an echo caused by a normal structure may mimic a gallstone. The most common example is folding of the gallbladder wall. A fold of the wall protruding into the lumen of the gallbladder can mimic a small gallstone or polyp. By moving the transducer head in a fan-shaped fashion or by changing the angle of observation, the fold can be visualized as an elongated continuous structure. Echoes from intestinal gas adjacent to the gallbladder can also mimic gallstones.

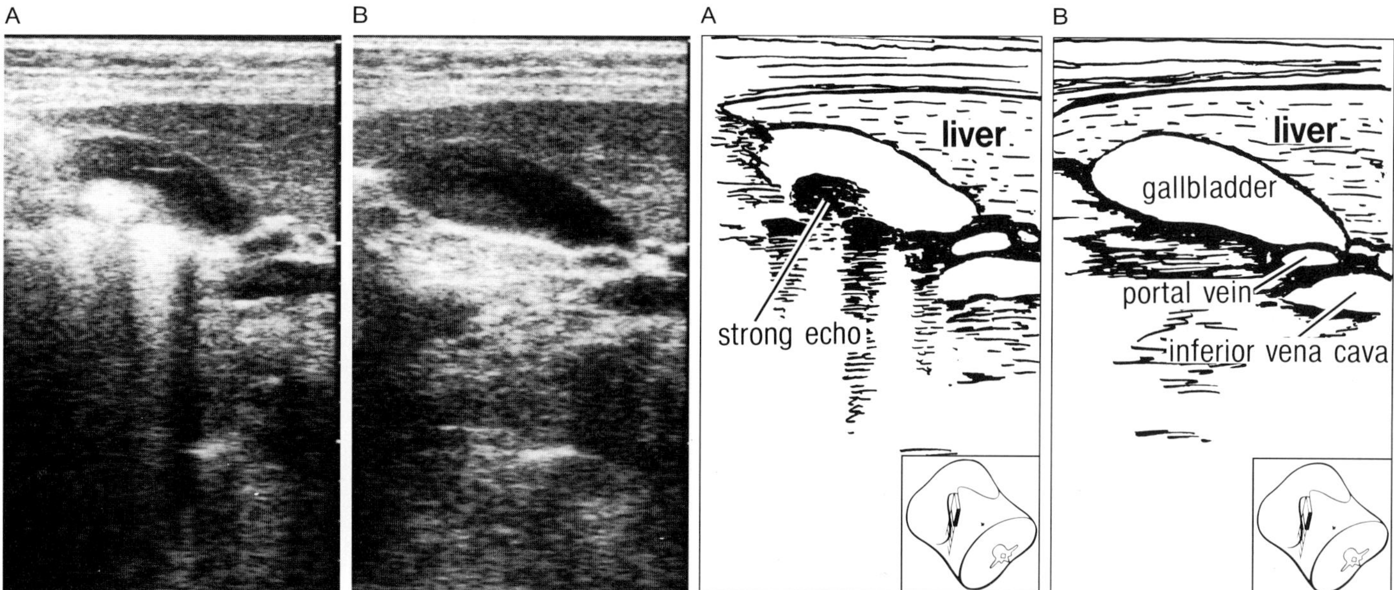

Fig. 4.36 A, B. *Case 1.* A hyperechoic structure, measuring 15 mm in dimension and associated with weak posterior acoustic shadowing, is demonstrated along the posterior wall of the gallbladder (**A**). This image simulates cholelithiasis, although there is no evidence of gall- stones within the gallbladder lumen on the image obtained from a slightly different angle (**B**). The hyperechoic complex simulating a gallstone in **A** was, in actuality, a strong echo from intestinal gas adjacent to the gallbladder

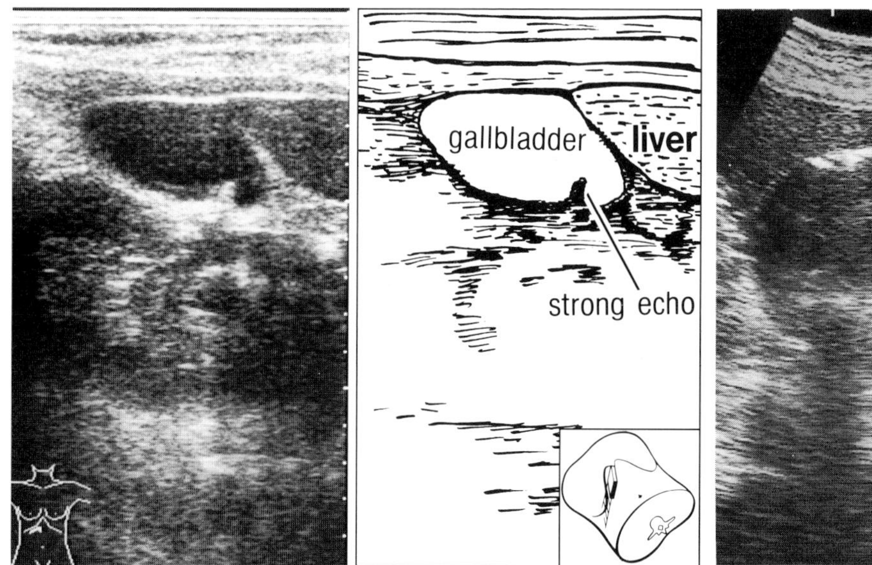

Fig. 4.37. *Case 2.* There is a hyperechoic area on the posterior wall of the neck of the gallbladder which is protruding into the lumen. There is no associated acoustic shadowing. This is a fold of the gallbladder wall

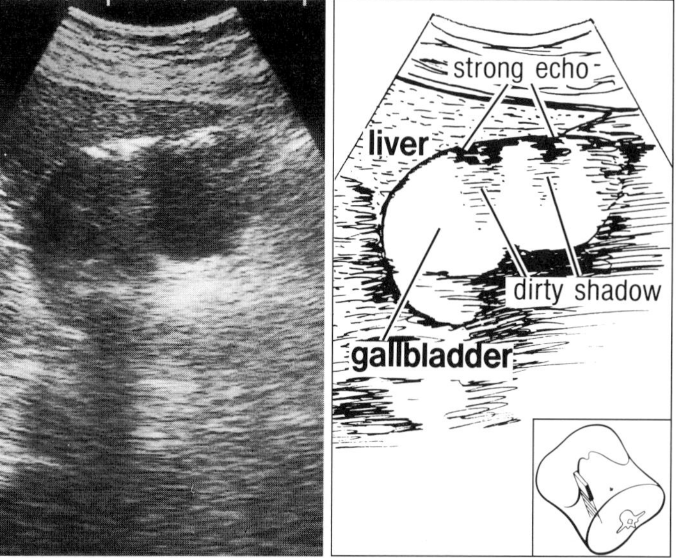

Fig. 4.38. *Case 3.* There are hyperechoic areas along the anterior wall of the gallbladder associated with dirty shadowing (see p. 102). This echo pattern is secondary to gas bubbles within the lumen of the gallbladder

Acute Cholecystitis

In acute cholecystitis, there is thickening of the gallbladder wall. The normal thickness of the wall of the gallbladder is less than 2 mm on ultrasonography. A hypoechoic layer is sometimes seen within the thickened wall, and thus the wall appears to consist of three layers. This hypoechoic layer is thought to represent subserosal edema or necrosis. Other findings sometimes seen in acute cholecystitis include strong echoes from the wall of the gallbladder, indistinct margins of the wall, and dilatation of the gallbladder (in association with an incarcerated gallstone at the neck).

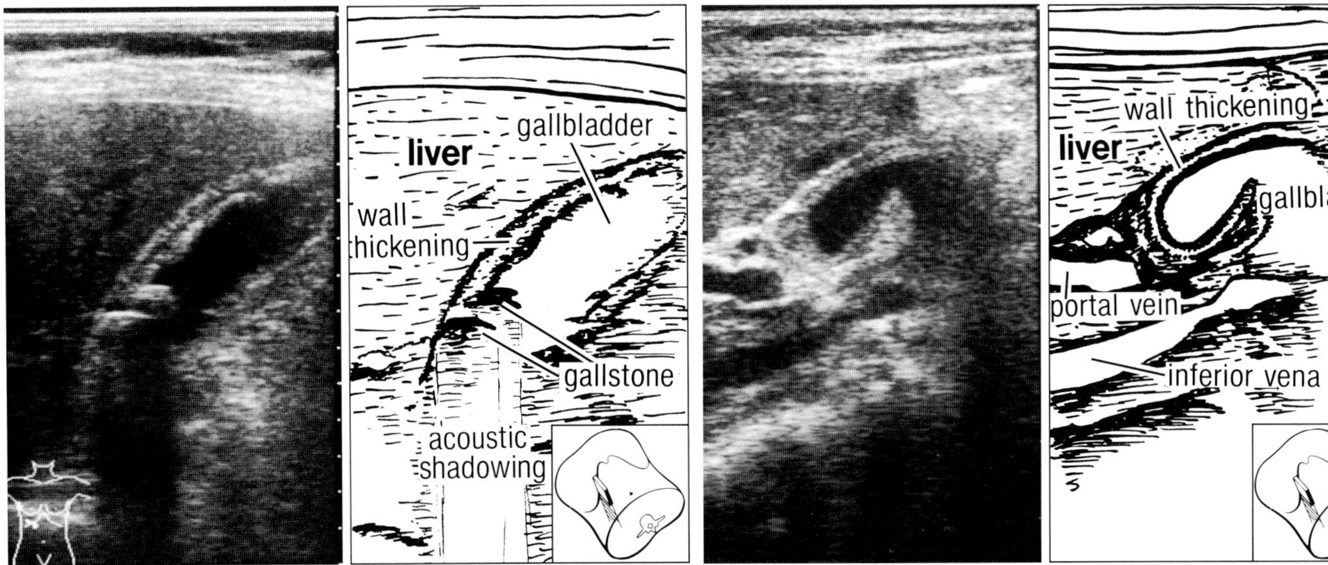

Fig. 4.39. *Case 1*. The gallbladder wall is thickened, measuring approximately 10 mm. There is a hypoechoic layer within the wall. This finding represents either edema of the wall secondary to inflammation or partial desquamation of the gallbladder wall. There are at least two gallstones present, measuring 15–20 mm in size

Fig. 4.40. *Case 2*. This patient had had gastric resection for carcinoma with postoperative fever and abdominal pain. The gallbladder wall is thick with a hypoechoic layer suggesting edema. There is also a hypoechoic area within the liver substance adjacent to the gallbladder, suggesting inflammation

Change in the Gallbladder Wall After TAE

TAE has been frequently utilized as a treatment for hepatocellular carcinoma. Part of the embolizing material injected into the hepatic artery may reach the cystic artery, and consequently the gallbladder may show severe ischemic changes. In this situation, the wall of the gallbladder becomes markedly thickened, and a hypoechoic layer develops within the wall, suggesting edema. When there is desquamation of the mucosa, fine echoes resembling bile sludge are seen within the lumen of the gallbladder.

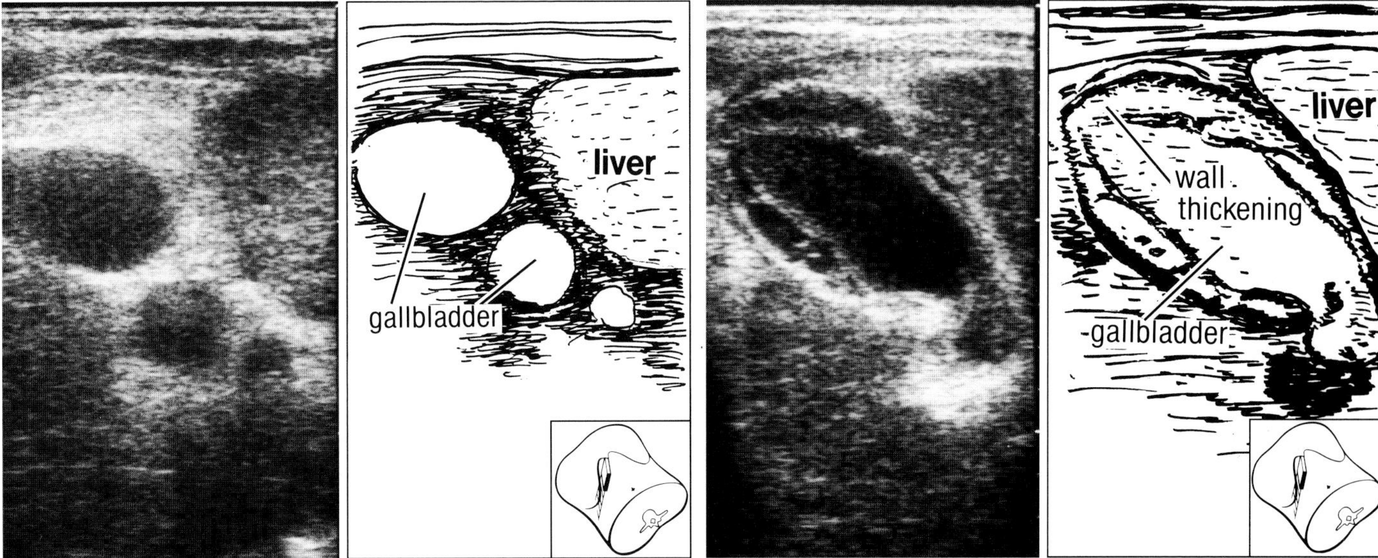

Fig. 4.41. *Case 1, gallbladder before TAE.* There is atrophy of the liver in the region of the gallbladder bed secondary to cirrhosis of the liver. The gallbladder is surrounded by liver parenchyma

Fig. 4.42. *Case 1, 8 days after TAE.* There is mild thickening of the gallbladder wall, and the central layer of the gallbladder appears relatively anechoic

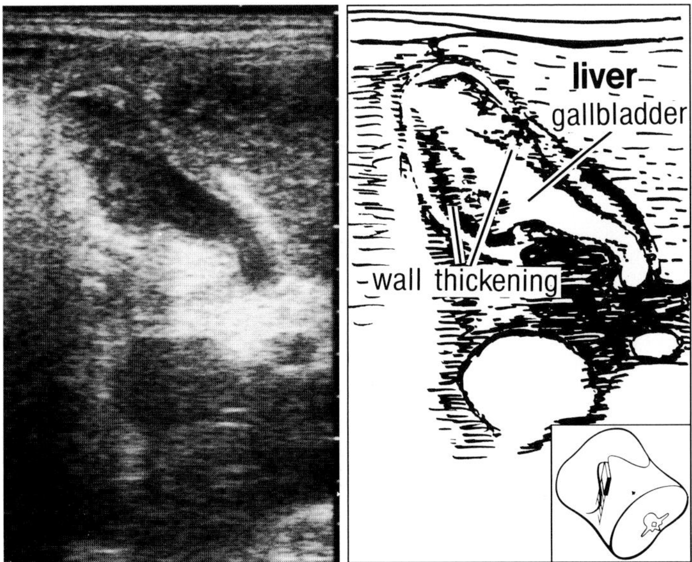

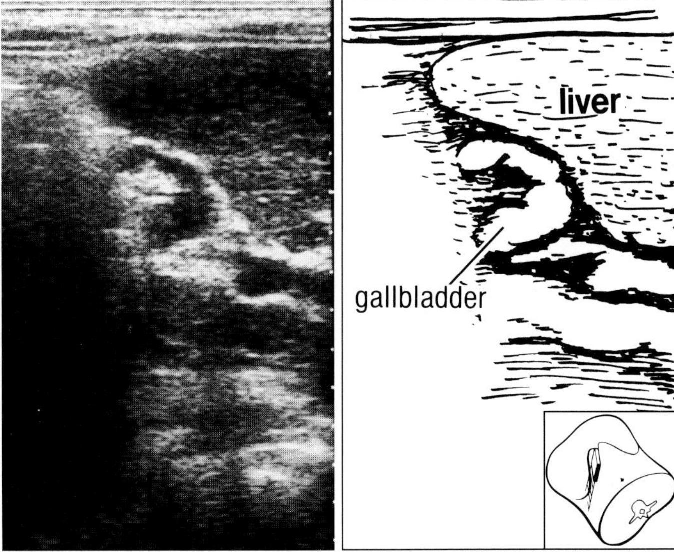

Fig. 4.43. *Case 1, 18 days after TAE.* The thickened gallbladder wall shows slight regression, but there is evidence of desquamation of the mucosa

Fig. 4.44. *Case 1, 2 months after TAE.* The gallbladder wall thickening has disappeared, but the gallbladder is severely deformed and contracted

Cancer of the Gallbladder   Few cancers of the gallbladder are found at an early stage. The survival rate is poor because of rapid extension into the liver parenchyma. Only the polypoid form of the tumor, which protrudes into the lumen of the gallbladder, can be surgically cured, but these small cancers are difficult to differentiate from cholesterol polyps or adenomas. Polypoid lesions of the gallbladder which are larger than 1 cm in size should be surgically excised because of the possibility of malignancy.

**Four Patterns
of Gallbladder Carcinoma**

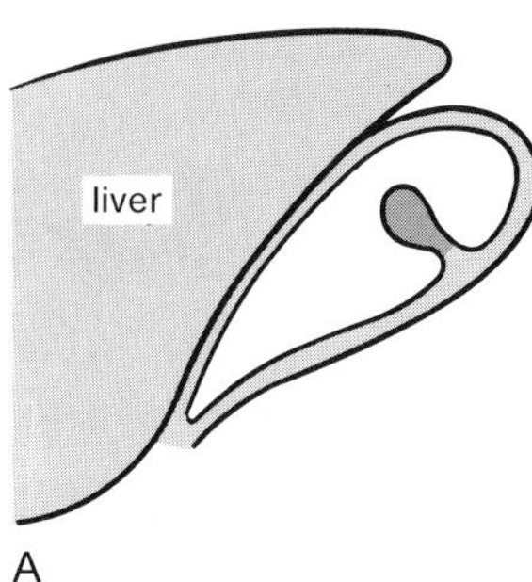

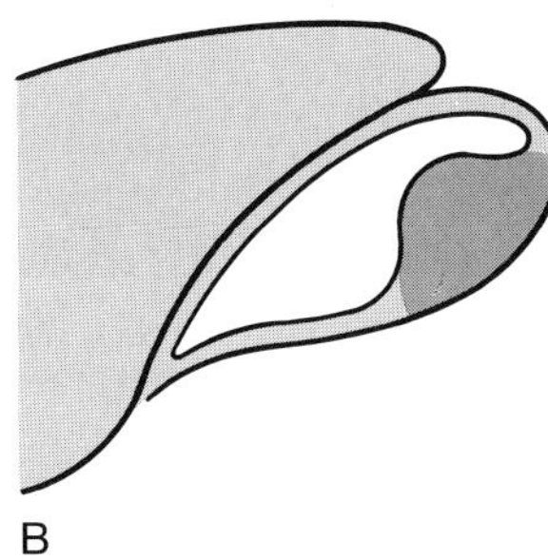

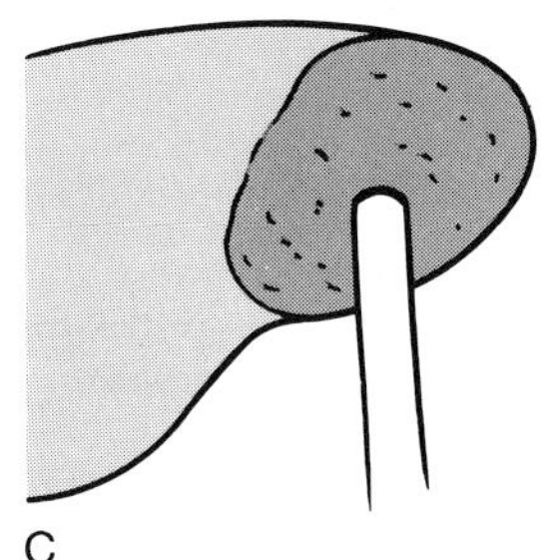

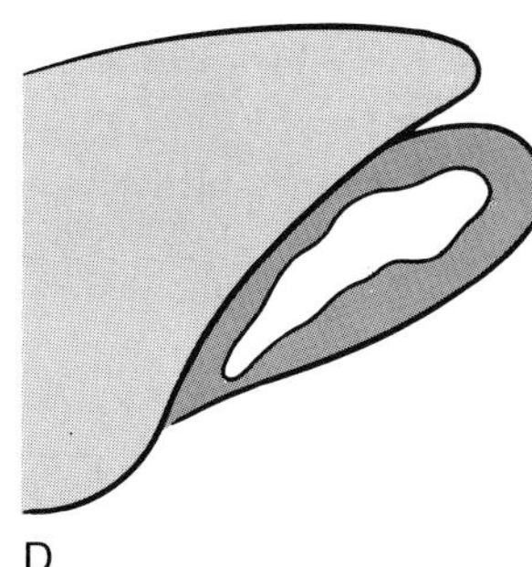

A   B   C   D

Fig. 4.45 A–D. Gallbladder carcinoma can be grossly divided into mass-forming types (**A, B, C**) and an infiltrating type (**D**). The former includes the polypoid (**A**), the localized mass type (**B**) in which a focal mass in the wall projects into the lumen of the gallbladder, and the massive tumor type (**C**) in which the entire gallbladder is involved and becomes a large solitary mass. The infiltrating type (**D**) presents with diffuse thickening of the gallbladder wall. All four types of gallbladder cancer are frequently associated with gallstones. Differential diagnoses of gallbladder carcinoma include benign polyp, bile sludge, cholecystitis and adenomyomatosis

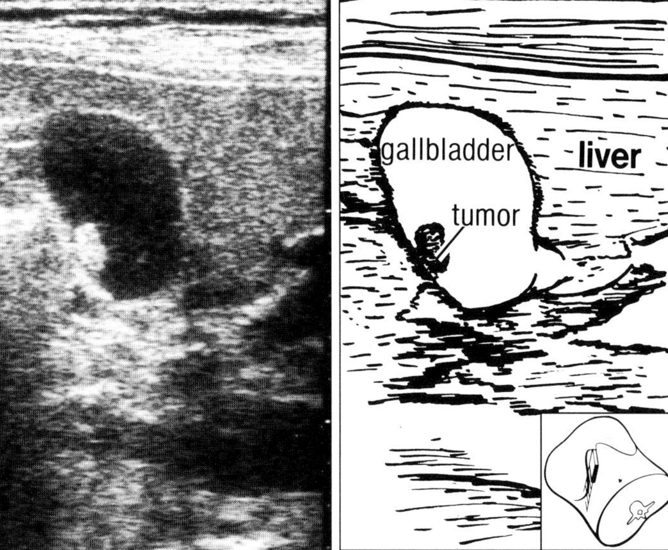

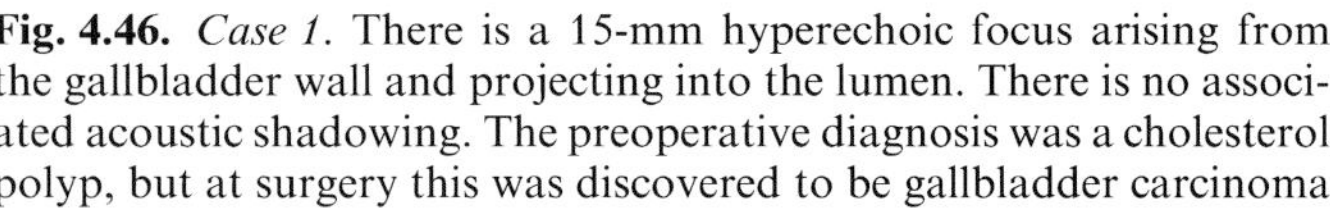

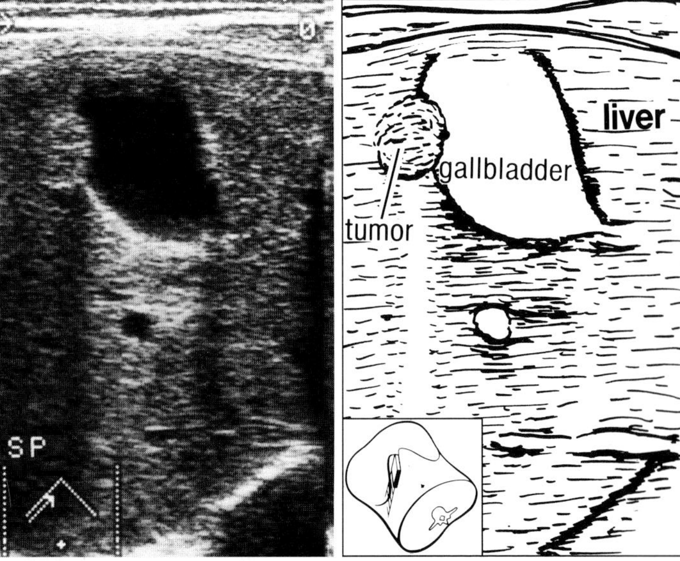

Fig. 4.46. *Case 1.* There is a 15-mm hyperechoic focus arising from the gallbladder wall and projecting into the lumen. There is no associated acoustic shadowing. The preoperative diagnosis was a cholesterol polyp, but at surgery this was discovered to be gallbladder carcinoma

Fig. 4.47. *A case for comparison.* There is a well-defined 18 × 28-mm mass on the gallbladder wall. This finding resembles a cancer of the gallbladder, but the tumor has a high echo level. This turned out to be a hemangioma of the liver with compression of the gallbladder

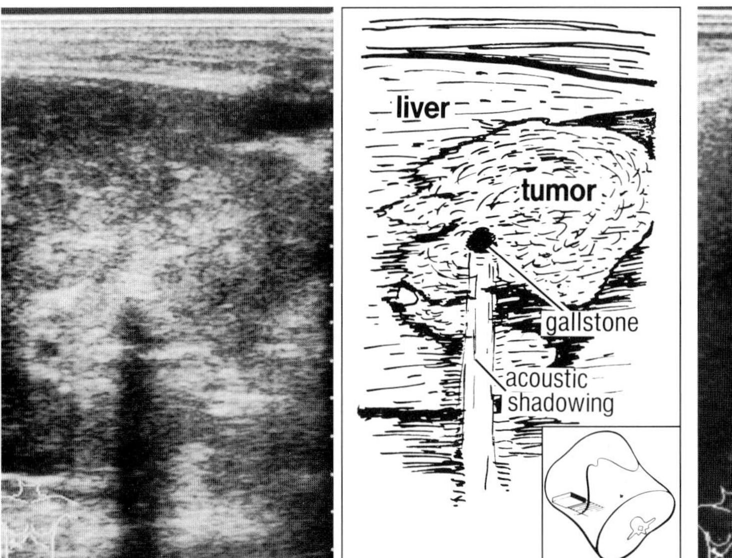

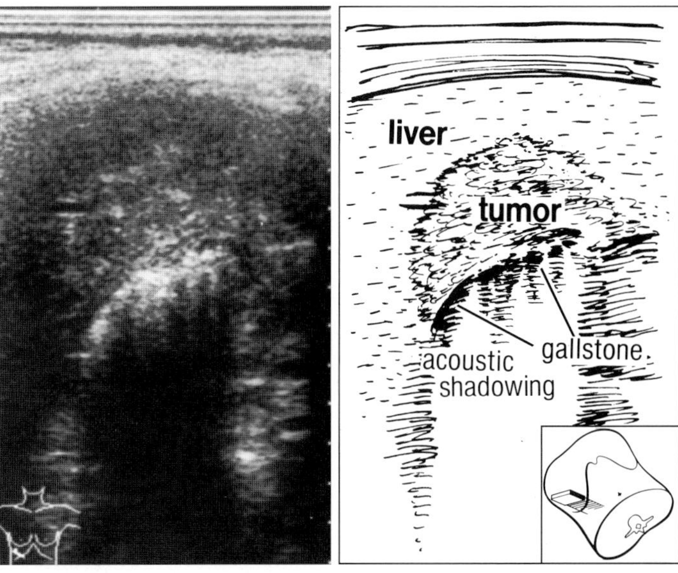

Fig. 4.48. *Case 2.* Scanning in the region of the inferior surface of the right lobe of the liver failed to visualize a normal cystic gallbladder. Instead, there is a solid mass with irregular margins in the expected region of the gallbladder. There is a strong echo, measuring 10 mm and associated with acoustic shadowing in the central portion of the solid mass. The presence of a gallstone strongly suggests the possibility of carcinoma of the gallbladder

Fig. 4.49. *Case 3.* There is a solid mass in the region of the porta hepatis containing several hyperechoic foci. A solid mass is also seen within the liver parenchyma, indicating tumor invasion. In this case, gallbladder carcinoma with invasion into the liver has created one large abnormal mass

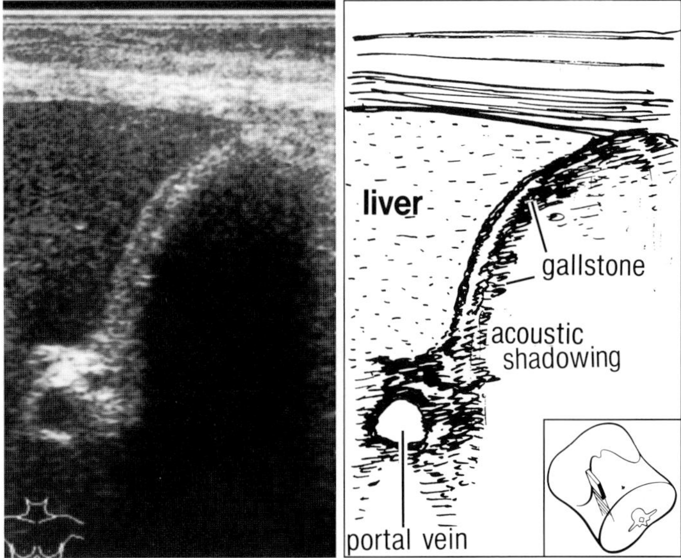

Fig. 4.50. *A case for comparison.* A case of cholelithiasis with multiple stones filling the lumen of the gallbladder. Initially, this case appears similar to case 3 (Fig. 4.49), but gallbladder wall thickening is clearly visualized, and there is good demarcation between the liver cancer the gallbladder. In addition, the echo pattern of the adjacent liver is normal

Cholesterol Polyp

Cholesterol polyps represent focal accumulation of foam cells containing phagocytosed cholesterol ester on the gallbladder wall. This is a benign process without malignant potential. These lesions are often multiple and manifest as hyperechoic foci, measuring 2–3 mm, projecting from the gallbladder wall without associated acoustic shadowing.

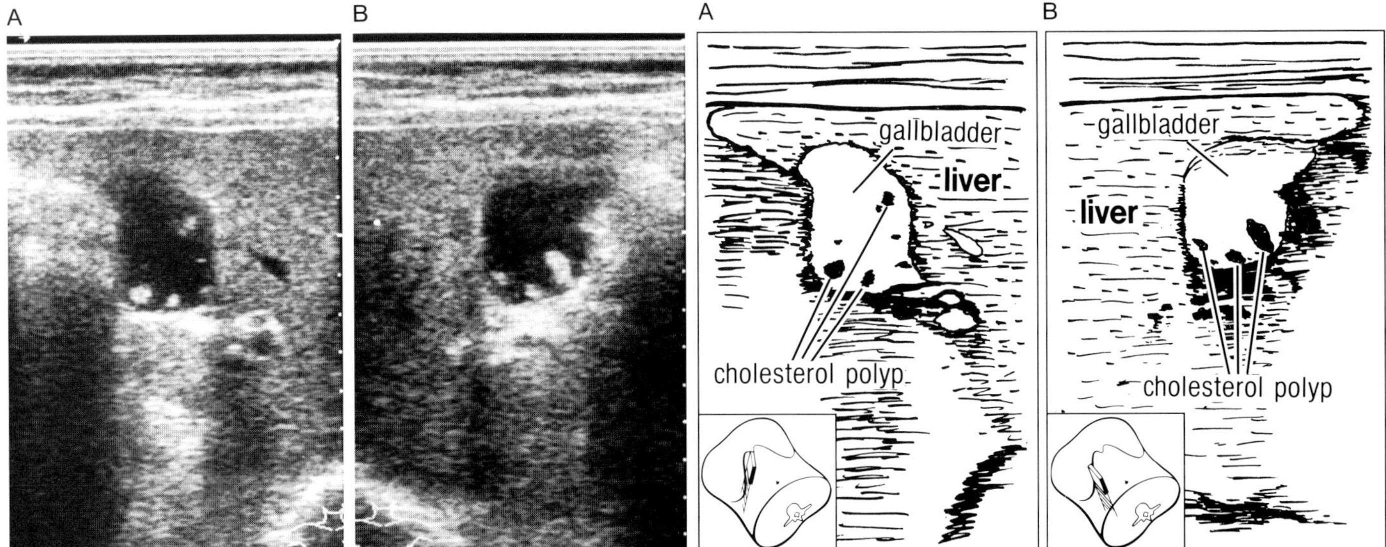

Fig. 4.51 A, B. *Case 1.* There are several hyperechoic foci projecting into the gallbladder lumen. The largest measures 1 cm. There is no associated acoustic shadowing. This is a typical ultrasonographic appearance of cholesterol polyps. Note, though, that it is uncommon for multiple cholesterol polyps to be visualized on a single ultrasonographic section as seen in this case

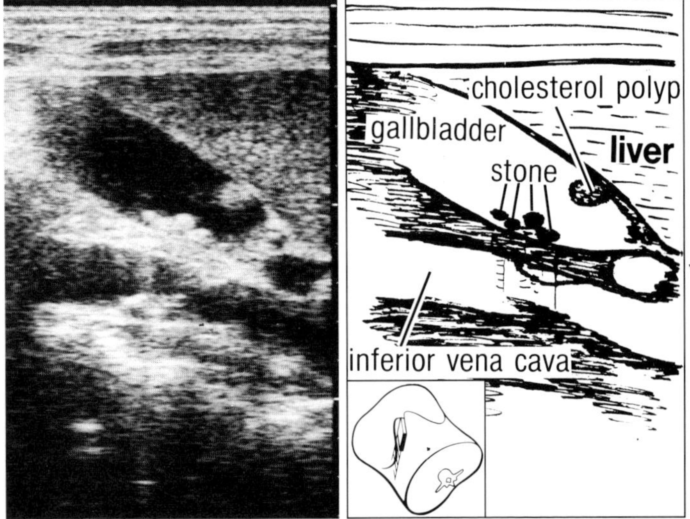

Fig. 4.52. *Case 2.* There are several hyperechoic lesions on the posterior wall of the gallbladder. Additionally, there is an abnormal echo, 8 mm in size, on the anterior wall of the gallbladder, near the neck, which did not move when the patient's position was changed. This echo is weaker when compared with the gallstones on the posterior wall and is approximately isoechoic with liver parenchyma

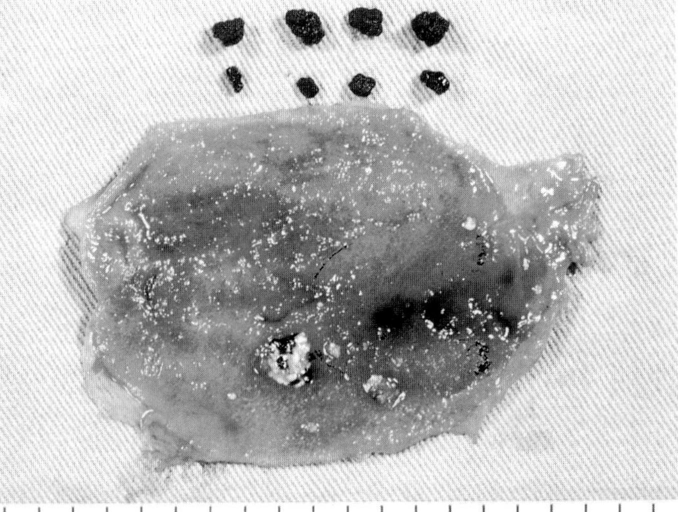

Fig. 4.53. *Case 2, surgical specimen.* There were eight bilirubin stones within the lumen of the gallbladder. Also present was a yellow-colored cholesterol polyp

Bile Sludge

A fine abnormal echo pattern with a horizontal fluid-fluid level is sometimes seen within the lumen of the gallbladder. This represents bile sludge. Sludge does not demonstrate acoustic shadowing. Sludge moves to the dependent portion of the gallbladder with changes in the patient's position. Side lobe artifacts can mimic this finding.

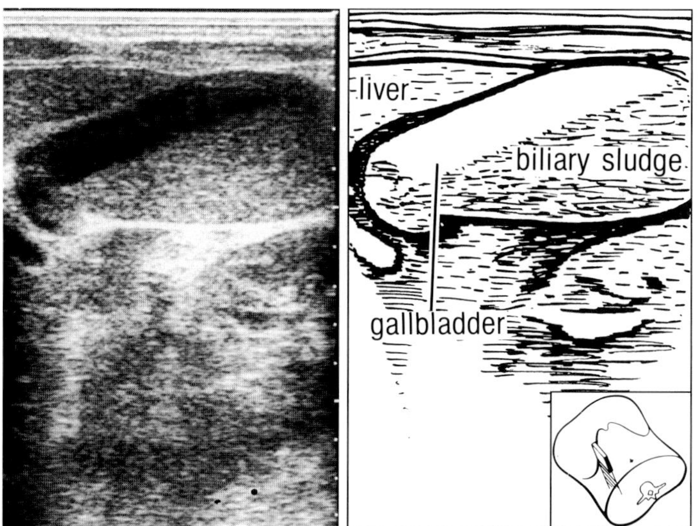

Fig. 4.54. *Case 1*. A patient with cancer of the pancreatic head. A collection of fine echoes is seen within the lumen of the gallbladder with a horizontal fluid-fluid level. Initially, this sludge was in the fundus of the gallbladder but, after changing the patient to the supine position, it moved toward the gallbladder neck

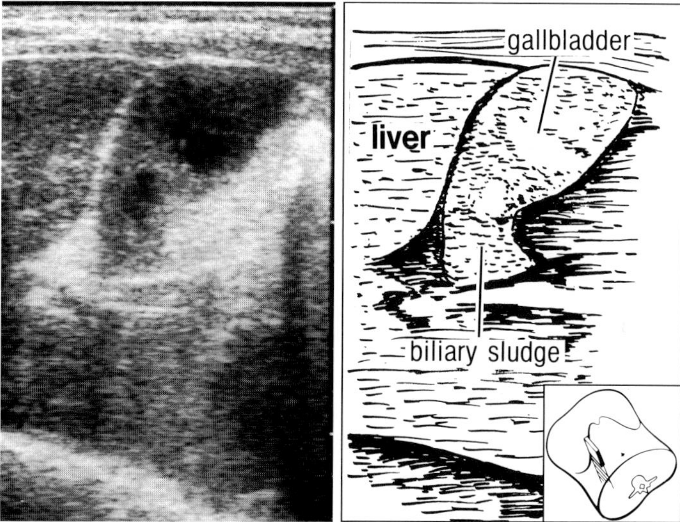

Fig. 4.55. *Case 2*. A patient who had had gastrectomy for gastric carcinoma 3 weeks earlier. Within the gallbladder lumen, there is an abnormal echo collection with a somewhat irregular contour. This moved to the dependent portion when the patient's position was changed

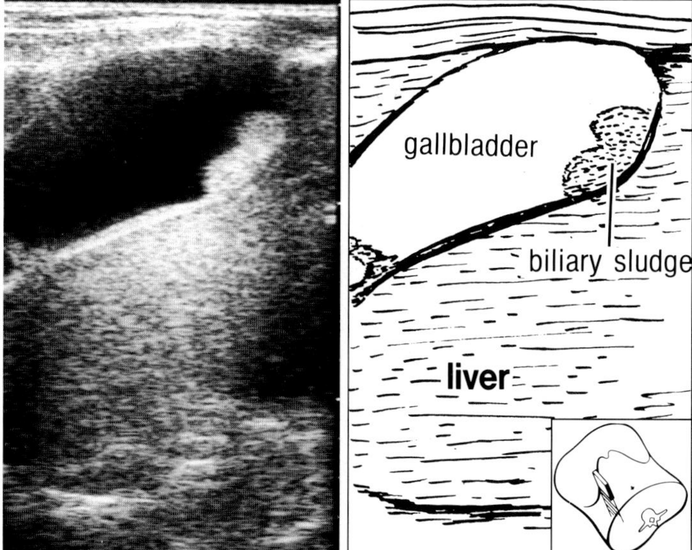

Fig. 4.56. *Case 3*. The gallbladder is enlarged, and there is a rounded abnormal echo collection in the fundus, resembling a polypoid lesion. However, when the patient's position was changed, this moved to the dependent portion of the gallbladder, confirming that this is bile sludge. This patient had obstructive jaundice

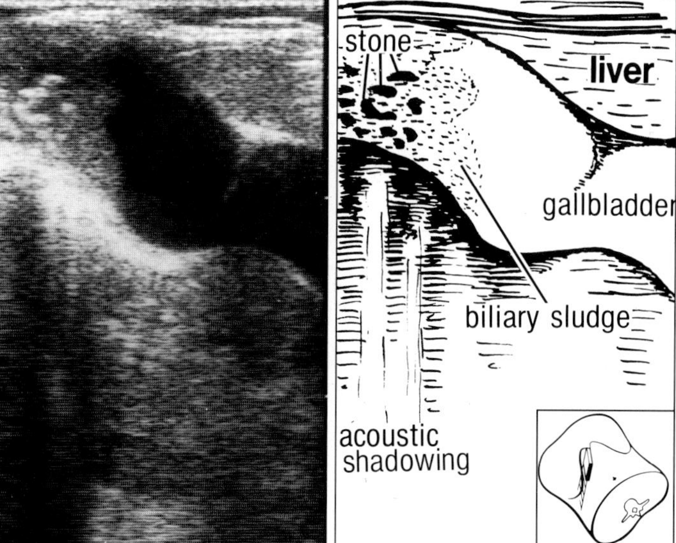

4.57. *Case 4*. A patient with hepatocellular carcinoma. The lumen of the gallbladder is significantly enlarged, and within the fundus there is a large echo collection containing several small hyperechoic foci, suggesting small gallstones within bile sludge

Adenomyomatosis

Adenomyomatosis is a condition in which there is hypertrophy of the mucosal and muscular layers of the gallbladder associated with formation of Rokitansky-Aschoff sinuses. This entity is divided into three different types (Fig. 4.58). Ultrasonographically, there is thickening of the gallbladder wall and associated deformity. Rarely, small stones within the Rokitansky-Aschoff sinus or comet-like echoes arising from these small stones can be visualized.

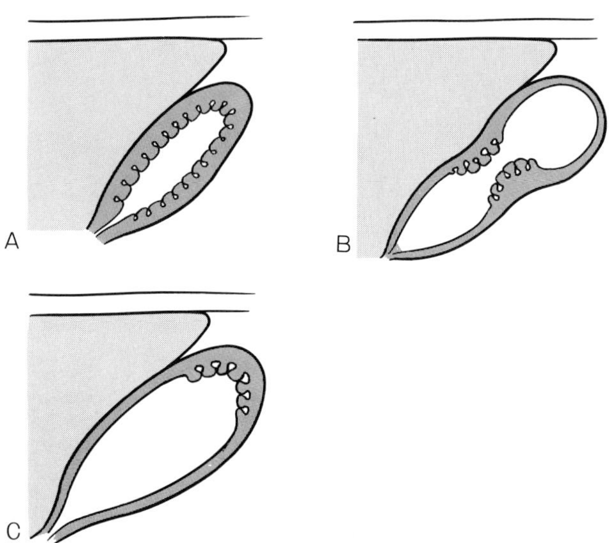

Fig. 4.58 A–C. *Classification of adenomyomatosis.* **A** Generalized type; **B** segmental type; **C** fundal type

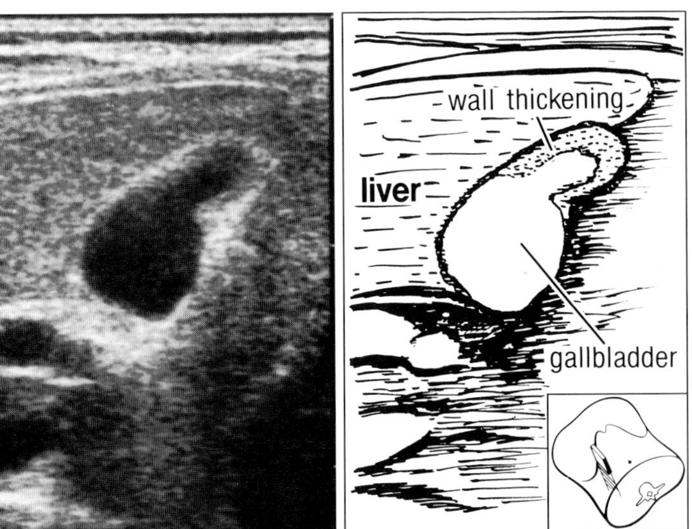

Fig. 4.59. *Case 1.* There is localized thickening of the wall of the fundus, and the gallbladder lumen is small. This is a typical example of the segmental type of adenomyomatosis. The patient had occasional right upper quadrant pain

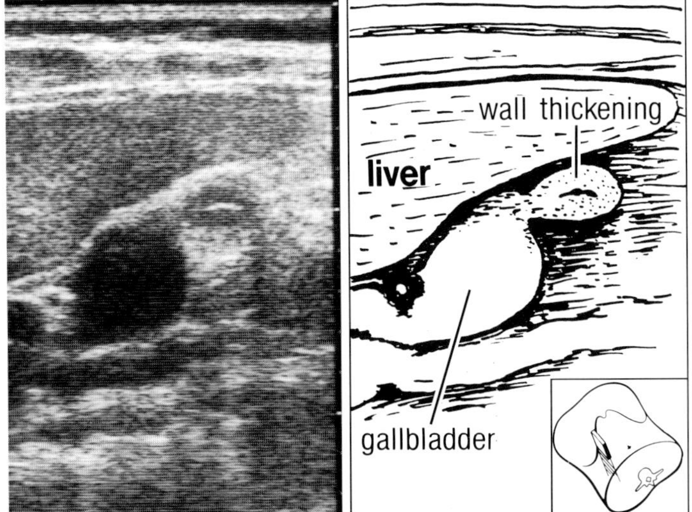

Fig. 4.60. *Case 2.* Another example of the segmental type of adenomyomatosis. The lumen appears obliterated in the region of the fundus

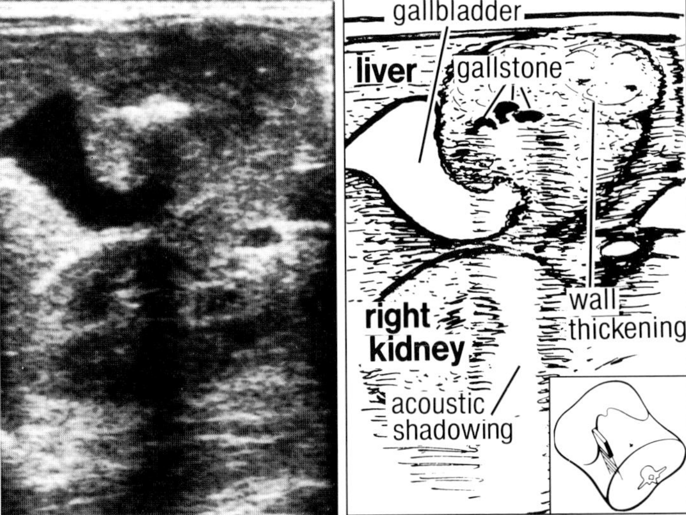

Fig. 4.61. *Case 3.* The wall of the gallbladder fundus is markedly thickened, and no lumen is visualized. There are hyperechoic areas suggesting stones in the central portion of the thickened wall. Punctate strong echoes are seen within the thickened wall, suggesting stones within the Rokitansky-Aschoff sinuses

Cirrhosis of the Liver and Thickening of the Gallbladder Wall

Thickening of the wall of the gallbladder is often seen in patients with severe hepatic dysfunction (see p. 81). This is thought to be secondary to increased portal venous pressure as the cystic vein is part of the portal system. Gallbladder wall thickening can be clearly visualized in patients with ascites, as a portion of the wall is in contact with the ascites. When ascites is secondary to peritoneal carcinomatosis, renal disease, or cardiac failure, the thickness of the gallbladder wall is normal.

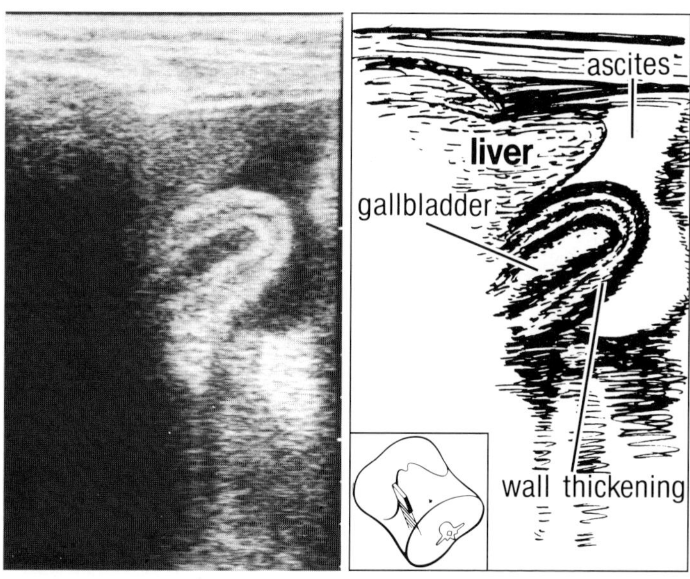

Fig. 4.62. *Case 1.* The gallbladder wall is thickened to 1 cm. There is a hypoechoic central layer in the wall creating the appearance of three layers. Some investigators suggest that ascites can cause apparent thickening of the gallbladder wall on ultrasonography, but thickening to this extent cannot be explained simply by the presence of ascites

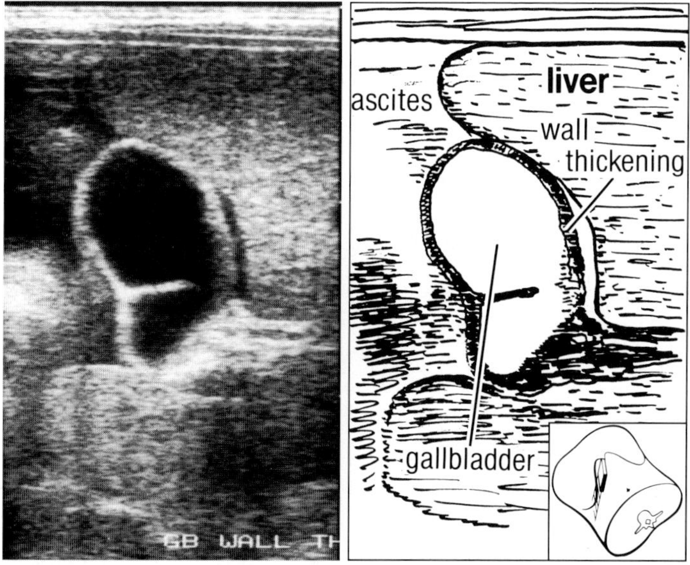

Fig. 4.63. *A case for comparison.* A patient with ascites secondary to malignant lymphoma. Although the gallbladder wall is within normal limits in thickness, it appears slightly thickened due to increased gain of the ultrasound beam through the ascites. In order to accurately measure the thickness of the gallbladder wall, the gain should be lowered so that only the wall of the gallbladder can be visualized

Folded Gallbladder

The typical gallbladder is pear shaped and elongated, but a folded gallbladder is not infrequently encountered. The reason for the folding may include cholecystitis, adenomyomatosis, deformity of the liver secondary to cirrhosis of the liver, and postsurgical change.

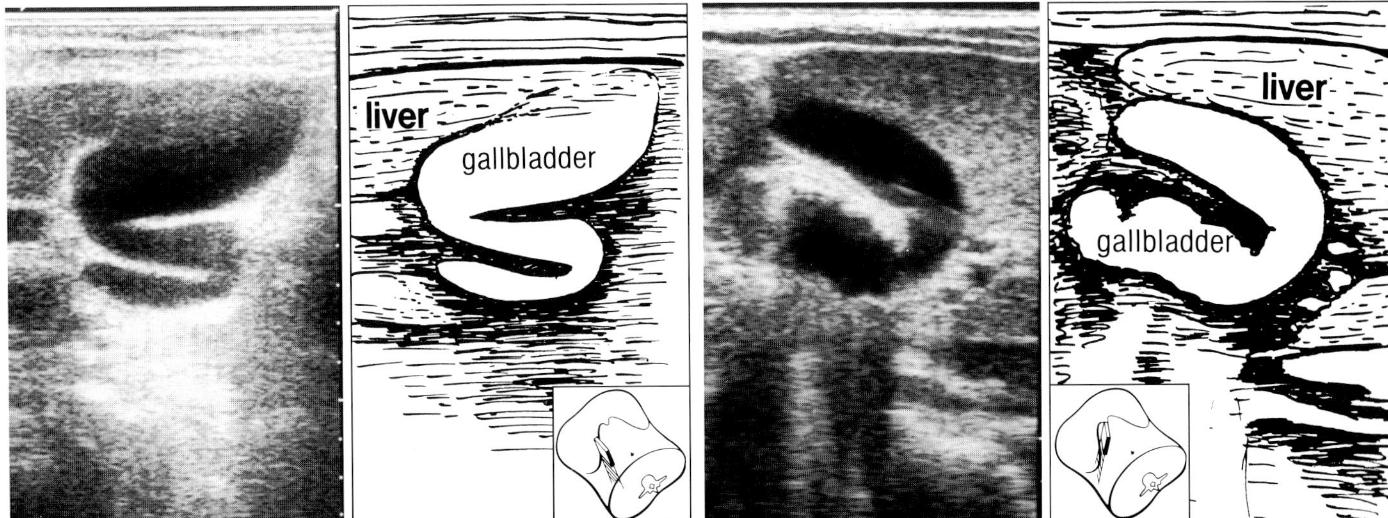

Fig. 4.64. *Case 1.* The gallbladder is deformed and S-shaped. This deformity is secondary to atrophy of the liver in the region of the gallbladder fossa in a patient with hepatic cirrhosis

Fig. 4.65. *Case 2.* A patient following gastrectomy for gastric cancer. There were liver metastases, and abdominal lymph node enlargement was present. The gallbladder is severely deformed

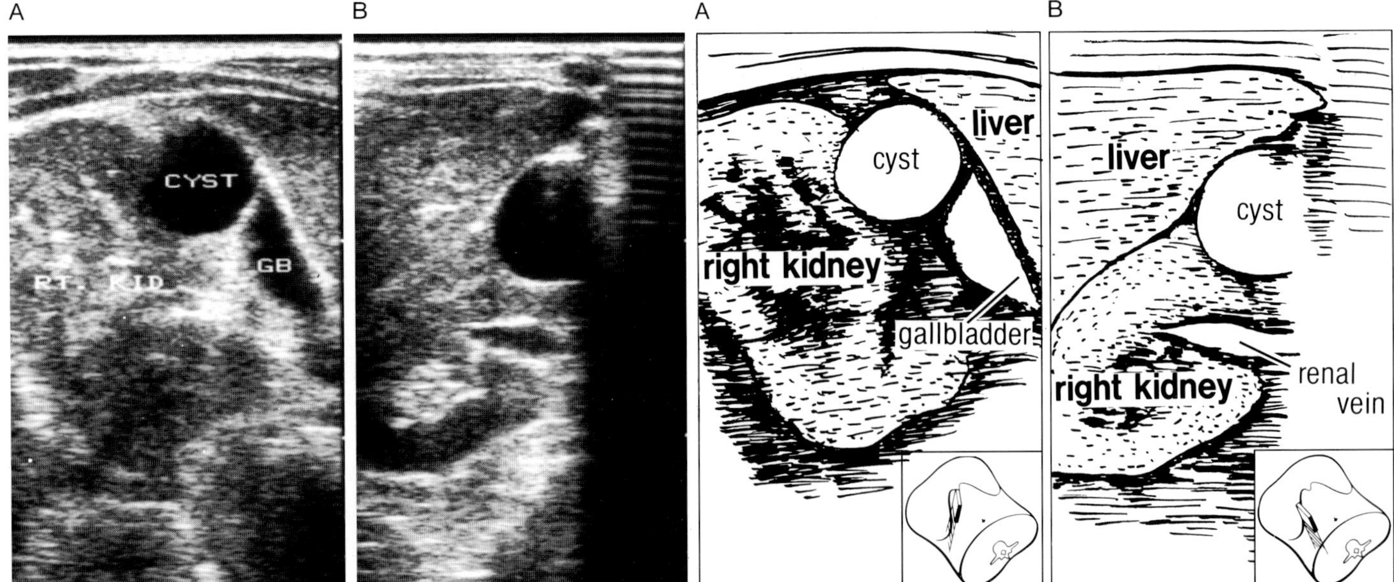

Fig. 4.66 A, B. *A case for comparison.* The gallbladder appears folded on itself, apparently having two chambers on the subcostal scan (**A**). However, the intercostal scan (**B**) reveals a cyst from the lower pole of the right kidney, projecting toward the liver. By changing the direction of observation, it is obvious that the right renal cyst is adjacent to the gallbladder, simulating a folded gallbladder

Choledocholithiasis

Although ultrasonographic examination is very accurate in detecting gallstones within the gallbladder, the accuracy is not very high in detecting stone formation within the extrahepatic bile duct. This is particularly true when a stone is located in the lower portion of the extrahepatic bile duct, secondary to artifacts from intestinal gas. However, even in these cases, the biliary dilatation secondary to stone formation can easily be visualized.

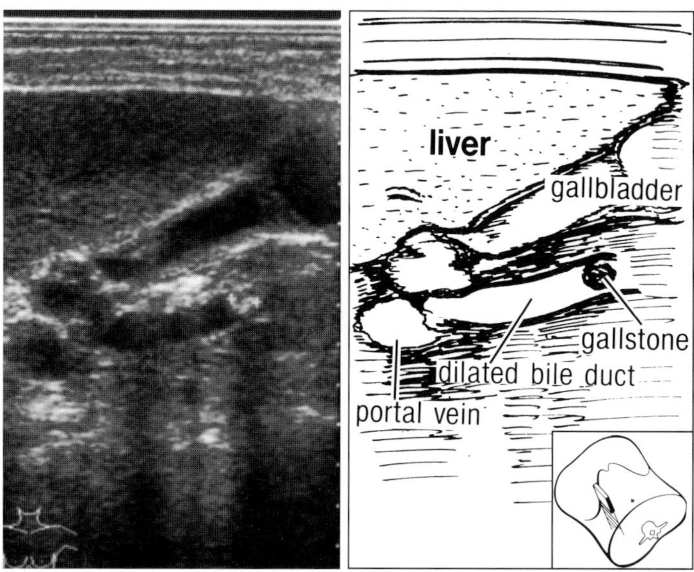

Fig. 4.67. *Case 1*. There is an 8-mm stone within the superior portion of the extrahepatic bile duct. The extrahepatic bile duct is dilated to 9 mm. Similar findings were seen on endoscopic retrograde cholangiopancreatography

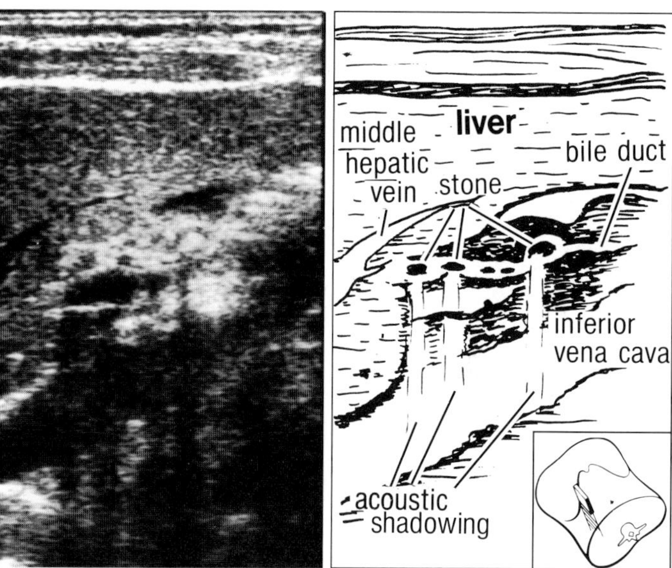

Fig. 4.68. *Case 2*. There are four or five hyperechoic foci within the lumen of the extrahepatic bile duct. There is no significant dilatation of the biliary system

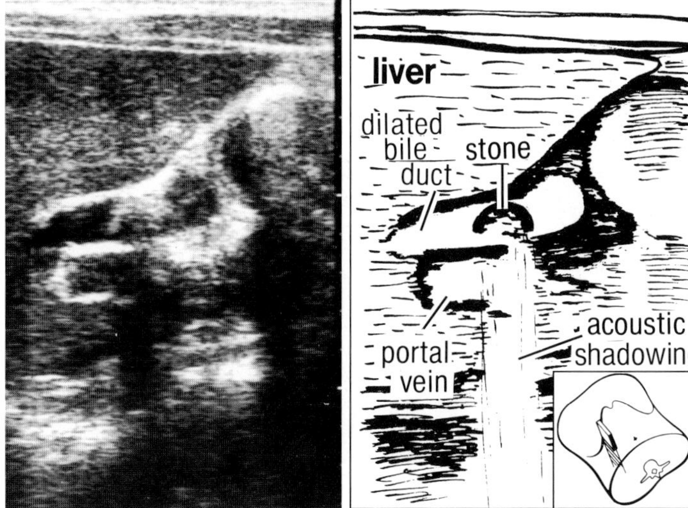

Fig. 4.69. *Case 3*. There is a stone measuring 15 mm within the superior portion of the extrahepatic bile duct. During the examination, only three stones were detected, whereas four bilirubin stones were removed at the time of surgery

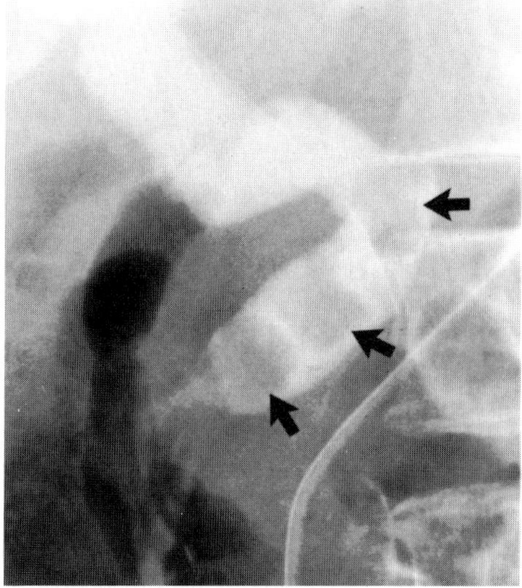

Fig. 4.70. *Case 3*. Radiograph of the extrahepatic bile duct following contrast injection via the percutaneous transhepatic cholangiography drainage (PTCD) tube. There are three filling defects (*arrows*) within the inferior portion of the extrahepatic bile duct

Compression of the Common Bile Duct

The differential diagnoses of ultrasonographic biliary dilatation include cancer of the pancreatic head, gallstone within the common bile duct, inflammatory stenosis of the common bile duct, and extrinsic compression of the common bile duct. Enlargement of the lymph nodes in the region of the porta hepatis or pancreatic head secondary to malignancy of other organs may compress the common bile duct and cause obstructive jaundice.

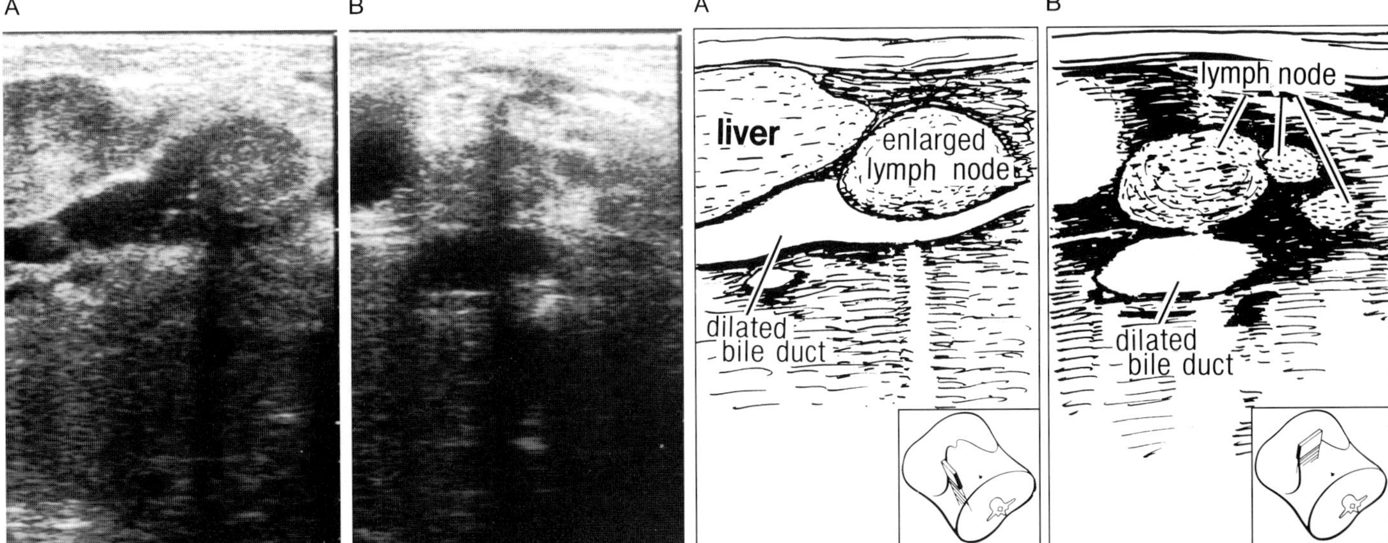

Fig. 4.71 A, B. *Case 1.* The longitudinal section of the porta hepatis (**A**) shows dilatation of the extrahepatic bile duct and a 25 × 40-mm homogeneous solid tumor in its lower segment. The transverse section (**B**) shows two additional solid masses. These masses represent enlarged lymph nodes secondary to metastatic gastric carcinoma

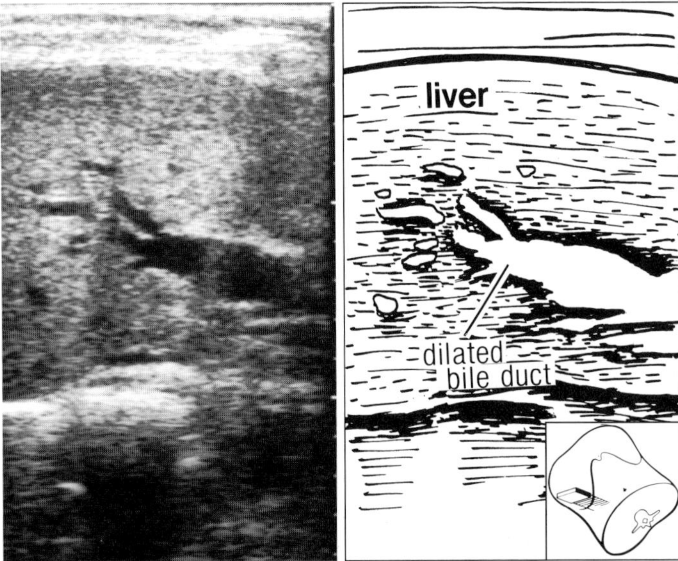

Fig. 4.72. *Case 1.* An intercostal scan demonstrates dilatation of the right branch of the intrahepatic biliary duct

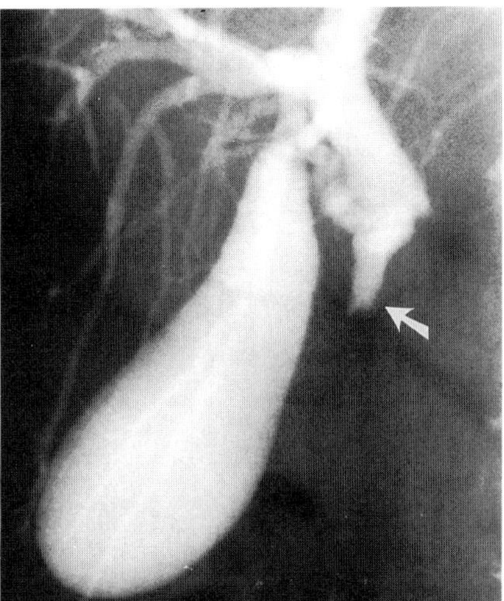

Fig. 4.73. *Case 1, percutaneous transhepatic cholangiogram.* There is mild dilatation of the intrahepatic bile ducts and the gallbladder. The proximal portion of the extrahepatic bile duct is also dilated. There is progressive narrowing of the lumen from the region of the confluence of the cystic duct and the common duct with complete occlusion distally (*arrow*)

Stenosis of the Common Bile Duct

Dilatation of the biliary system can be caused by narrowing of the distal portion of the extrahepatic bile duct without the presence of tumor or stones. In these cases, the intrahepatic bile ducts show only mild dilatation. The bile sludge within the gallbladder typically seen in a patient with acute obstructive jaundice, is usually absent.

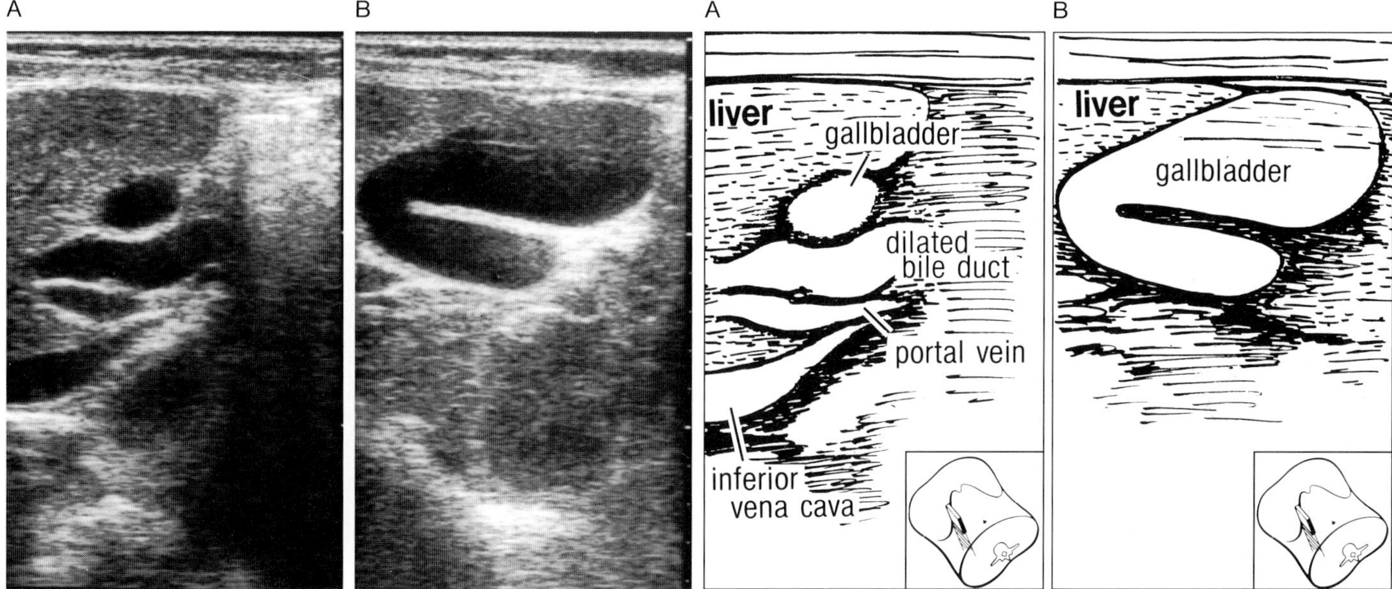

Fig. 4.74 A, B. *Case 1.* **A** The longitudinal section shows marked dilatation of the extrahepatic bile duct which is larger in diameter than the portal vein. **B** The longitudinal section of the gallbladder gives the impression that the gallbladder is under pressure, although accurate size determination of the gallbladder is difficult due to its folding. There is no evidence of bile sludge

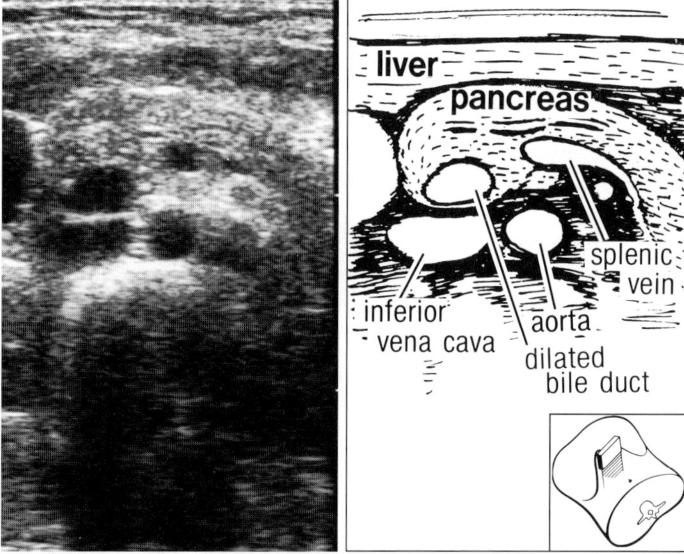

Fig. 4.75. *Case 1, transverse section of the pancreas.* There is dilatation of the distal portion of the common bile duct where it passes through the pancreatic head. This finding suggests that the abnormality is in the region of the papilla of Vater. A normally sized main pancreatic duct is visualized in the pancreatic body

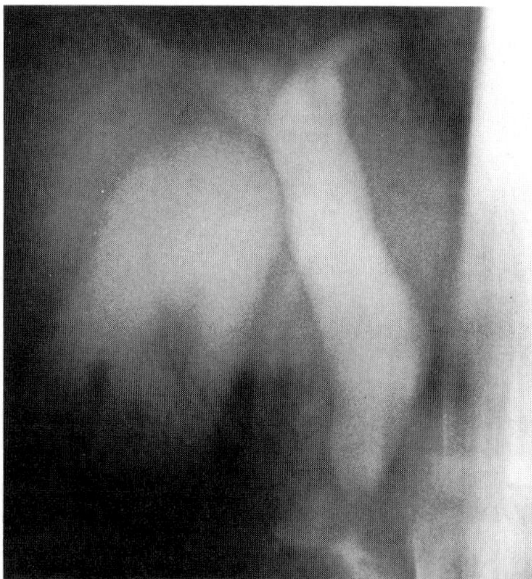

Fig. 4.76. *Case 1, drip infusion cholangiogram.* There is mild dilatation of the extrahepatic bile duct, but no definite tumor is visualized. Subsequent CT examination also failed to prove the presence of a mass. At the 1-year follow up, there was no interval change

Cancer of the Common Bile Duct

Cancer of the common bile duct results in obstruction of the biliary system with proximal biliary dilatation. Dilatation of the biliary system can easily be diagnosed by ultrasonography; but, when the tumor is small and is located in the distal portion of the common bile duct, the diagnosis of cancer may be difficult to make on the basis of ultrasonographic examination alone. As the tumor becomes larger, ultrasonography can visualize the tumor, but then differentiating a tumor of the common bile duct from a tumor of the pancreatic head becomes difficult.

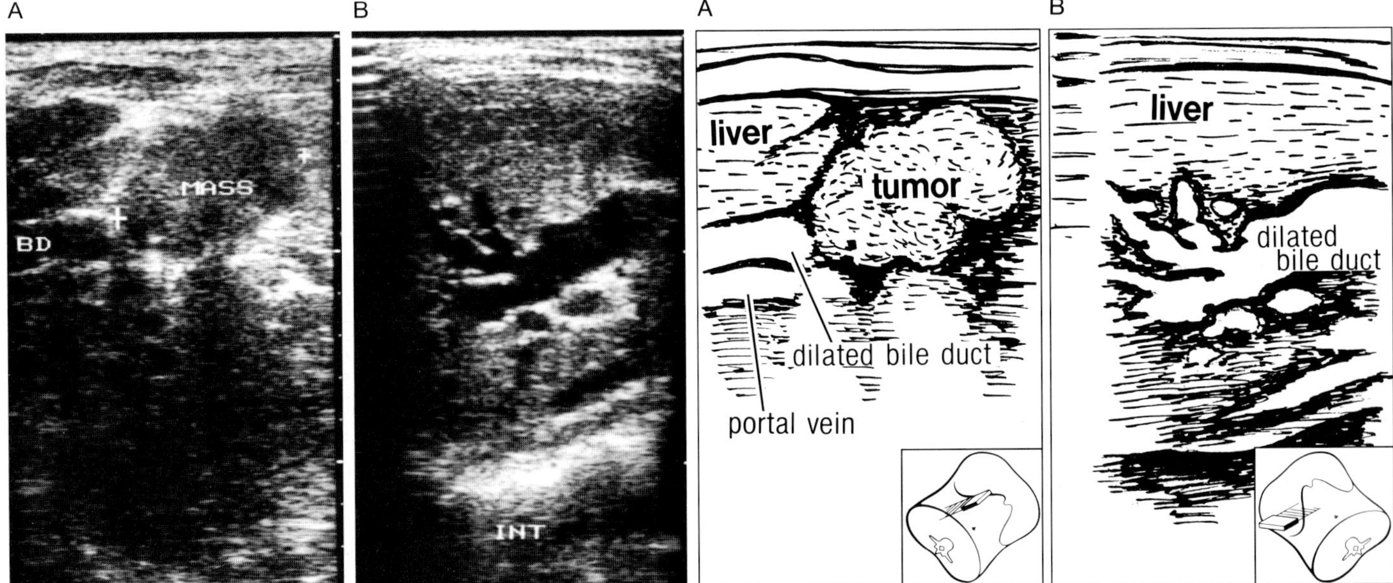

Fig. 4.77 A, B. *Case 1.* Cancer of the bile duct. The longitudinal section of the porta hepatis (**A**) demonstrates dilatation of the extrahepatic bile duct and a 4 × 5-cm solid mass below the dilated segment. On this image alone, differentiating cancer of the bile duct from cancer of the pancreatic head is difficult. The intercostal section of the liver (**B**) demonstrates severe dilatation of the intrahepatic bile ducts

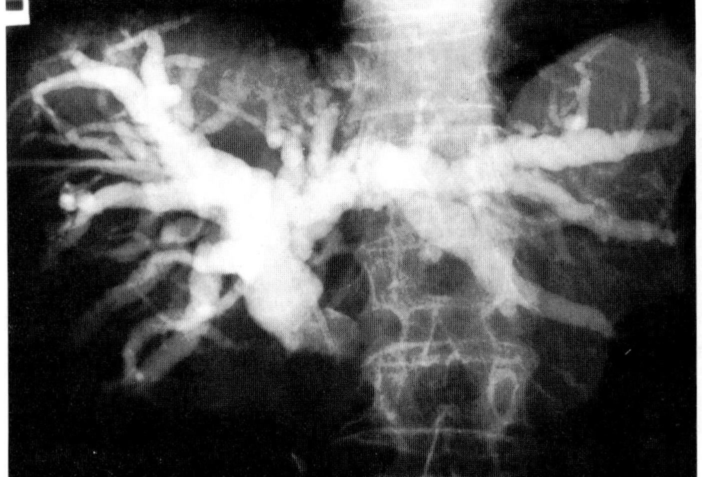

Fig. 4.78. *Case 1, percutaneous transhepatic cholangiogram.* There is marked dilatation of the intrahepatic and proximal extrahepatic bile duct. The gallbladder is not visualized

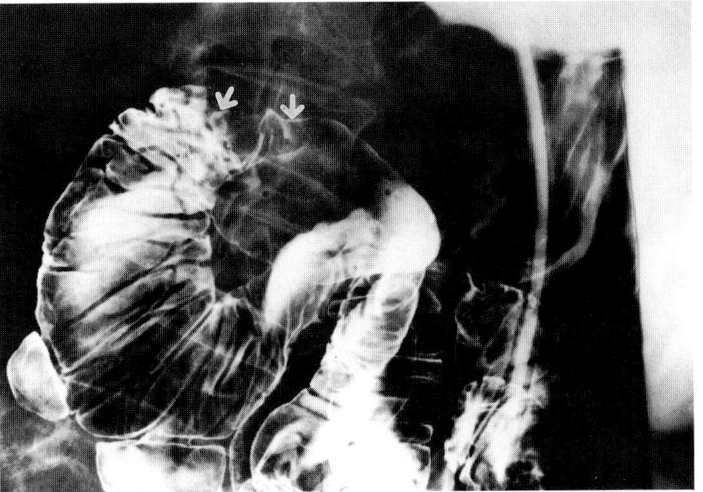

Fig. 4.79. *Case 1, hypotonic duodenography.* There are no significant abnormalities adjacent to the papilla of Vater, but there is poor distensibility of the gastric antrum and the duodenal bulb (*arrows*). This represents extrinsic compression

Choledochal Cyst

Choledochal cyst is a disease entity with congenital dilatation of the extrahepatic bile duct. Classically, the presenting signs and symptoms include a mass in the right upper quadrant, abdominal pain, and jaundice; but few cases have all three findings. This disease has a higher association than normal with cholelithiasis and cholangiocarcinoma.

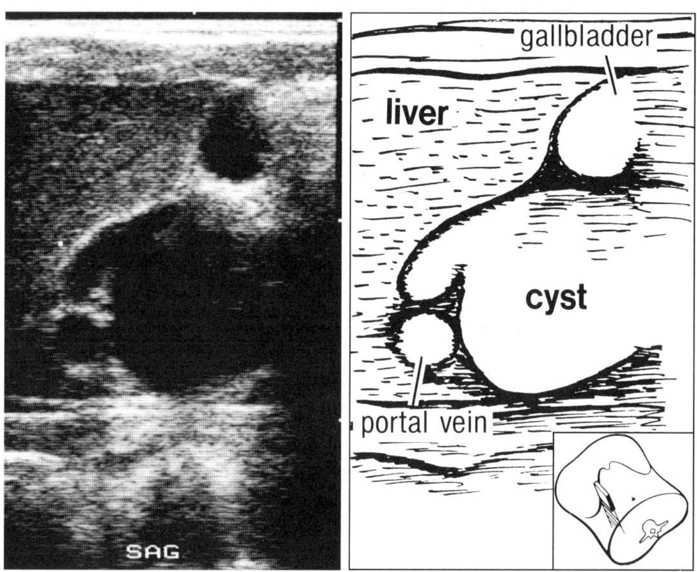

Fig. 4.80. *Case 1.* Proximally, the bile duct is approximately 1 cm in diameter with subsequent severe saccular dilatation of the lumen in its distal portion. The gallbladder is displaced anteriorly and is pushed against the abdominal wall

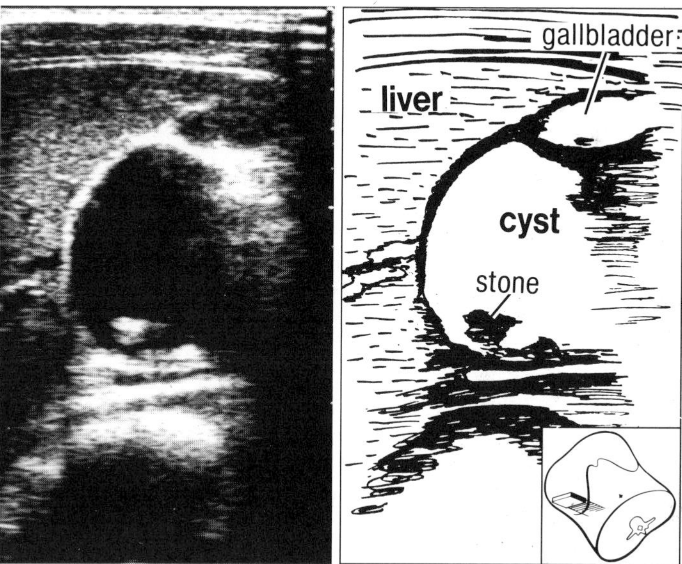

Fig. 4.81. *Case 1.* There is a 1-cm hyperechoic area in the posterior aspect of the dilated portion of the bile duct. This represents a stone which moved to the dependent aspect when the patient's position was changed

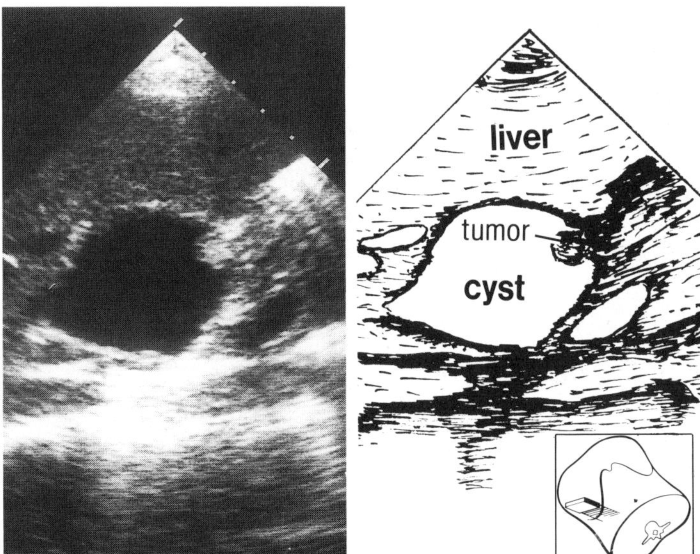

Fig. 4.82. *Case 1.* There is a 1-cm pedunculated polypoid structure arising from the wall of the portion of the bile duct which has a saccular dilatation. This was a surgically proven cancer

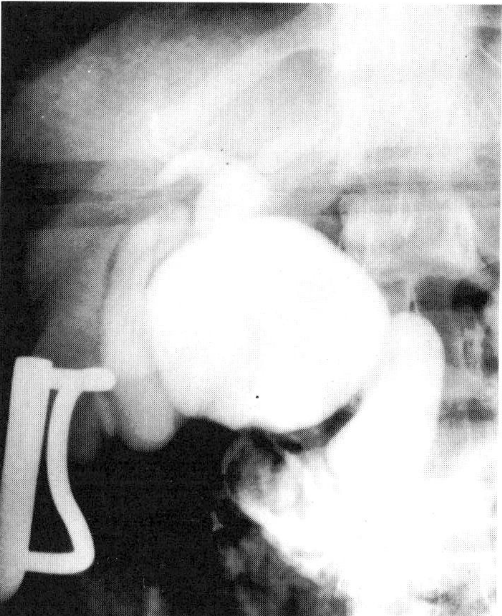

Fig. 4.83. *Case 1, intraoperative cholangiogram.* Saccular dilatation of the bile duct with gallbladder compression

5 Pancreas

Anatomy of the Pancreas

The pancreas lies obliquely in the upper abdomen with the main pancreatic duct in its center. From right to left the pancreas is divided into the head, body, and tail. Sometimes the portion between the head and body is called the pancreatic neck. The pancreatic head is folded inferiorly along the medial aspect of the second portion of the duodenum. The tip of the pancreatic head, which is curved and pointing to the left, is called the uncinate process. Anterior to the pancreatic head lie the gastric antrum and duodenal bulb, and posteriorly the inferior vena cava. The splenic vein runs transversely, posterior to the body of the pancreas. This vein joins the superior mesenteric vein behind the neck of the pancreas to form the portal vein. The junction of these two veins is called the splenoportal confluence. The pancreatic tail is located anterior to the left kidney, and its tip approaches the splenic hilum. Anterior to the pancreatic tail are the body of the stomach and the splenic flexure of the large intestine.

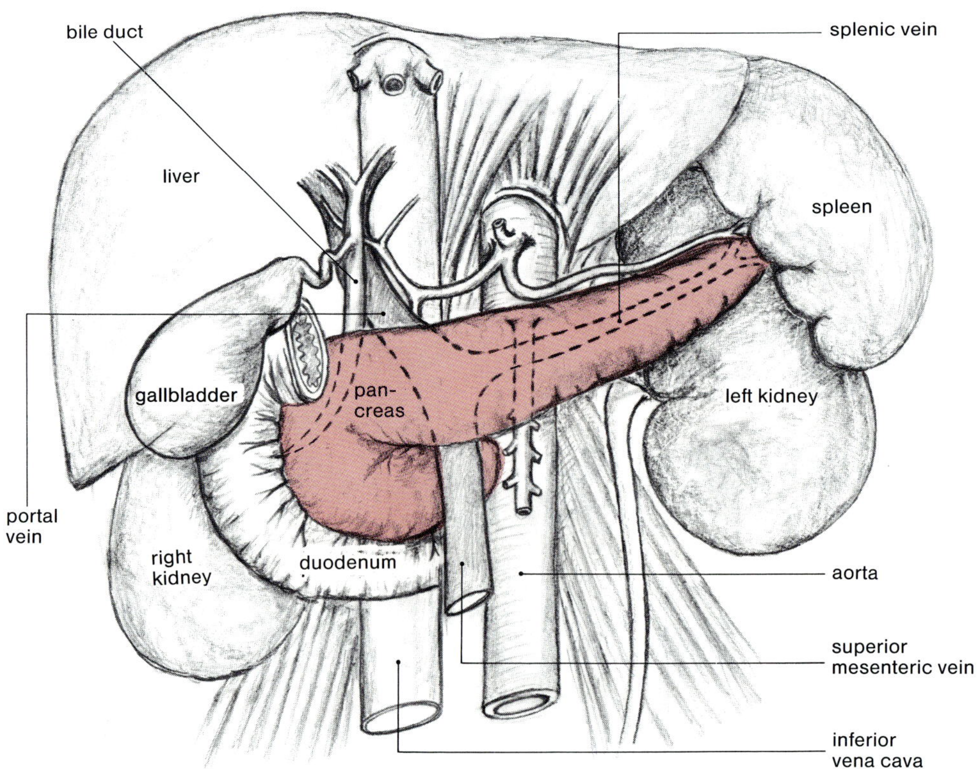

Fig. 5.1. Anatomy of the pancreas

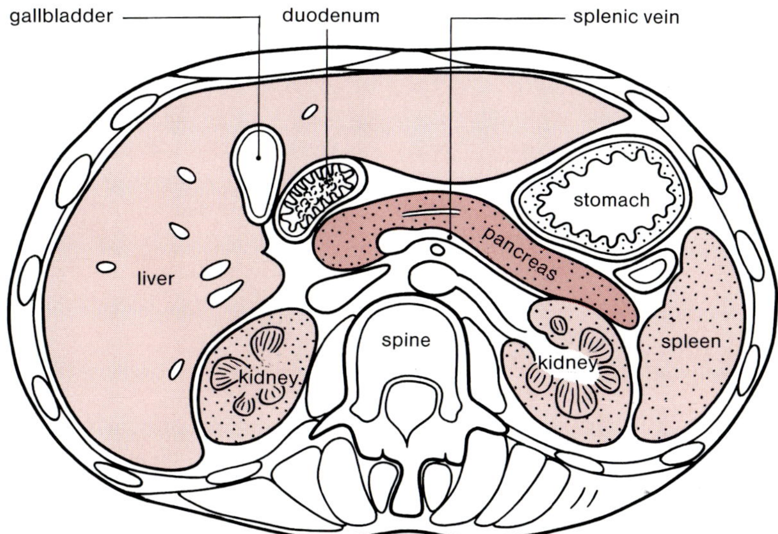

Fig. 5.2. *Transverse section of the pancreas and surrounding organs*. In order to visualize the entire pancreas from head to tail, it is necessary to obtain a slightly oblique angle on transverse scanning because the long axis of the pancreas has a slightly oblique position with the tail more cephalad than the head. On this diagram, the entire pancreas, from head to tail, is illustrated on one transverse section, but in practice one section can visualize only one segment of the pancreas. The stomach and the intestine cannot be well demarcated on ultrasonographic examination unless they are filled with fluid. Gas within the gastrointestinal tract often limits visualization of the pancreas

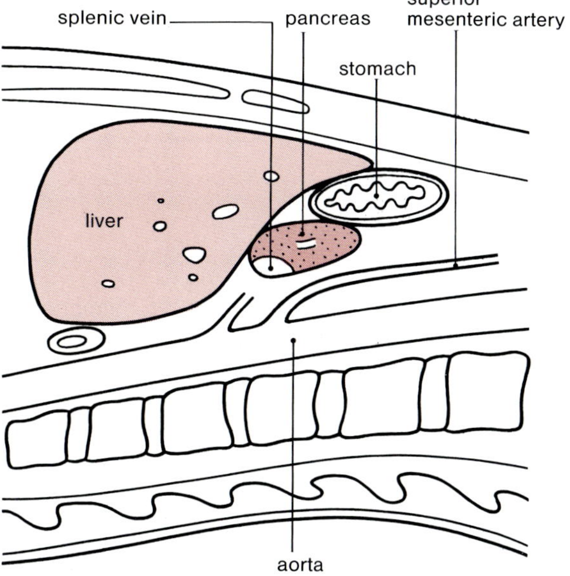

Fig. 5.3. *Longitudinal section of the pancreas and surrounding organs*. This is a longitudinal section of the abdomen through the pancreatic body along the abdominal aorta. The splenic vein often mildly indents the posterior surface of the pancreas. There is a wide variation in the relationship of positions of the pancreas, liver, and spleen. In a subject with an average body habitus, the body of the pancreas can easily be visualized in deep inspiration using the liver as an acoustic window. In a subject with a heavy body habitus, the pancreas may not be visualized at all since the left lobe of the liver is usually small and there is overlapping intestinal tract or thick fatty tissue of the omentum. In this situation, where the liver cannot be utilized as an acoustic window, the pancreas may be better visualized during expiration as there is less interposition of intestinal gas and fat

Ultrasonographic Appearance of a Normal Pancreas

The pancreatic contour is composed of smooth, curved lines. The body has the smallest diameter, measuring 6–17 mm in thickness. The pancreatic tail is slightly thicker than the body, and the pancreatic head is the thickest portion of the pancreas. The diameter of the pancreas changes with age. It is largest in the 3rd decade and becomes atrophic after the age of 50. The normal thickness of the pancreas varies greatly according to the measuring technique. For example, measurements of the body of the pancreas through the splenic vein on the transverse section are usually smaller than on sagittal sections of the same segment. In addition, the size and shape of the pancreas change with inspiration and expiration. The echogenicity of the pancreas is usually greater than or almost equal to that of the left lobe of the liver. In normal cases, the pancreas is never hypoechoic relative to the liver.

Transverse Scanning

The splenic vein can be visualized by careful movement of the transversely placed transducer head in the epigastrium. During slow deep respiration, a phase of respiration in which the splenic vein is most clearly visualized should be found. Generally, the splenic vein is better visualized during expiration. The pancreas is visualized anterior and adjacent to the splenic vein. As the pancreatic head curves caudally, the pancreatic head is usually visualized 2–4 cm caudal to the level of the pancreatic body. Because of gas within the gastric antrum and duodenal bulb, the pancreatic head may not be adequately visualized. The tail of the pancreas is difficult to visualize with the patient in a supine position because of gas within the gastric body and the splenic flexure of the large intestine. The pancreas has a slightly oblique axis, with its head caudal with respect to its tail. Slightly oblique transverse sections can visualize the pancreatic head and body well. In our experience, tilting the transducer head approximately 20° gives the best results.

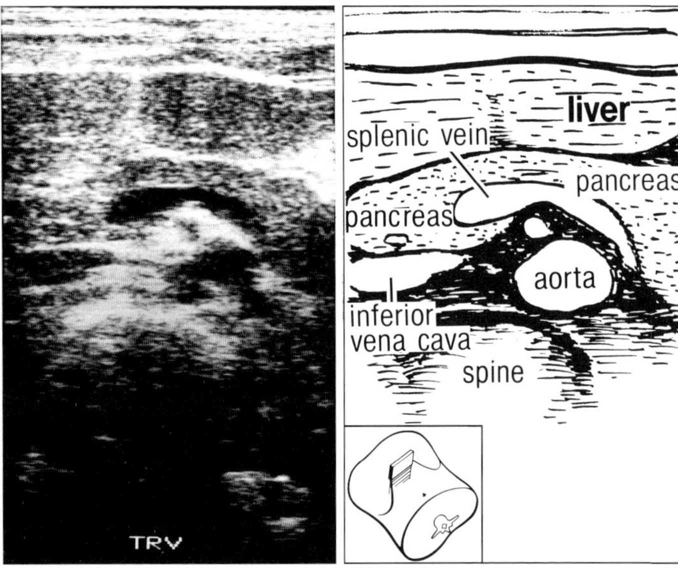

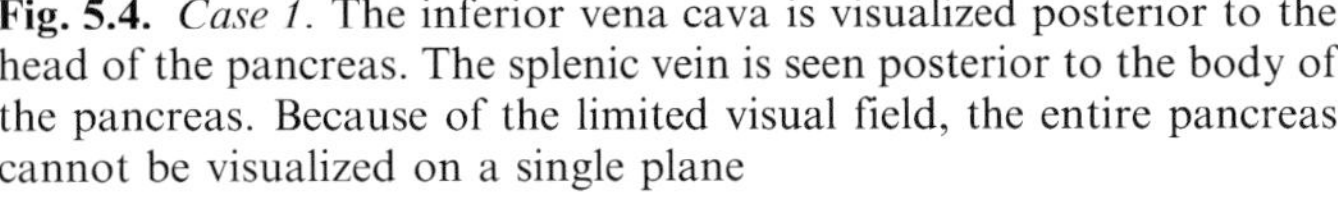

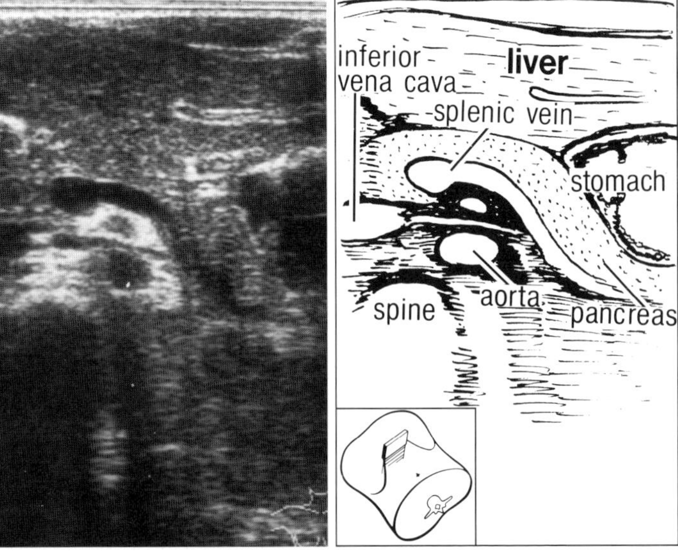

Fig. 5.4. *Case 1.* The inferior vena cava is visualized posterior to the head of the pancreas. The splenic vein is seen posterior to the body of the pancreas. Because of the limited visual field, the entire pancreas cannot be visualized on a single plane

Fig. 5.5. *Case 2.* This transverse section was obtained in an erect position following oral administration of 300 ml water. The tail of the pancreas is clearly visualized

Longitudinal Scanning

A longitudinal section in the midline of the upper abdomen demonstrates a cross-section of the body of the pancreas adjacent to the inferior surface of the liver. A cross-section of the splenic vein is also visualized on the posterior surface of the pancreas. Once the location of the pancreas is determined in the midline, a wider area of the pancreas should be observed by moving the transducer head to the right and left. The pancreatic head and tail may be difficult to evaluate because of gas within the stomach.

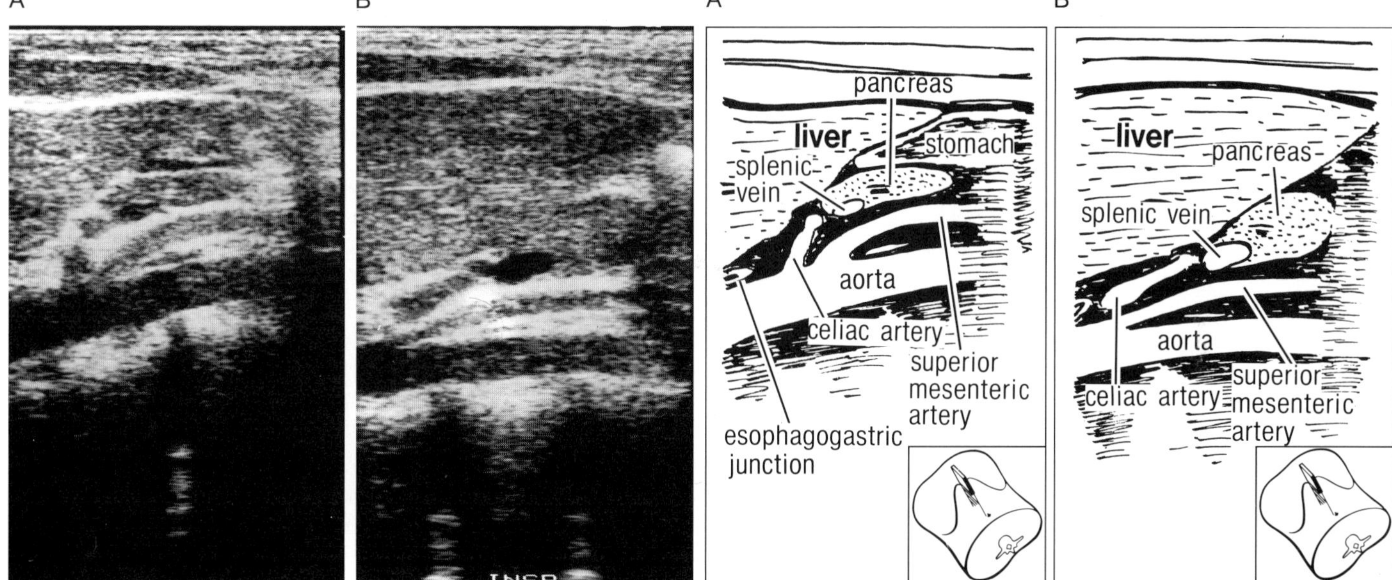

Fig. 5.6 A, B. *Case 1.* With the patient in a supine position, these images were obtained in expiration (**A**) and inspiration (**B**). The great differences in the shape and position of the pancreas according to the respiratory phase can be appreciated on these images. This example clearly illustrates the difficulty in accurately measuring the thickness of the body of the pancreas on transverse section through the splenic vein as only part of the pancreas is included. On inspiration (**B**), the location of the abdominal aorta and pancreas appears deep compared to expiration (**A**). This is because the abdomen is more distended on inspiration

Erect Position and Oral Administration of Water

The pancreas is often well visualized in the erect position. In the supine position, the area of the gastric angle overlaps the pancreatic body, whereas in the erect position the stomach descends and thereby minimizes overlapping of the pancreas. This effect is more prominent in a thin patient whose stomach has a greater excursion when assuming the erect position.

When there is persistent overlapping of the stomach with the pancreas, oral administration of 300–500 ml water may be helpful. By this method, gas within the stomach is replaced by water to create an acoustic window through which the pancreas can be visualized. Using this method, the pancreatic tail, which is located posterior to the body of the stomach, can also be visualized. Juice, tea, or other noncarbonated beverages can be used instead of water. Although air bubbles are seen within the fluid in the stomach immediately after drinking, the larger bubbles disappear within 4–5 min. The amount of water necessary for visualization of the pancreas varies in individual cases; the air-fluid level in the gastric body should be higher than the pancreatic tail. With the legs dangling over the side of the bed, the patient can comfortably assume the sitting position.

Normal Appearance
of the Pancreas
by Contact Compound Scanner

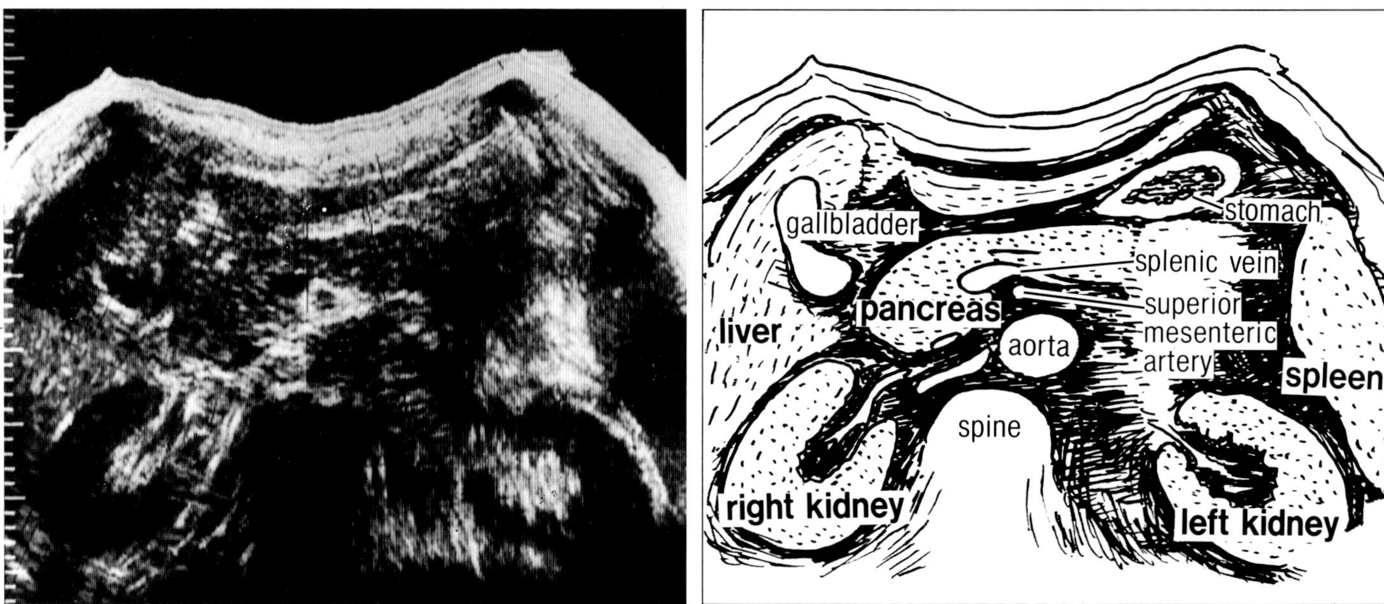

Fig. 5.7. *Transverse section.* On this image, the pancreatic head and body are visualized. The pancreatic tail is not well visualized because of gas within the stomach. This image was obtained by slightly tilting the transducer head along the long axis of the pancreas

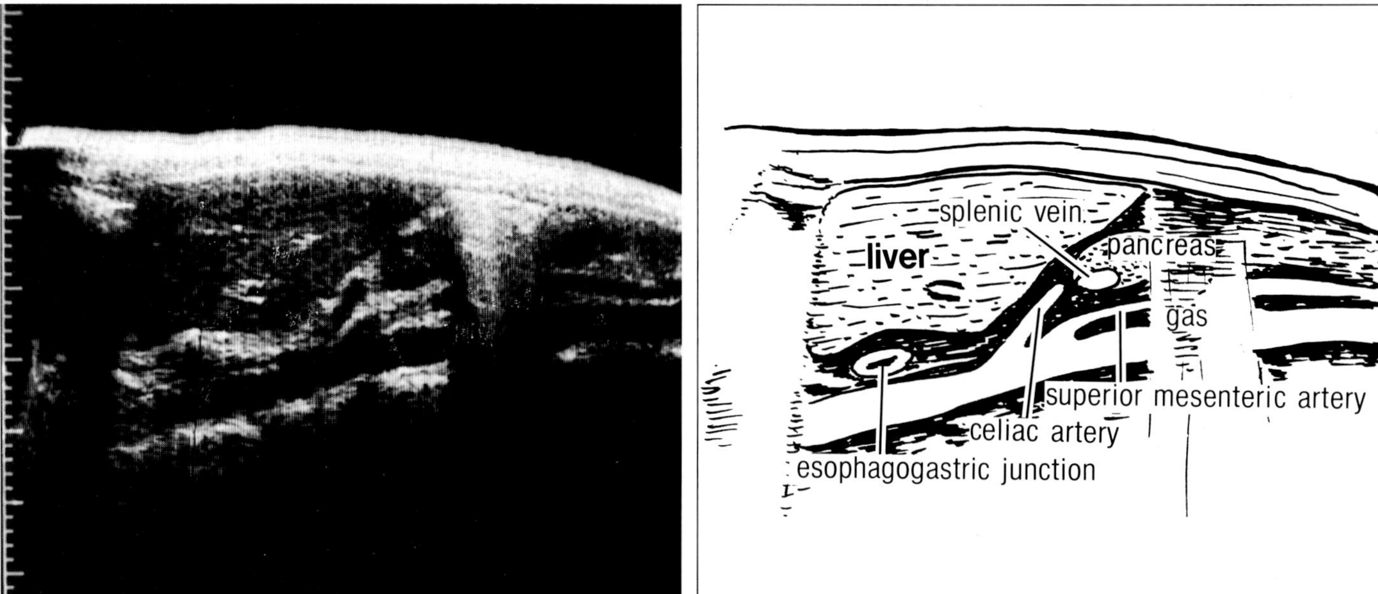

Fig. 5.8. *Longitudinal section.* The pancreatic body is well visualized posterior to the left lobe of the liver and anterior to the superior mesenteric artery

Liver Configuration Affecting Ultrasonographic Visualization of the Pancreas

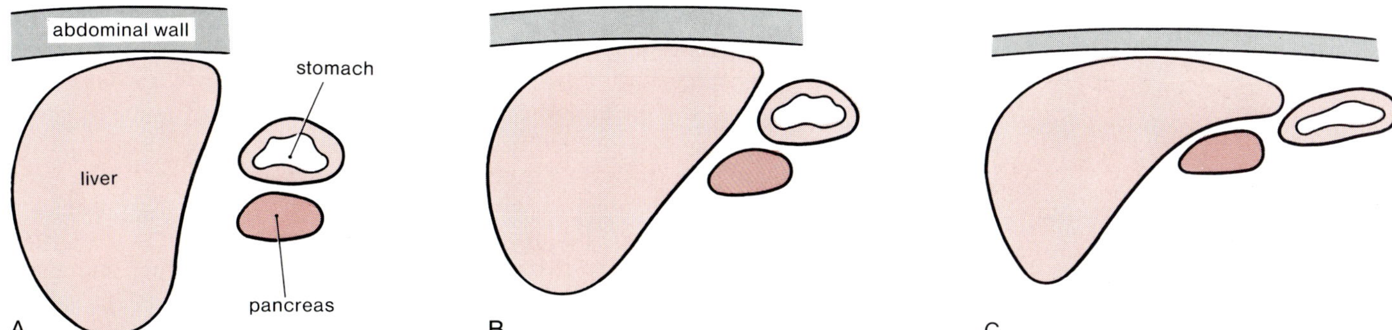

Fig. 5.9 A–C. Successful visualization of the pancreas by ultrasonography depends greatly on the patient's body habitus. **B** Visualization in an average patient. It is well known that in an obese patient, visualization of the pancreas is limited due to the positional relationship of the liver and pancreas. This figure illustrates longitudinal sections in the midline. In an obese patient, the left lobe of the liver usually resembles **A**. In this situation, there is gas-containing stomach and fat anterior to the pancreas which limit visualization of the pancreas. In addition, in the obese patient, the location of the pancreas is relatively deep in the abdomen, and the abdominal wall is thick, hence there is poor penetration of the ultrasound beam. In contrast, in a thin patient, the left lobe of the liver extends caudally directly covering the pancreas as in **C**. In this situation, only the liver, which transmits the ultrasound beam well, lies between the abdominal wall and the pancreas. A relatively superficial location of the pancreas and a thin abdominal wall also aid visualization of the pancreas

Normal Thickness Range of the Pancreatic Body

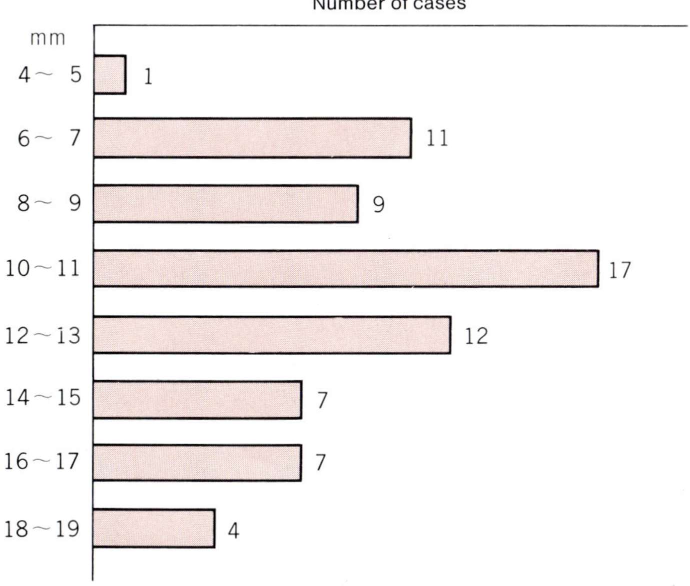

Fig. 5.10. Normal thickness range of the pancreatic body is measured on the transverse section of the body of the pancreas through the splenic vein. As mentioned before, the transverse scan may not necessarily provide an accurate thickness measurement of the pancreas, but this is the imaging plane which is most often used in ultrasonography. The thickness of the pancreatic body is most commonly 6–17 mm. When the thickness of the pancreatic body is over 20 mm on the transverse section through the splenic vein, the pancreas is considered to be enlarged

Pancreatic Cancer

Pancreatic cancer is visualized as a solid hypoechoic mass when compared to normal pancreas. In cases of pancreatic cancer, strong inflammatory changes often exist around the tumor. On ultrasonographic examination, the tumor and the surrounding inflammatory areas can be visualized as a single solid mass. Generally, the internal echo texture of pancreatic cancers is heterogeneous, but this finding is not always very prominent, and homogeneously visualized cancers are occasionally encountered. The contour of pancreatic cancer is typically irregular; but this finding can also be seen with inflammatory masses of chronic pancreatitis, and exact differentiation is not possible. Pancreatic cancer most frequently arises in the head of the pancreas. With pancreatic head cancer, dilatation of the intra- and extrahepatic biliary ducts and enlargement of the gallbladder can be clearly visualized in addition to the solid mass. Because of the obstruction of the main pancreatic duct in the pancreatic head by the tumor, dilatation of the main pancreatic duct can be seen in the pancreatic body. These findings are indirect signs of pancreatic cancer, but are not specific to cancer and can be visualized in any condition in which there is obstruction of the common bile duct and main pancreatic duct in the region of the pancreatic head.

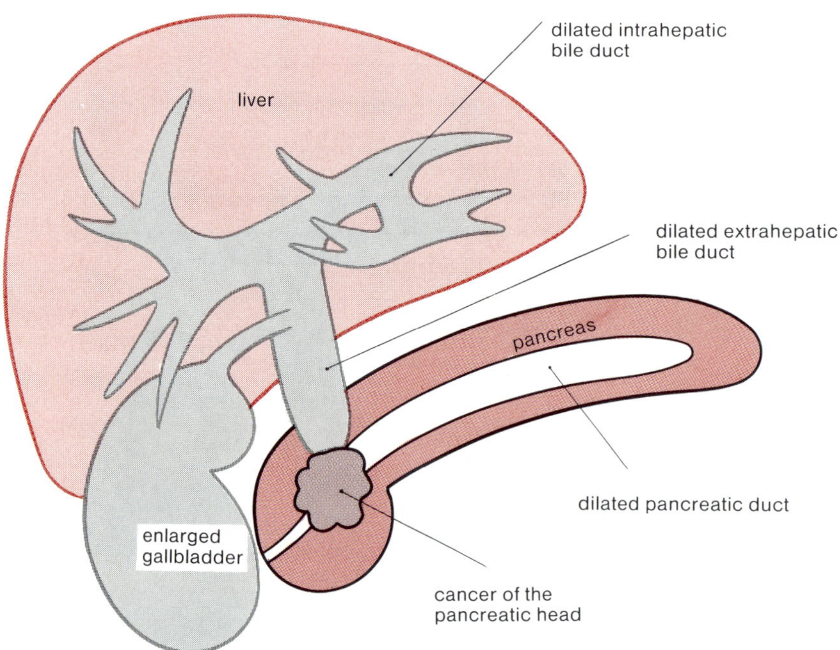

Fig. 5.11. Pancreatic cancer

Cancer of the Head
of the Pancreas

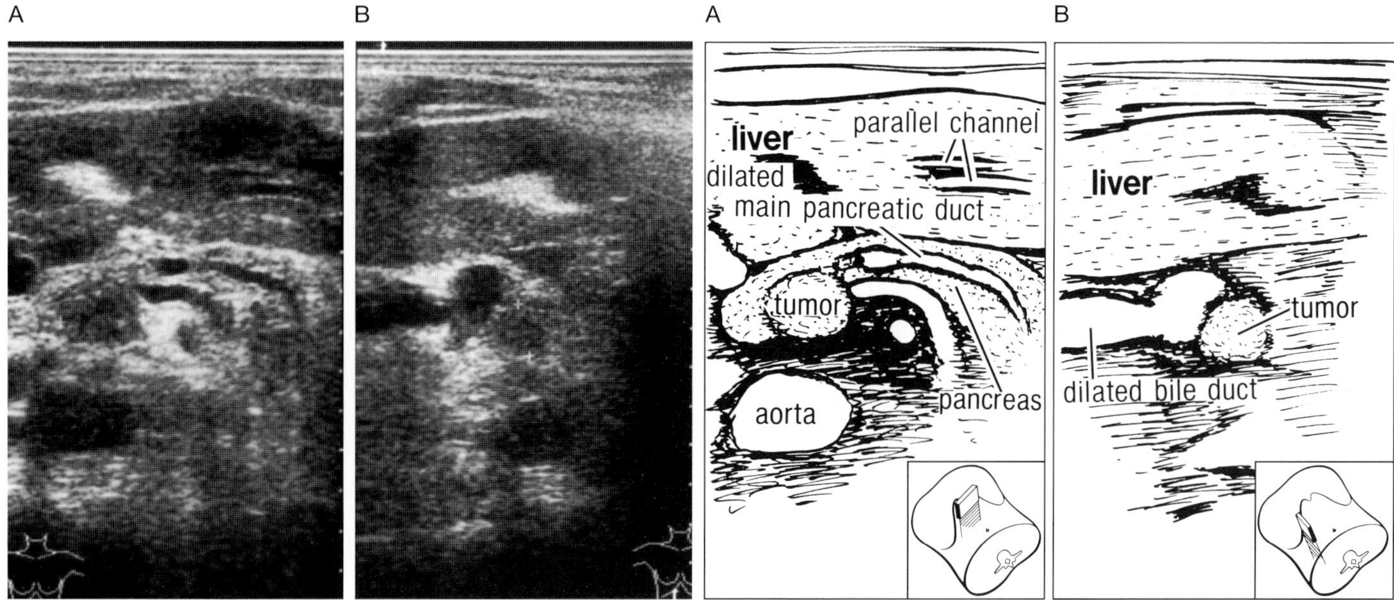

Fig. 5.12 A, B. *Case 1*. The transverse section across the long axis of the pancreas (**A**) shows a 20 × 17-mm solid tumor in the region of the pancreatic head. There is mild dilatation of the main pancreatic duct in the pancreatic body. The longitudinal section through the pancre- atic head (**B**) shows dilatation of the extrahepatic biliary duct to 13 mm. There is a 15-mm hypoechoic mass at the site of the abrupt occlusion of the extrahepatic bile duct, representing a tumor of the pancreatic head

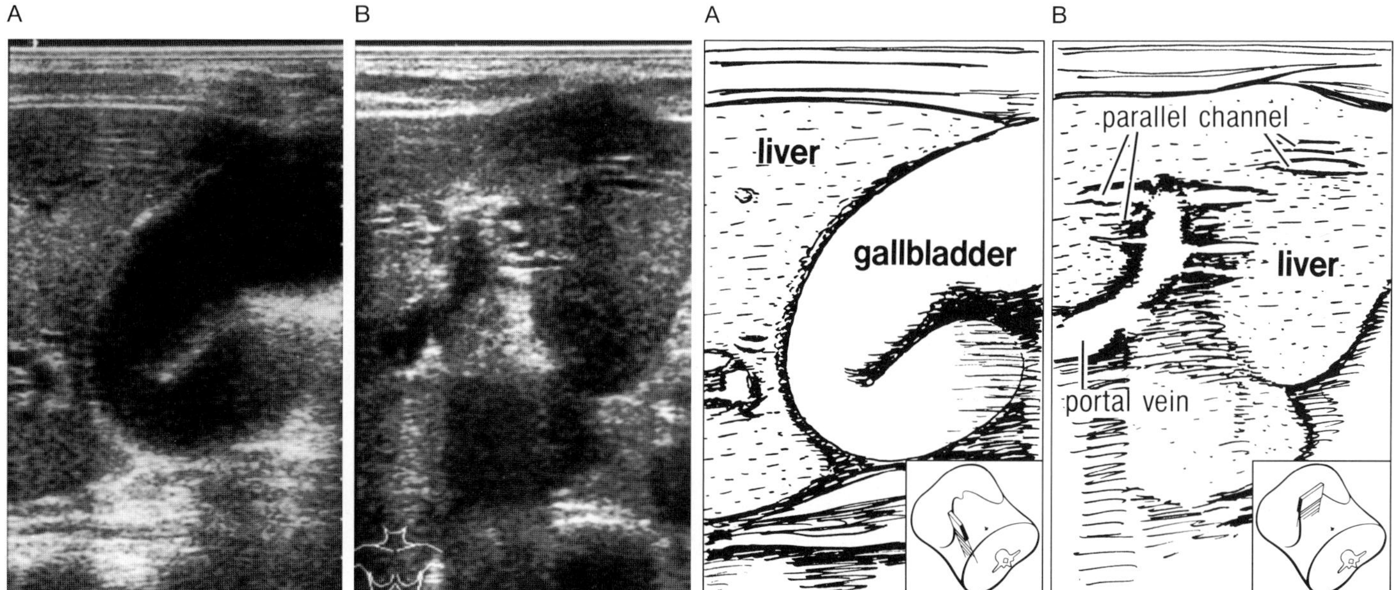

Fig. 5.13 A, B. *Case 1*. The longitudinal section of the gallbladder (**A**) and transverse section of the left lobe of the liver (**B**) show enlargement of the gallbladder and mild dilatation of the intrahepatic bile ducts (parallel channel sign). Both of these findings are seen with obstructive jaundice

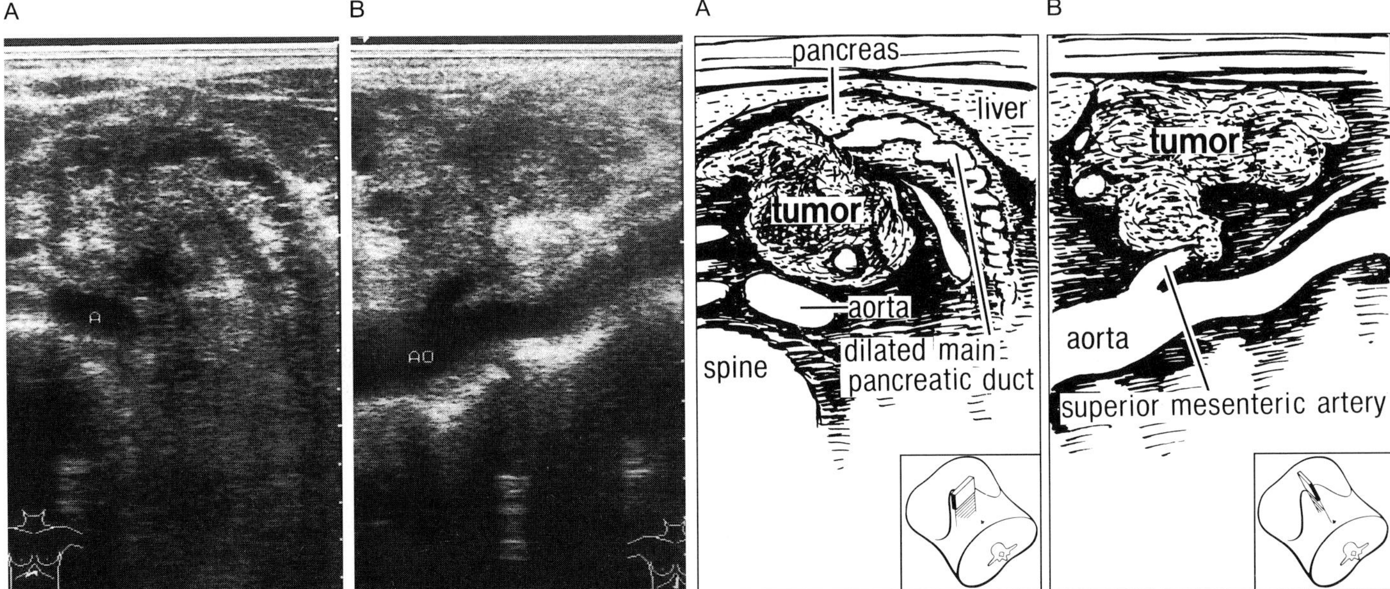

Fig. 5.14 A, B. *Case 2.* The transverse section across the long axis of the pancreas (**A**) demonstrates a 5-cm solid mass in the region of the pancreatic head. The internal echo texture is inhomogeneous with mixed strong and weak echoes. The main pancreatic duct is dilated with a beaded appearance. On the longitudinal section of the abdominal aorta (**B**), tumor in the region of the pancreatic head is visualized directly anterior to the abdominal aorta because the entire pancreas is deviated to the left. The tumor has a markedly irregular surface. The origin of the superior mesenteric artery is encased in tumor. In this case, there was dilatation of the intra- and extrahepatic bile ducts, and there was enlargement of the gallbladder with bile sludge. There were multiple hypoechoic masses in the liver measuring approximately 2 cm in size, suggesting metastatic disease

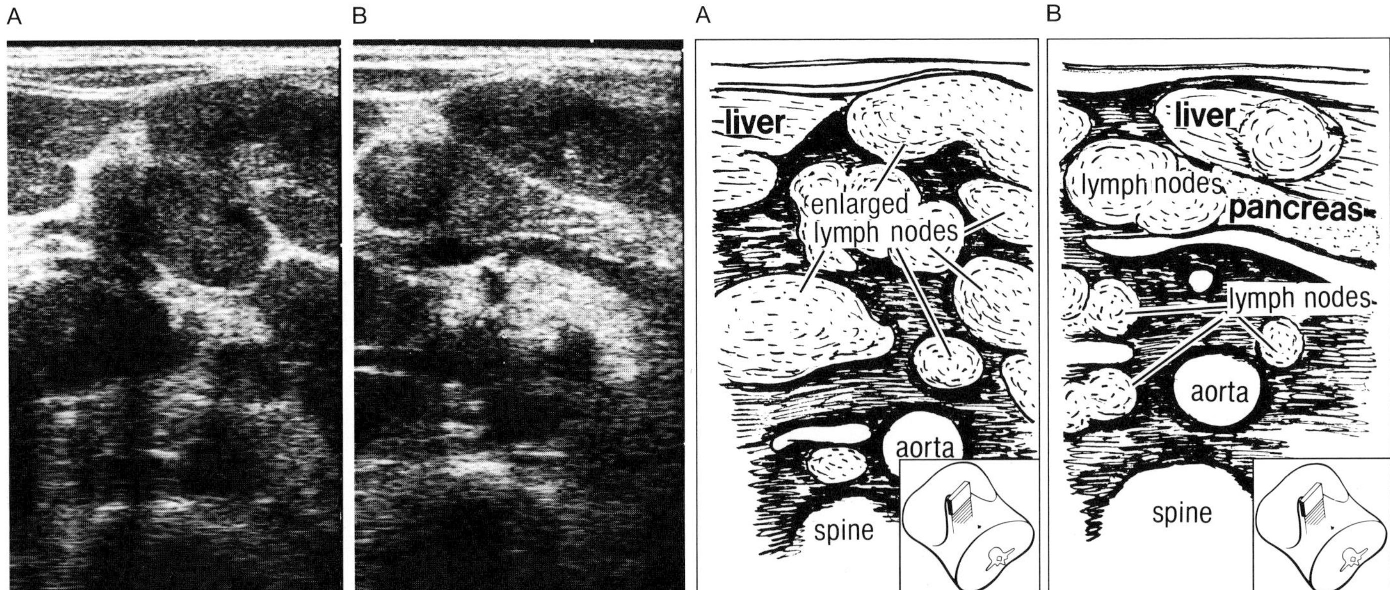

Fig. 5.15 A, B. *Case for comparison.* The transverse section across the long axis of the pancreas demonstrates a 24 × 35-mm well-defined solid mass in the region of the pancreatic head. The internal echo texture is relatively homogeneous. This simulates a mass in the region of the pancreatic head, but actually represents an enlarged peripancreatic lymph node in a patient with hepatocellular carcinoma

Cancer of the Uncinate Process
of the Pancreas

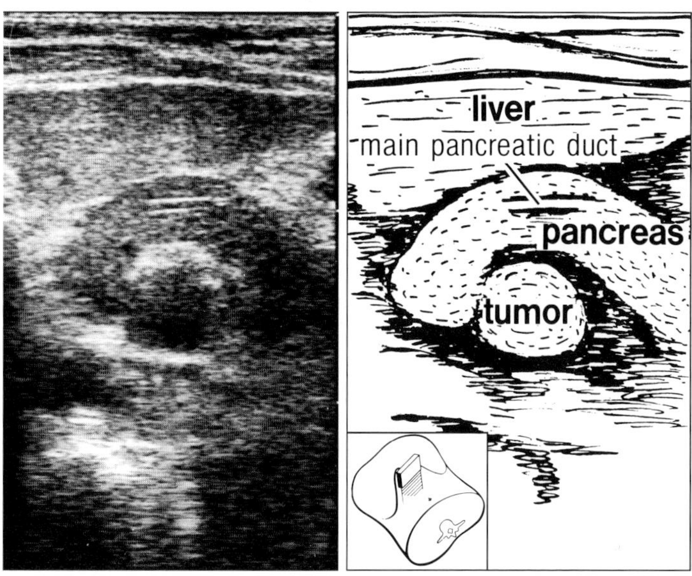

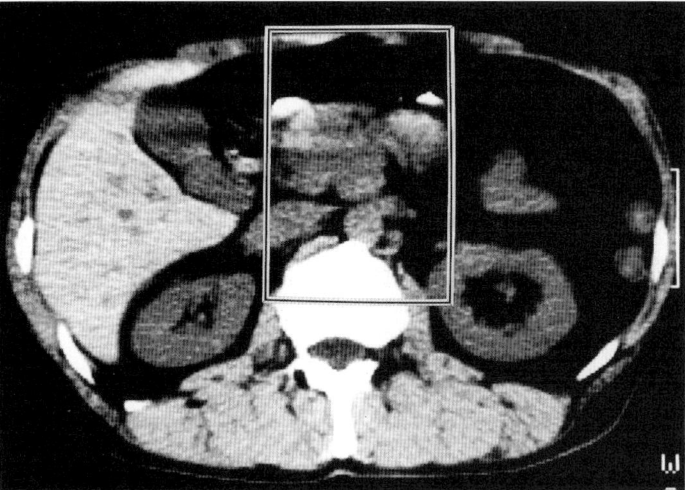

Fig. 5.16. *Case 1.* There is a 25 × 33-mm solid mass in the region of the uncinate process of the pancreas. The size of the main pancreatic duct is within normal limits. There is no dilatation of the biliary system

Fig. 5.17. *Case 1, CT scan.* There is a solid mass in the uncinate process. The pancreas is otherwise normal. The *outlined area* grossly corresponds to the ultrasonographic field shown in Fig. 5.16

Cancer
Involving the Entire Pancreas

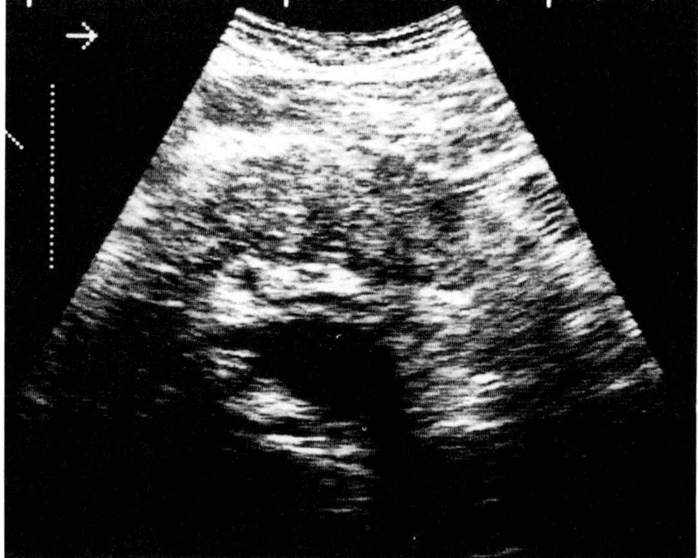

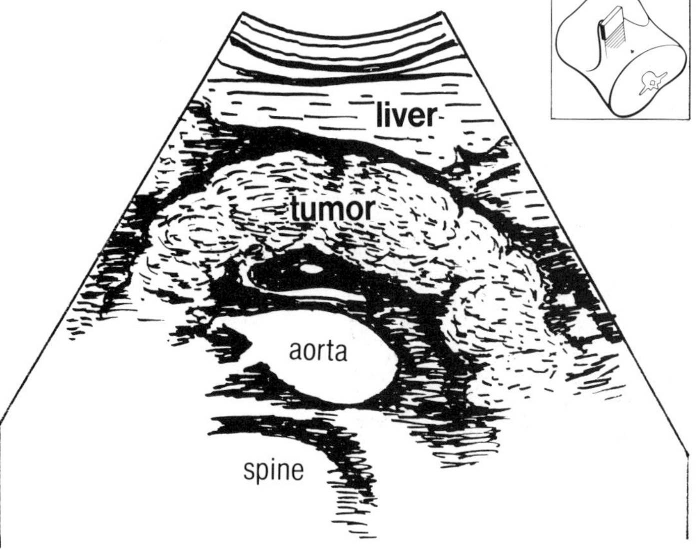

Fig. 5.18. *Case 1.* There is diffuse enlargement of the pancreas from the head to the tail together with an irregular contour and inhomogeneous internal texture. The splenic vein was not identified and was thought to be infiltrated by cancer

Cancer of the Pancreatic Tail

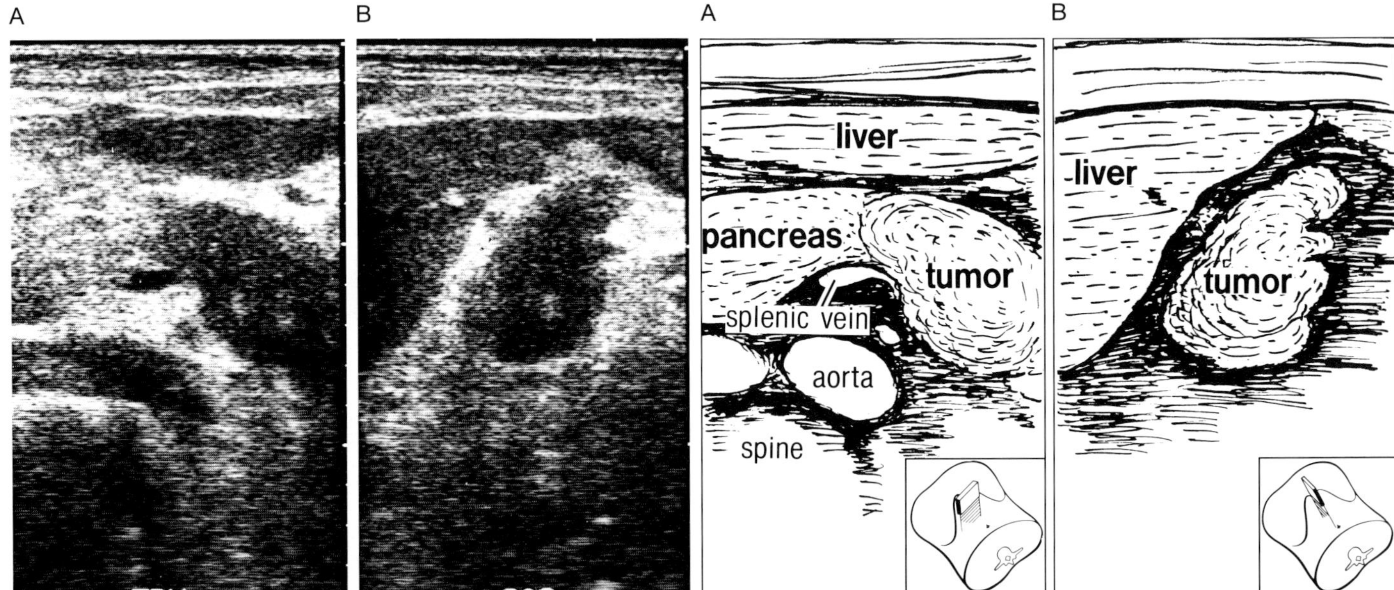

Fig. 5.19 A, B. *Case 1.* The transverse section of the pancreas (**A**) shows that there is diffuse enlargement of the pancreas from the body to the tail with decreased internal echoes. The main pancreatic duct is not dilated. The splenic vein was not visualized in the region of the pancreas. The longitudinal section through the pancreatic tail (**B**) documents a hypoechoic solid mass inferior to the left lobe of the liver. There were multiple solid masses, ranging in size from 2 to 3 cm, in both lobes of the liver, suggesting metastases

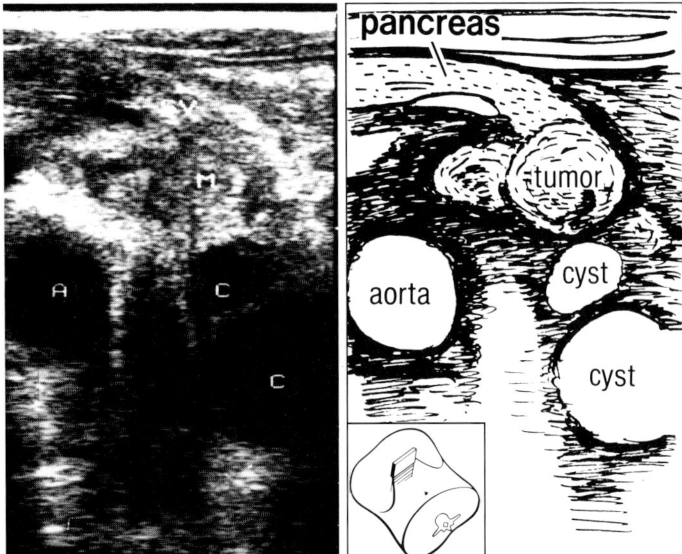

Fig. 5.20. *Case 2.* The tail of the pancreas is irregularly enlarged with an inhomogeneous internal echo pattern. There are at least two cystic masses, 3 cm in size, at the tip of the pancreatic tail. The splenic vein was not identified and was thought to be occluded by tumor. There were tortuous vascular structures behind the stomach, representing collateral circulation secondary to splenic vein obstruction

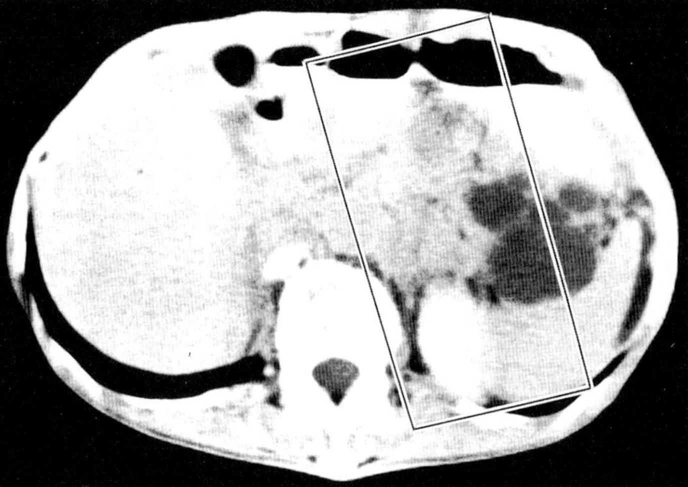

Fig. 5.21. *Case 2, CT scan.* The solid mass in the region of the pancreatic tail is not clearly visualized, but cystic masses at the tip of the tail are clear. The cystic masses are thought to represent secondary pseudocysts caused by the obstruction of the main pancreatic duct. The *outlined area* grossly corresponds to the ultrasonographic field in Fig. 5.20

Pancreatic Cystadenoma

Pancreatic cystadenoma is a benign tumor of the pancreas. It is divided into two large groups. One is mucinous cystadenoma with relatively large cystic structures containing septations. The other is serous cystadenoma with a fine network pattern within the cystic spaces, which simulates a solid tumor on ultrasonographic examination because of the presence of internal echoes. Malignant degeneration of a mucinous cystadenoma results in a cystadenocarcinoma.

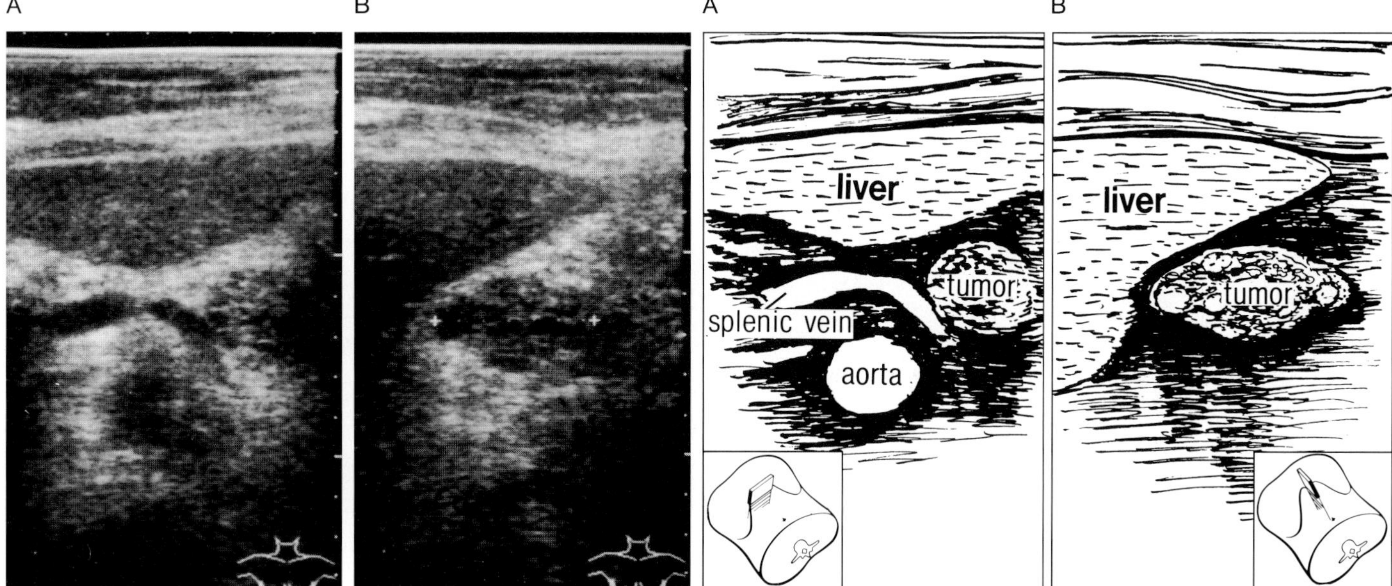

Fig. 5.22 A, B. *Case 1.* The transverse section across the long axis of the pancreas (**A**) demonstrates a 35-mm solid mass with an inhomogeneous internal echo texture at the junction of the pancreatic body and tail. The main pancreatic duct is not dilated. The surface of the tumor is relatively smooth. The longitudinal section through the tumor (**B**) shows similar findings. When compared with the typical appearance of the pancreas, the surface of the mass is relatively smooth. This is a case of serous cystadenoma with a network pattern within the cystic spaces simulating a solid tumor

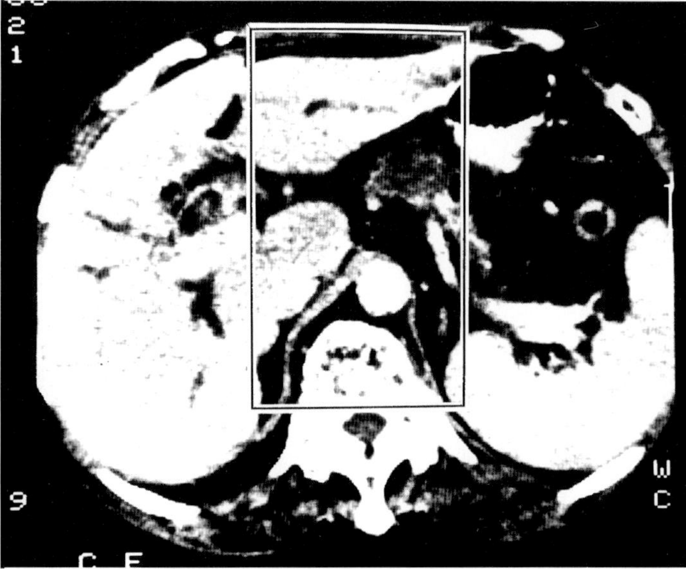

Fig. 5.23. *Case 1, CT scan through a section of the pancreatic tumor.* The cystadenoma is visualized as a low-density mass. The *outlined area* grossly correlates with the ultrasonographic images in Fig. 5.22

Acute Pancreatitis

Although ultrasonographic examination is sensitive in cases of pancreatic tumors, it is not as good in inflammatory diseases of the pancreas. However, as pancreatitis advances, the pancreas changes in configuration and internal texture, presenting characteristic ultrasonographic findings. No definite abnormality is detected in cases of relatively mild acute pancreatitis. In severe cases of acute pancreatitis, however, the pancreas appears enlarged, and the internal echogenicity is decreased relative to the liver parenchyma. Formation of pseudocysts may be visualized during the course of acute pancreatitis. Rarely, dilatation of the main pancreatic duct is visualized. Inflammatory changes of the surrounding tissues may also be visualized. Note that enlargement of the pancreas in cases of acute pancreatitis persists for a certain length of time after the serum amylase returns to normal.

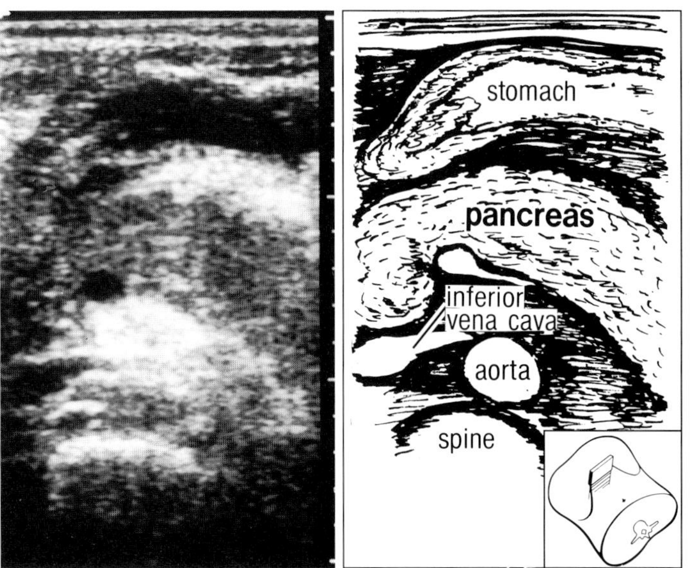

Fig. 5.24. *Case 1.* The pancreas is diffusely enlarged, and the contour is slightly indistinct

Fig. 5.25. *Case 1, CT scan.* Diffuse enlargement of the pancreas

Can Acute Pancreatitis Be Diagnosed on Ultrasonography?

The clinical diagnosis of acute pancreatitis will usually be evident on the basis of the patient's symptoms and the serum and urine amylase, but the ultrasonographic examination does not always show characteristic findings. Diffuse enlargement of the pancreas and a decreased internal echogenicity are seen only in advanced cases of acute pancreatitis. It must be said that typical (mild) acute pancreatitis cannot be detected by ultrasonographic examination, and therefore a normal ultrasonographic examination of the pancreas cannot exclude this entity.

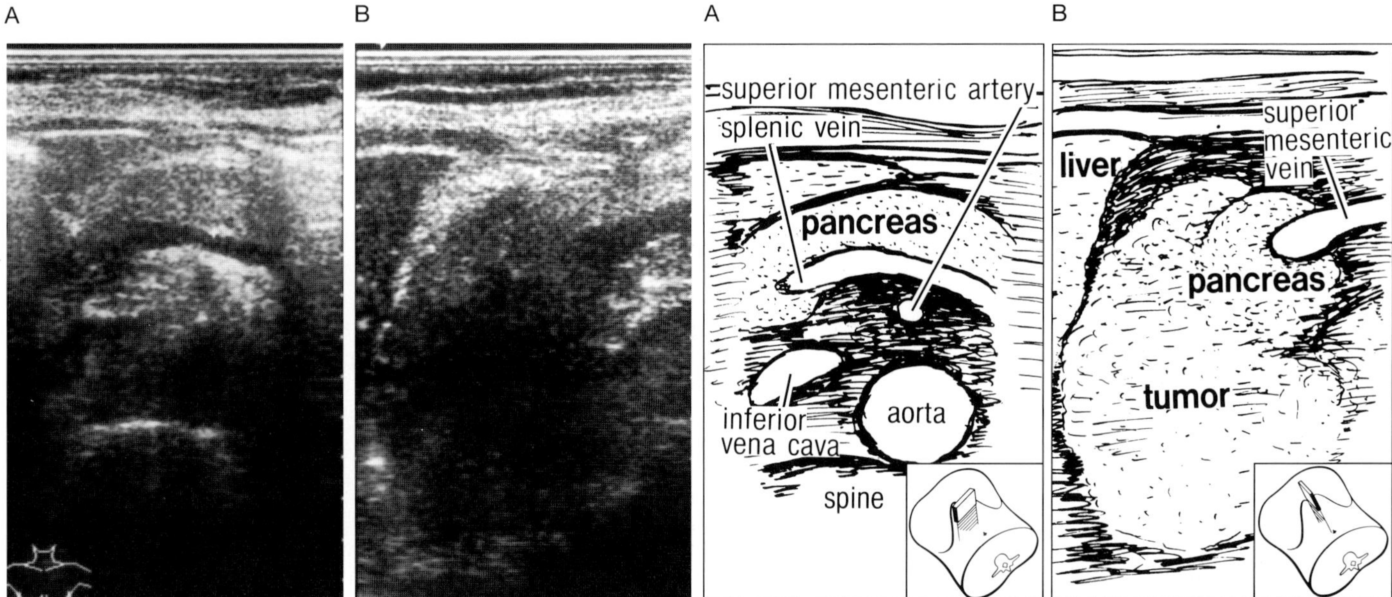

Fig. 5.26 A, B. *Case 2.* Acute pancreatitis. The transverse section (**A**) shows a pancreas with an anteroposterior dimension of 17 mm, which is at the upper limits of normal. However, this patient had had an ultrasonographic examination 3 years earlier, and at that time the pancreas had been 8 mm in diameter. In addition, after clinical resolu-tion of the pancreatitis, the thickness of the pancreas was only 10 mm (shown in Fig. 5.27). The longitudinal section of the pancreas (**B**) shows a large solid mass adjacent to the superoposterior aspect of the pancreas; this is an inflammatory mass secondary to a pancreatic fluid leak. This patient also had a left pleural effusion

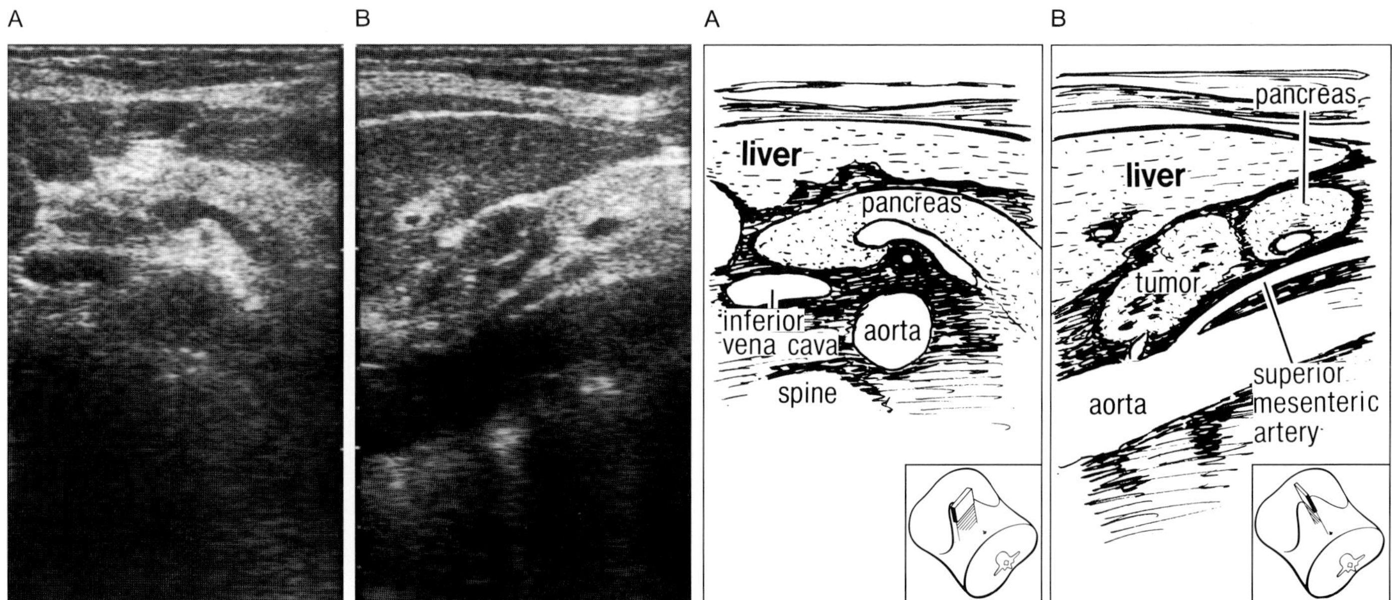

Fig. 5.27 A, B. *Case 2.* Ultrasonographic examination performed 55 days after the initial examination shows that the pancreas has returned to normal size. The longitudinal section (**B**) shows that the previously seen inflammatory mass has significantly decreased in size

Chronic Pancreatitis

In chronic pancreatitis, the pancreas shows either atrophy or localized enlargement (tumor-forming pancreatitis). In cases with localized enlargement, differentiation from pancreatic cancer is difficult. Dilatation of the main pancreatic duct is often seen. In chronic pancreatitis, the pancreatic duct may be easily visualized because it is usually more than 3 mm in caliber, whereas a normal main pancreatic duct is less than 2 mm. Radiologic examination of the abdomen may demonstrate calcifications in the pancreas in a patient with chronic pancreatitis. The ultrasonographic examination may visualize some of these calcifications, although the sensitivity for calcifications in a solid organ is not as high as in the case of gallstones due to smaller differences in acoustic impedance between the calcifications and the surrounding tissues. As seen with acute pancreatitis, pseudocyst formation may be visualized during the course of chronic pancreatitis. However, it is not unusual for the pancreas to appear normal on ultrasonography in a patient with a clinical diagnosis of chronic pancreatitis.

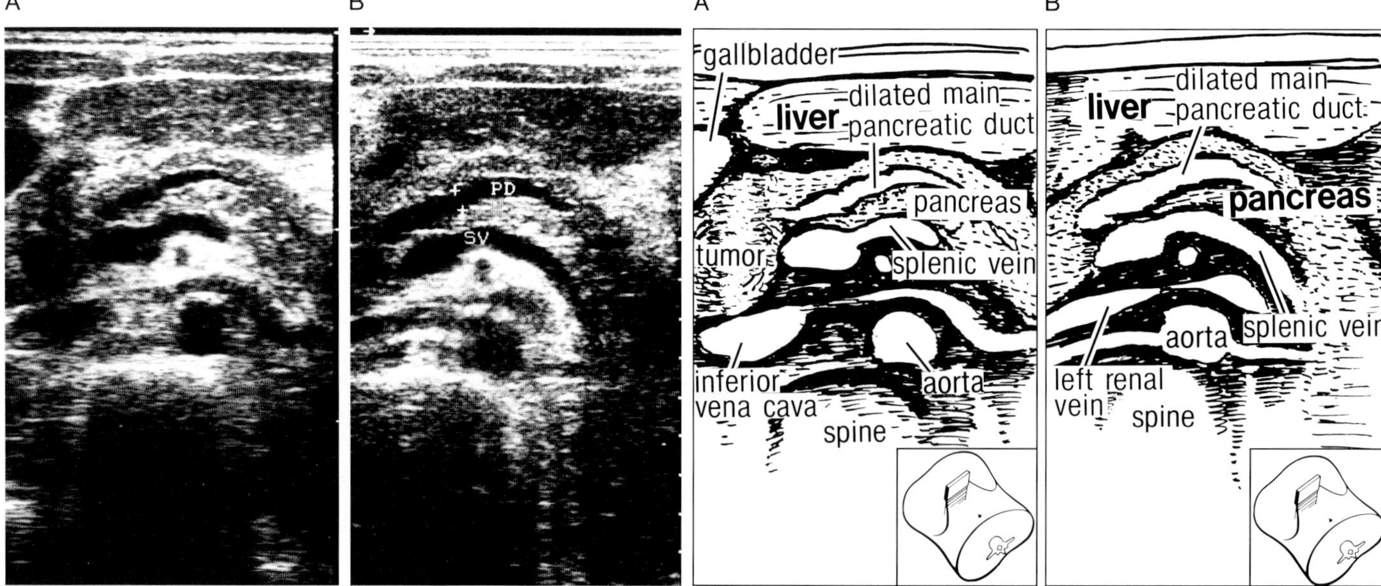

Fig. 5.28 A, B. *Case 1.* This patient had had severe upper abdominal pain 2 months prior to this examination and had been diagnosed as having acute pancreatitis because of increased levels of serum and urine amylase. The transverse section of the pancreas (**A**) shows dilatation of the main pancreatic duct, measuring 4 mm in its maximal dimension. Visualization of the pancreatic head is somewhat limited because of intestinal gas, but there appears to be mild enlargement.

Image **B** was obtained several months after the initial examination. The findings are similar, but on the second examination the maximal diameter of the main pancreatic duct is 5 mm, and there was an 8-mm cystic lesion in the area of the pancreatic head (not shown), suggesting a pseudocyst. This patient has occasional severe upper abdominal pain and clinically carries a diagnosis of chronic recurrent pancreatitis

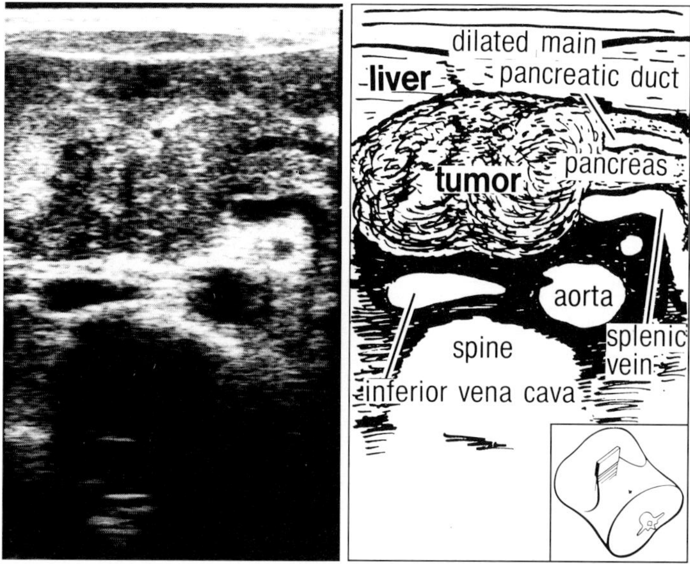

Fig. 5.29. *Case 2*. This patient had had upper abdominal pain after meals for 5 years and was clinically diagnosed as having pancreatitis. Recently, a high serum amylase had been detected on screening blood, and an ultrasonographic examination was performed. This showed a mass in the pancreatic head. Following treatment, this mass decreased in size. This is an example of an inflammatory mass of chronic pancreatitis

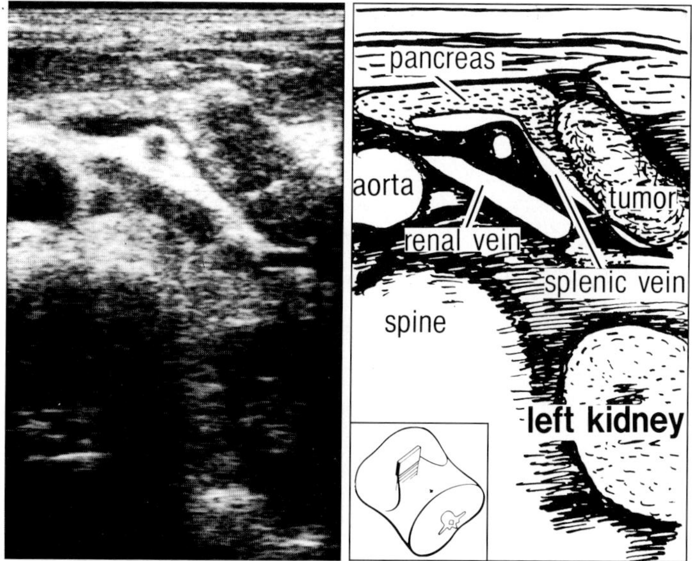

Fig. 5.30. *Case 3*. Chronic pancreatitis. There is a hypoechoic mass-like lesion in the pancreatic body and tail. Just as in Fig. 5.29 differentiation from pancreatic cancer was difficult

Pancreatolithiasis

Although pancreatic calcification is one of the findings seen in chronic pancreatitis and logically should be discussed in the section on chronic pancreatitis, it will be discussed independently here. Pancreatic calcifications are visualized in the upper quadrants on a radiograph of the abdomen. CT also clearly demonstrates pancreatic calcifications. In contrast, ultrasonography is not very sensitive for this condition. This problem is similar to the problem of identifying gallstones within a contracted gallbladder or stones within the intrahepatic bile ducts which are more difficult to visualize when compared to gallstones within the fluid-filled gallbladder.

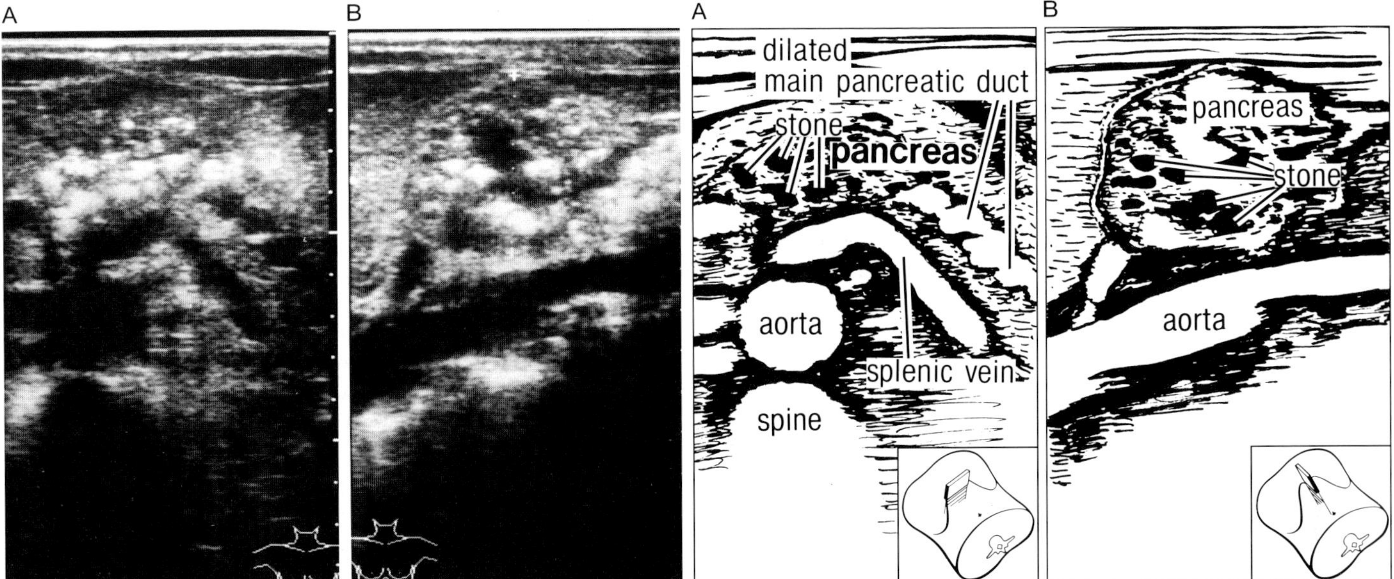

Fig. 5.31 A, B. *Case 1.* There are multiple coarse strong echoes throughout the pancreas. This is a typical example of pancreatic calcifications, but is only rarely seen. There is also dilatation of the main pancreatic duct

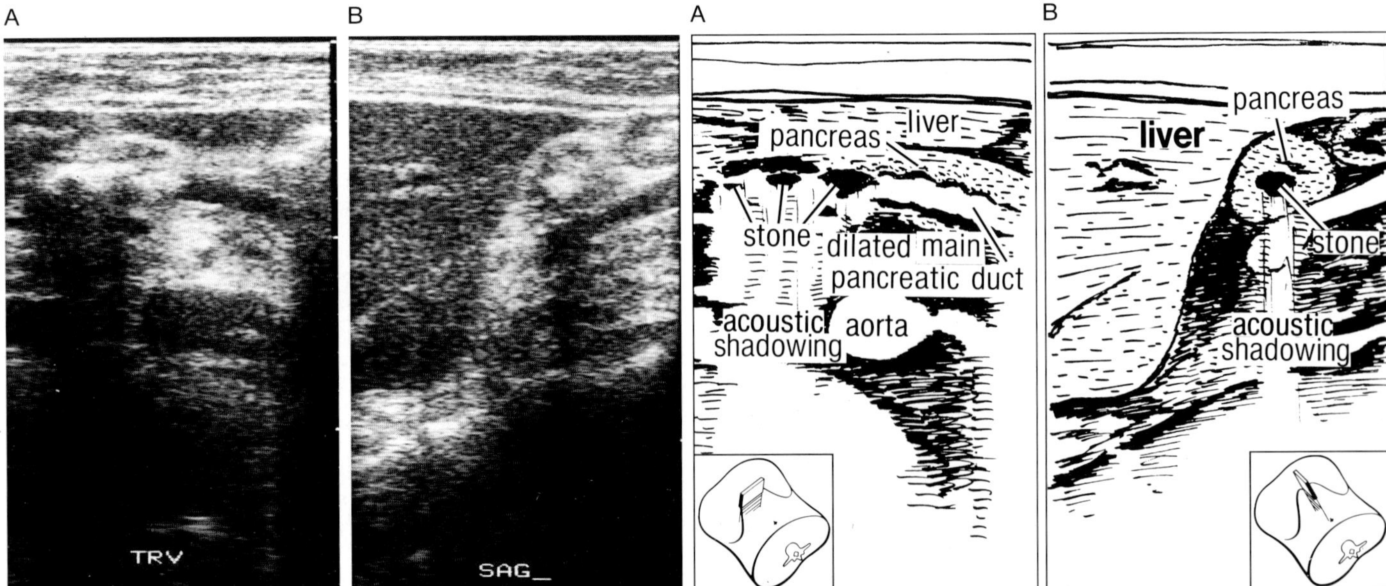

Fig. 5.32 A, B. *Case 2.* There is dilatation of the main pancreatic duct in the region of the pancreatic body. There are at least four hyperechoic areas within the pancreatic duct near the head of the pancreas.

This is an example of pancreatolithiasis within the main pancreatic duct. Calculi within the pancreatic ducts are more easily diagnosed than calcifications within the substance of the pancreas

Pancreatic Pseudocyst

Most pancreatic cysts are pseudocysts which lack an epithelial lining. Pancreatic pseudocyst can be secondary to acute pancreatitis, chronic pancreatitis, abdominal trauma, or stenosis or obstruction of the main pancreatic duct secondary to cancer or inflammation around the duodenal papilla. When a pseudocyst is small, it is visualized as a cystic mass within the pancreas, but as it becomes larger, it becomes difficult to determine which organ the giant cyst is arising from on ultrasonographic examination.

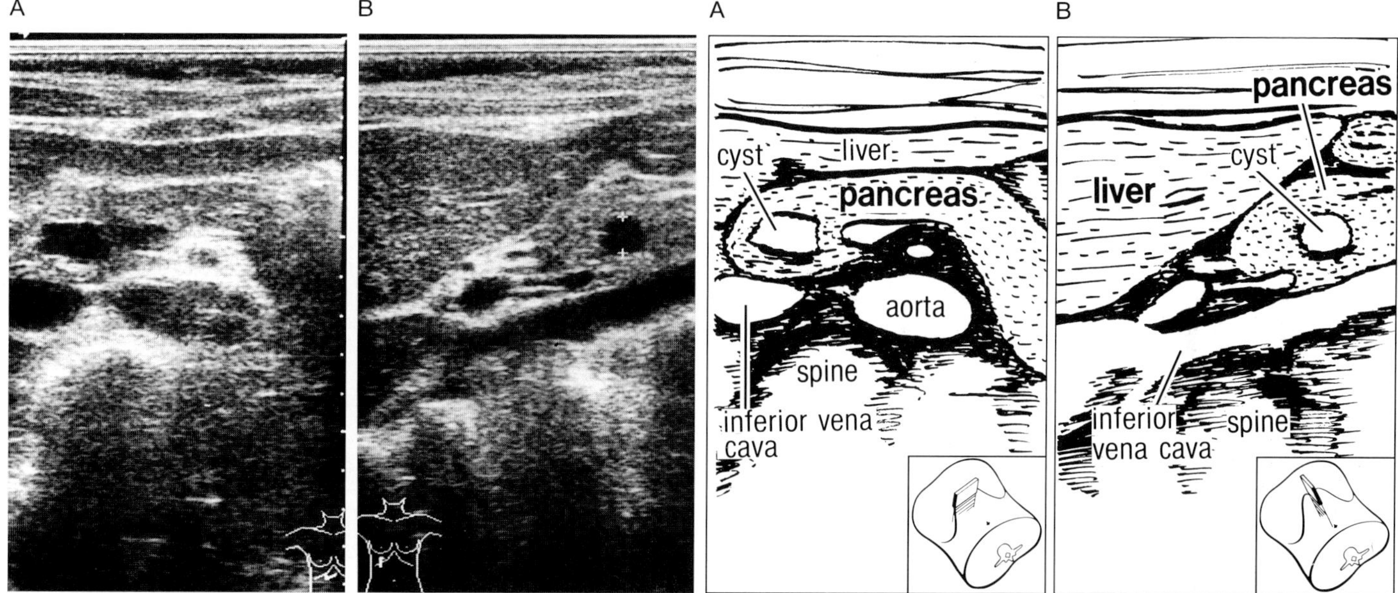

Fig. 5.33 A, B. *Case 1.* There is a 9 × 5-mm cystic mass in the region of the pancreatic head. There are no other significant abnormalities. The main pancreatic duct was within normal size limits. This patient had had a history of epigastric pain 4 years previously and was diagnosed as having gallstones. A follow-up study showed no change in the size of the cystic mass in the pancreatic head

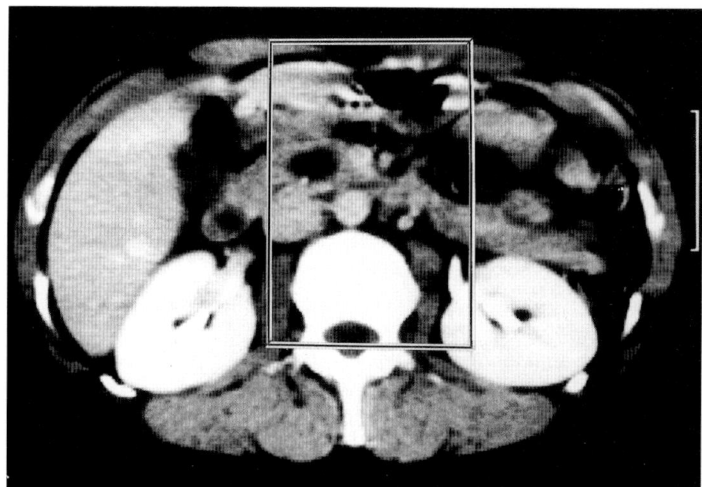

Fig. 5.34. *Case 1, CT scan.* There is a low-density mass in the pancreatic head. The *outlined area* corresponds to the ultrasonographic field in Fig. 5.33

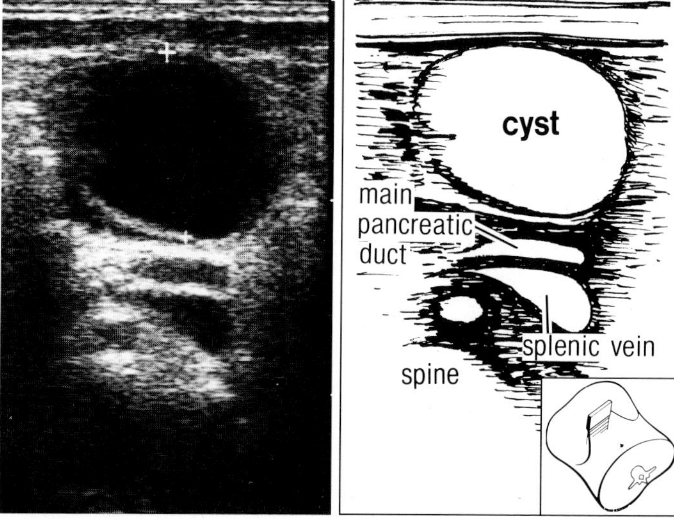

Fig. 5.35. *Case 2.* There is a 5-cm pancreatic pseudocyst arising from the body of the pancreas and extending anteriorly. There is mild dilatation of the main pancreatic duct

6 Spleen

Anatomy of the Spleen

Normally, the spleen is located under the left hemidiaphragm. Its upper pole is near the greater curvature of the gastric fundus. Its long axis is parallel to the left tenth rib, coursing anteroinferiorly. The lower pole of the spleen is on the mid-axillary line. The superior surface of the spleen is in contact with the left hemidiaphragm and is convex in contour; the medial surface is slightly concave. The splenic hilum is on the medial side of the spleen, and this is where the splenic artery and vein enter the spleen. Arteromedial to the spleen lie the stomach, pancreatic tail, and splenic flexure of the colon. Inferior to the spleen is the left kidney. The superior and lateral surface is in contact with the left hemidiaphragm and the left ninth to eleventh ribs. The lower pole of the left lung is in proximity.

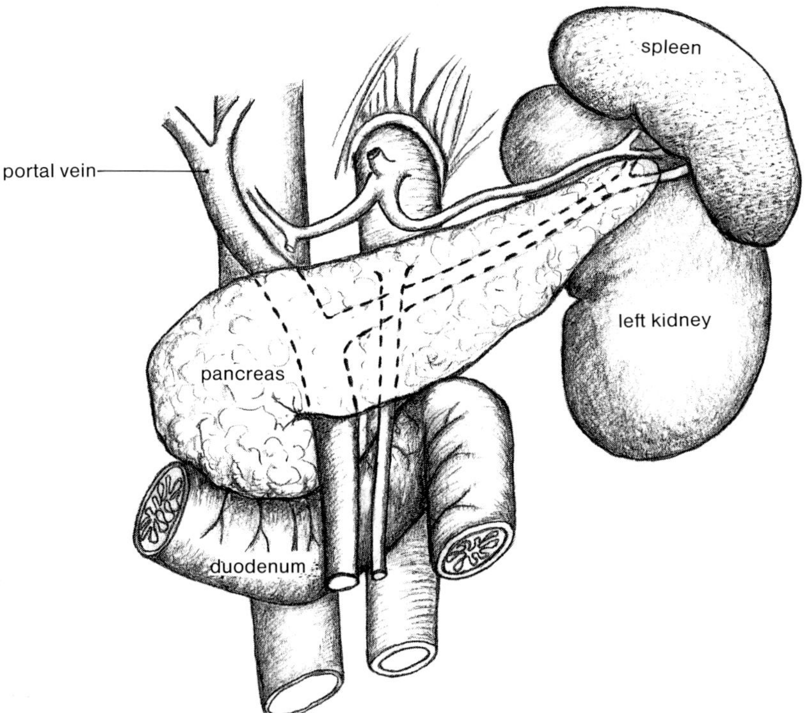

Fig. 6.1. Anatomy of the spleen

Scanning Techniques

The easiest way to visualize the spleen on ultrasonographic examination is to scan from the left tenth intercostal space with the transducer head posterior to the mid-axillary line, although only part of the spleen may be visualized because of overlapping lung. If the spleen is not visualized from the tenth intercostal space, adjacent intercostal spaces should be utilized. Usually, a larger portion of the spleen is visualized on expiration compared to inspiration. A normally sized spleen may be difficult to visualize because of overlapping lung. Most abnormal spleens are enlarged, and consequently evaluation of the spleen is relatively easy. A normal spleen has approximately the same echogenicity as the liver.

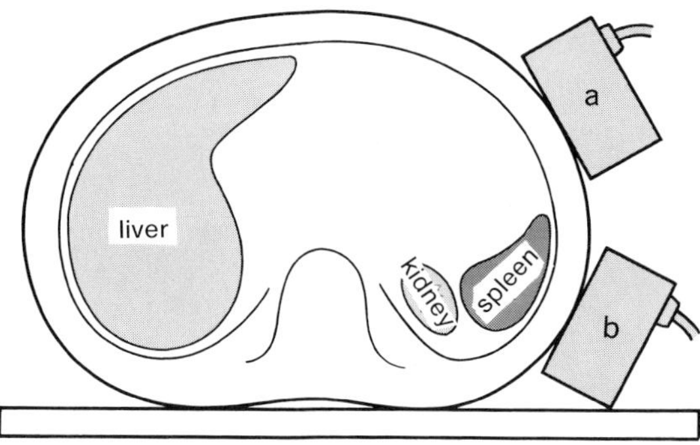

Fig. 6.2. *Technique of visualizing the spleen.* With the transducer head in an anterior position *a*, the spleen is not well visualized. The spleen is located posteriorly and it should be examined with the transducer head as in position *b*. With the patient in the right decubitus position, manipulation of the transducer head becomes easier, but a large portion of the spleen is covered by the left lung in this position

Ultrasonographic Appearance of a Normal Spleen

Except in the presence of massive ascites, there is always a blind spot when imaging the spleen with a linear-type transducer head. It is difficult to accurately measure the size of the spleen when it is not enlarged. Fortunately, focal abnormalities in the spleen are rare, and most splenic diseases are associated with diffuse enlargement. On ultrasono-

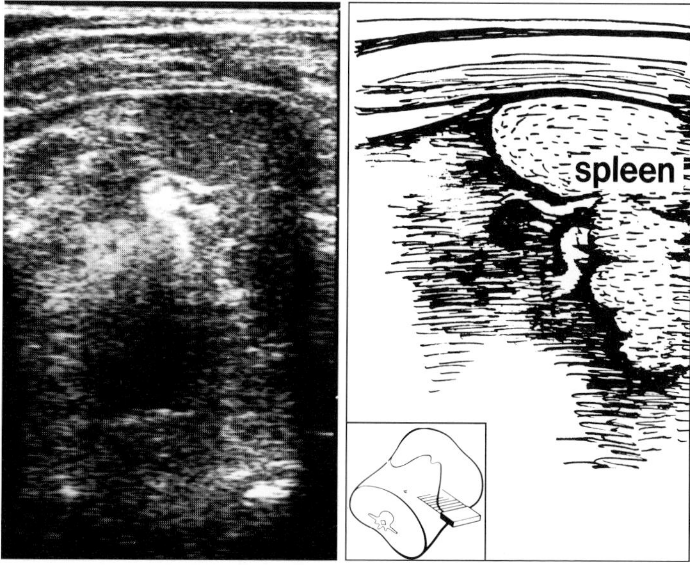

Fig. 6.3. *Case 1.* The upper margin of the spleen, immediately below the diaphragm, is not visualized because of air in the lung

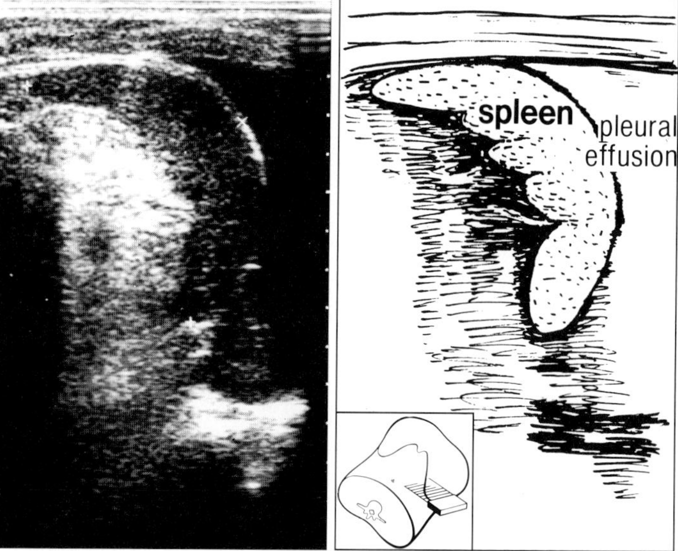

Fig. 6.4. *Case 2.* With a large amount of ascites or pleural effusion, the entire spleen can be visualized

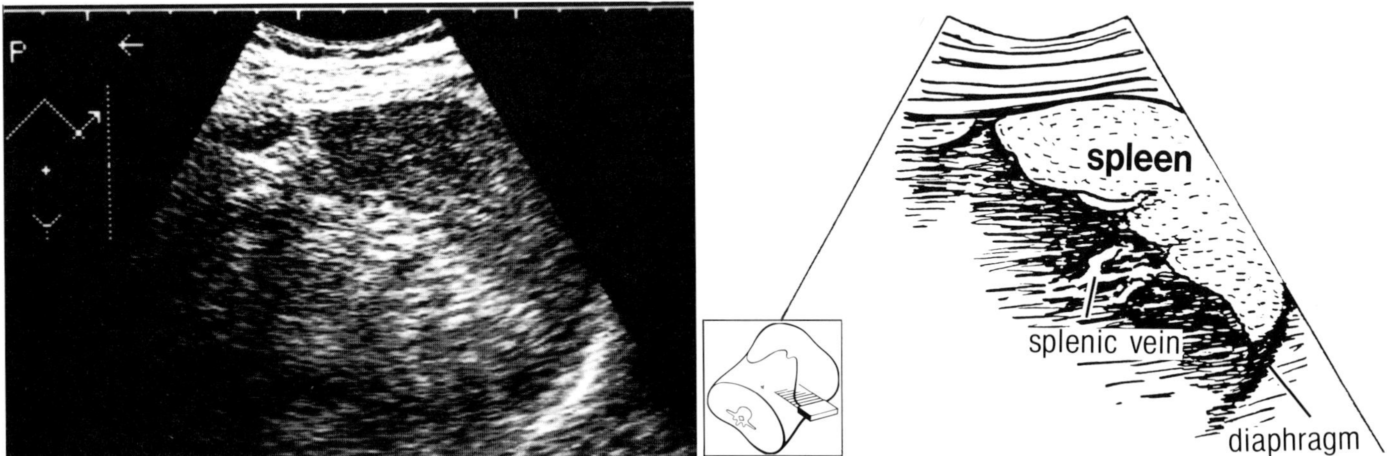

Fig. 6.5. *Case 3.* The curved linear- or sector-type transducer head reduces the size of the blind area when imaging the spleen

graphic examination, if there is no splenomegaly and there is a homogeneous echo pattern which is approximately the same as that of the liver, the spleen is diagnosed as being normal. When the spleen is visualized as being crescent shaped by intercostal scanning in expiration and the lower pole is within 3–4 cm of the lower edge of the lung (which is determined by the position of a gas shadow), the spleen is normal in size.

Splenomegaly

It is well known that the spleen enlarges in liver disease (see pp. 78–79) and hematologic diseases. Enlargement of the spleen is usually symmetric, and the lower pole of the spleen extends toward the umbilicus. It is important to try to visualize the entire spleen from a left intercostal position, but knowing only the location of the lower pole of the spleen suggests the splenic size. When there is marked splenomegaly, a dilated splenic vein and short gastric vein are visualized in the region of the splenic hilum.

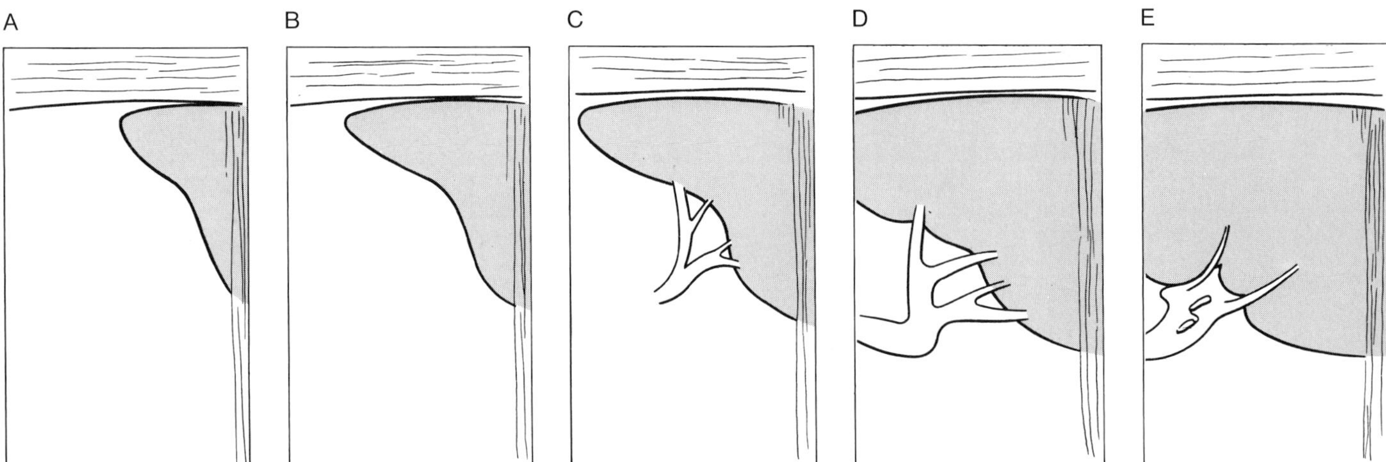

Fig. 6.6 A–E. Splenomegaly: **A** normal spleen; **B** minimal; **C** mild; **D** moderate; **E** marked

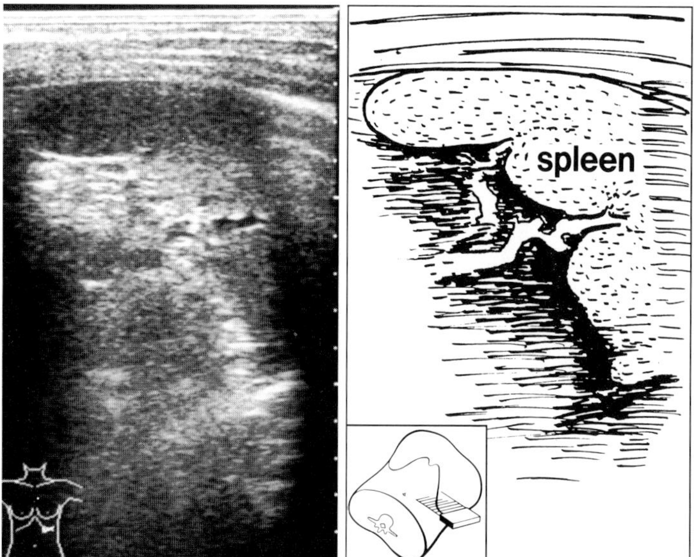

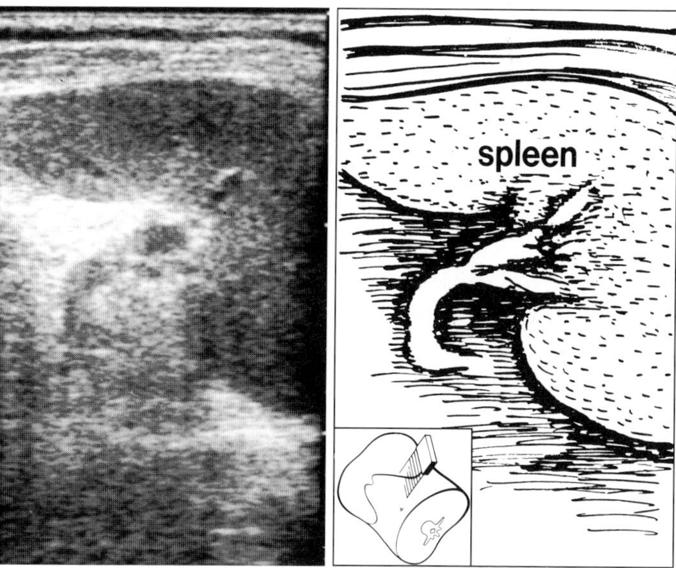

Fig. 6.7. *Minimal splenomegaly.* This study was performed using a transducer head with an 8-cm effective visual field. The overall length of the spleen adjacent to the abdominal wall is approximately two-thirds of the length of the transducer head. On close examination, there is a moderately enlarged splenic vein in the region of the splenic hilum

Fig. 6.8. *Mild splenomegaly.* This patient had chronic hepatitis. The visualized length of the spleen is approximately the same length as the transducer head. There is a dilated splenic vein in the region of the splenic hilum

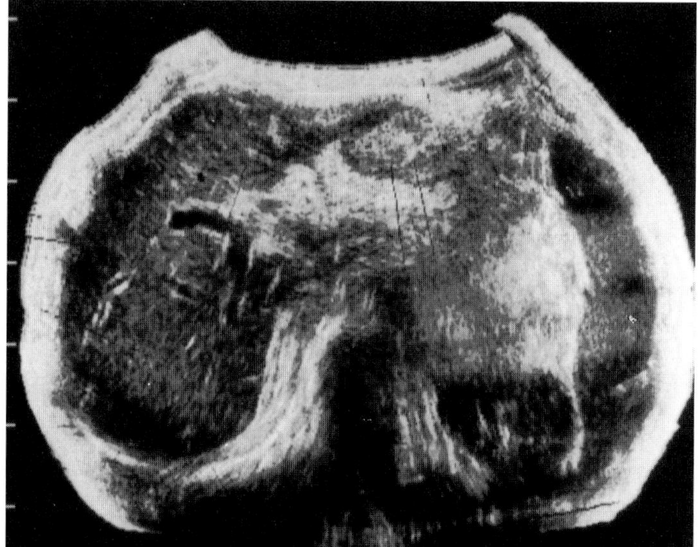

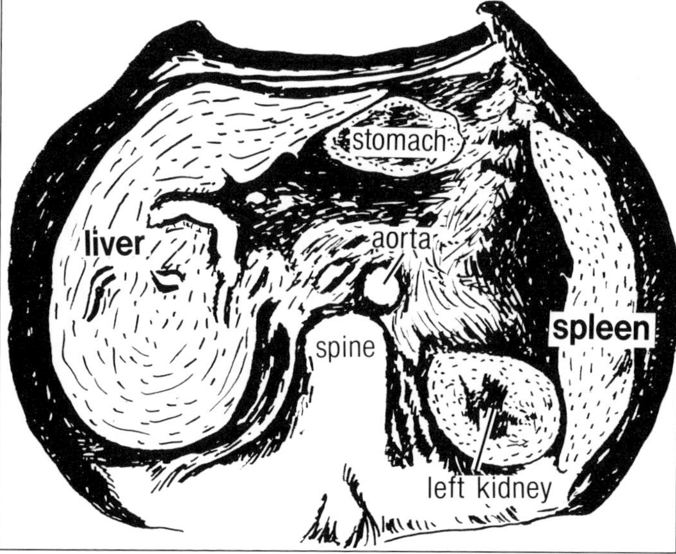

Fig. 6.9. Contact compound image of the same case as in Fig. 6.8. The spleen is enlarged, extending toward the anterior abdominal wall

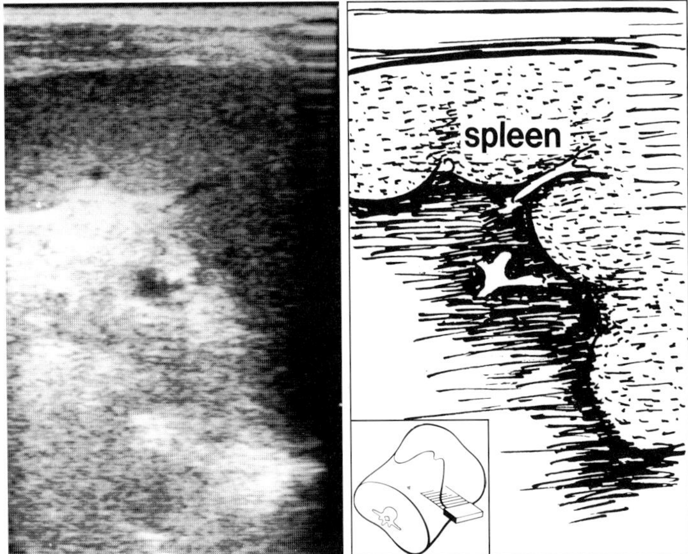

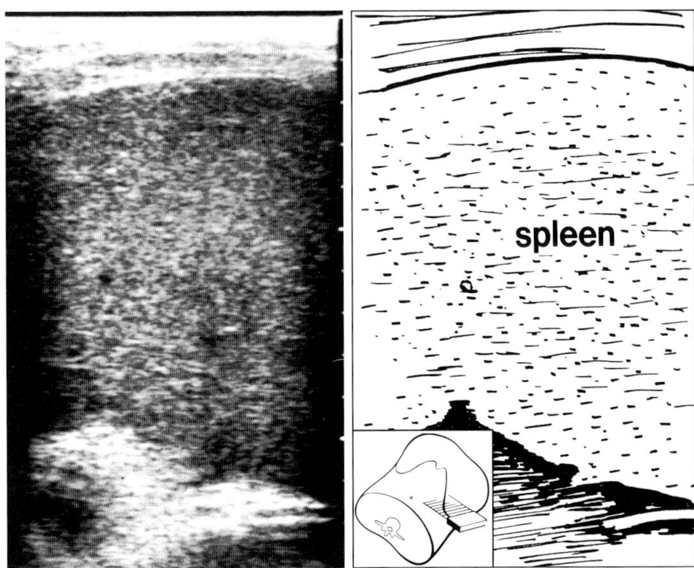

Fig. 6.10. *Moderate splenomegaly*. Ultrasonographic examination was performed to rule out cirrhosis of the liver. The liver was normal in size and shape. There was moderate splenomegaly with the length of the visualized portion of the spleen larger than the 8 cm transducer head

Fig. 6.11. *Marked splenomegaly*. This patient had aplastic anemia. The spleen is markedly enlarged, extending across the midline and below the level of the umbilicus. Marked splenomegaly is seldom seen in cases of cirrhosis of the liver, and hematologic diseases should be considered

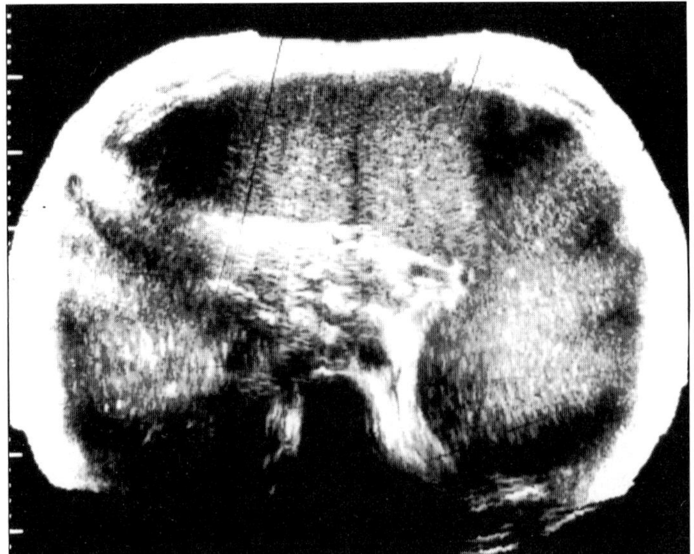

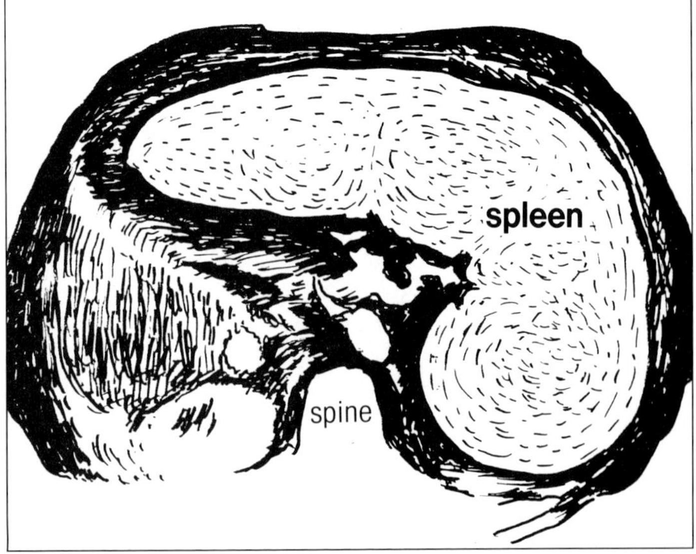

Fig. 6.12. Contact compound image of the same case as in Fig. 6.11. On the contact compound image, the entire spleen is visualized on a single slice as opposed to a linear-type scanner with which several different images are required to visualize the entire spleen

Causes of Splenomegaly

- Congestive disease of the spleen
  Primary hepatic disease: cirrhosis of the liver, chronic hepatitis, acute hepatitis
  Obstruction of the portal vein or splenic vein
- Hematologic disorders
  Hemolytic anemia, malignant lymphoma, idiopathic thrombocytopenic purpura, leukemia, myelofibrosis, polycythemia vera
- Infectious or inflammatory diseases
  Acute inflammation: sepsis, infectious mononucleosis, infectious endocarditis, psittacosis
  Chronic inflammation: tuberculosis, malaria, sarcoidosis
  Collagen disease: Felty's syndrome, systemic lupus erythematosus
- Miscellaneous
  Glycogen storage disease, Gaucher's disease, Niemann-Pick disease, Hand-Schüller-Christian disease, amyloidosis.

Accessory Spleen

If a rounded solid mass is visualized in the region of the splenic hilum in a patient with splenomegaly, accessory spleen should be considered. Most accessory spleens are located in the region of the splenic hilum and have approximately the same echogenicity as the spleen. As the spleen enlarges, accessory spleens also become larger, although most often they are approximately 1 cm in dimension. Accessory spleens are seen in 10% of autopsy cases. Ultrasonographic examination can only visualize an accessory spleen which is larger than 1 cm in a patient with splenomegaly.

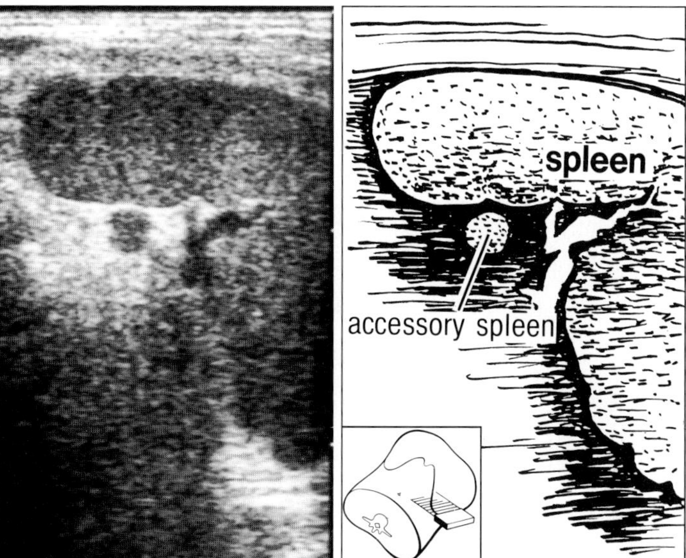

Fig. 6.13. *Case 1*. Patient with hepatic cirrhosis. There is a 1-cm solid, round mass in the region of the splenic hilum. The diagnosis of accessory spleen is made because of the similar echogenicity relative to the spleen. There is mild splenomegaly

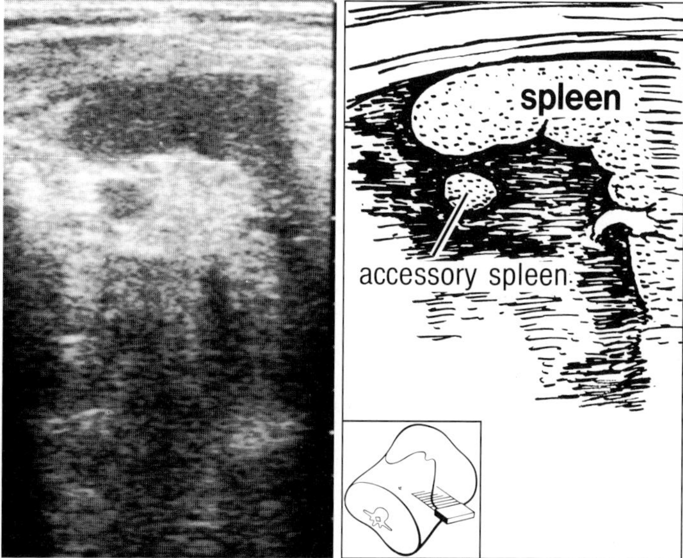

Fig. 6.14. *Case 2*. The visualized portion of the spleen is normal in size, but, judging from the distance between the lower pole and the splenic hilum (the location of the splenic vein), there is minimal to mild enlargement. This image may have been obtained in inspiration or in a patient with a large portion of the spleen covered by lung. Inferior to the splenic hilum, there is a 1.5-cm rounded mass which has the same echo pattern as the spleen, suggesting an accessory spleen

Solid Tumors of the Spleen

Primary tumors of the spleen are very rare. They include malignant lymphoma, fibroma, hamartoma, hemangioma, and lymphangioma. Metastatic tumor or direct invasion of tumor from adjacent organs is also seen.

Metastatic Tumors of the Spleen from Gastric Cancer

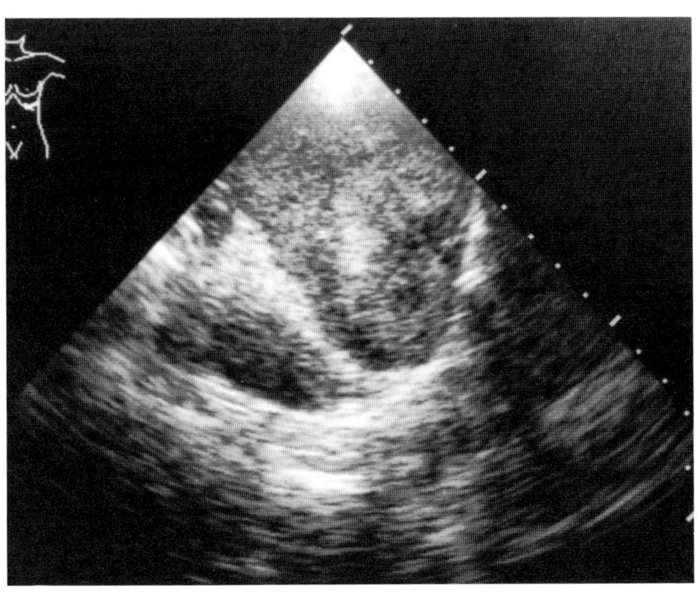

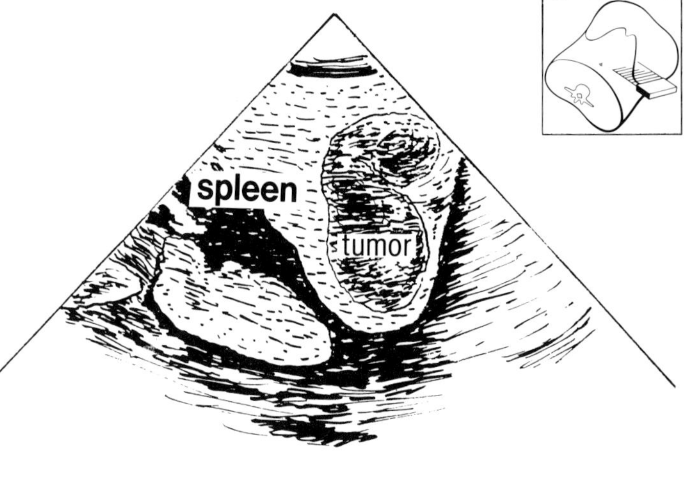

Fig. 6.15. *Case 1.* There is a 35 × 54-mm hyperechoic mass near the upper pole of the spleen. Its contour is irregular. There is mild splenic enlargement. With a linear-type transducer, only part of this tumor could be visualized because of its high location in the spleen. This patient had had a gastrectomy for gastric carcinoma 1.5 years previously and had had a progressive increase in carcinoembryonic antigen for the last 6 months

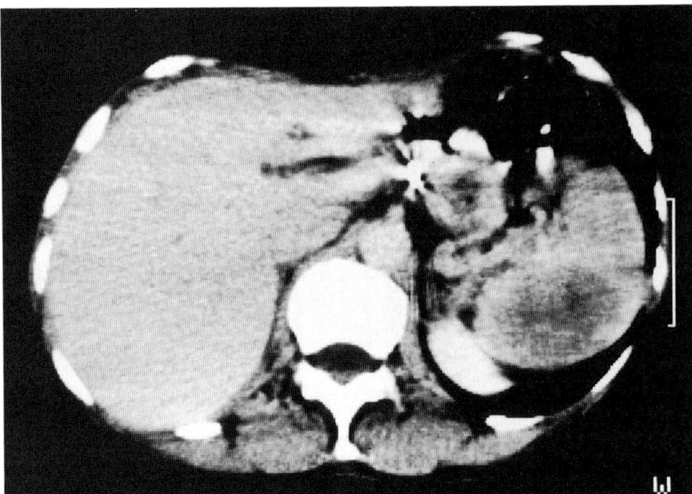

Fig. 6.16. *Case 1, CT scan.* There is a 35 × 15-mm inhomogeneous low-density mass in the posterior portion of the spleen

Cystic Tumors of the Spleen

True cysts of the spleen are usually congenital, and most of these are solitary. Cystic structures of various sizes can be formed by abnormal dilatation of lymphatic channels, blood vessels, or splenic sinuses. Other cystic lesions of the spleen include dermoid cyst, epidermoid cyst, echinococcosis, and those formed secondary to hematoma or abscess.

Splenic Cysts

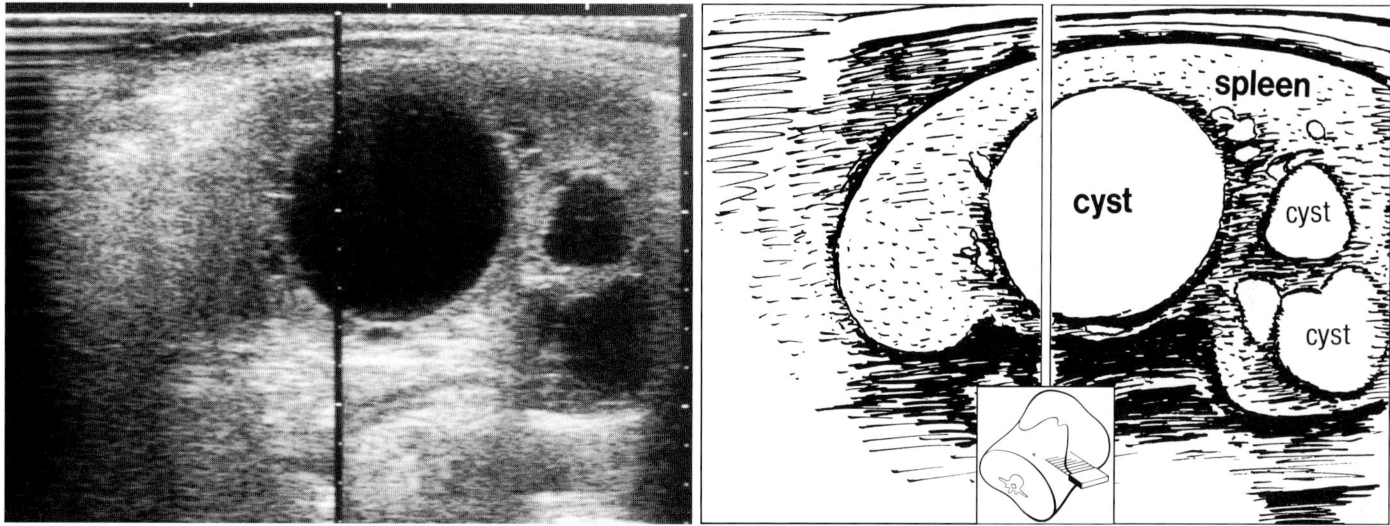

Fig. 6.17. *Case 1*. There was compression of the greater curvature of the stomach on a gastrointestinal study. Within the spleen there are several cysts of various sizes, with the largest measuring 6 cm

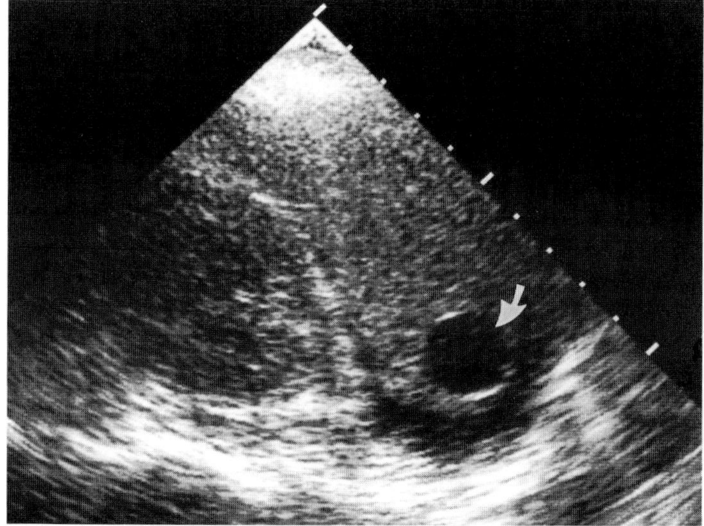

Fig. 6.18. *Case 2*. There is a 17-mm cyst in the upper pole of the spleen (*arrow*). This location is difficult to evaluate with a linear-type scanner. This patient had liver metastases from colon cancer

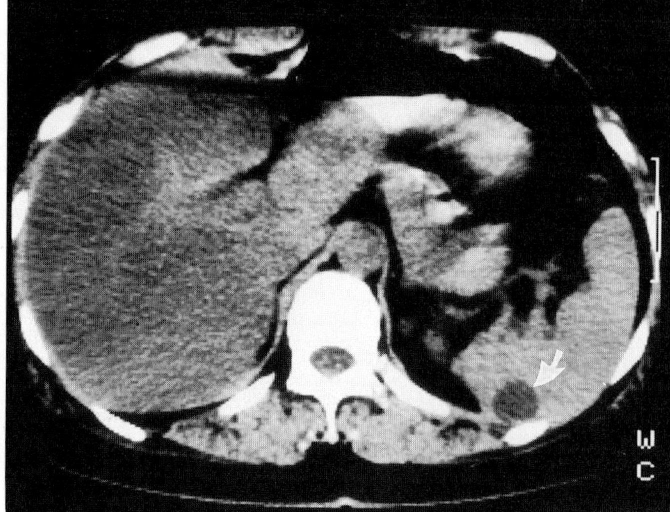

Fig. 6.19. *Case 2, CT scan*. There is a low-density mass in the posterior portion of the spleen (*arrow*)

7 Kidney

Renal Anatomy

The kidneys have a bean-shaped configuration. The central portion on the medial surface is concave and is called the renal hilum. Normal kidney length is approximately 12 cm. The surface of the kidney is bounded by a fibrous capsule. The kidney is fairly well surrounded by fat, and a fascia encases this perirenal fat. The kidney is grossly divided into the renal parenchyma in the periphery and the renal sinus in the center.

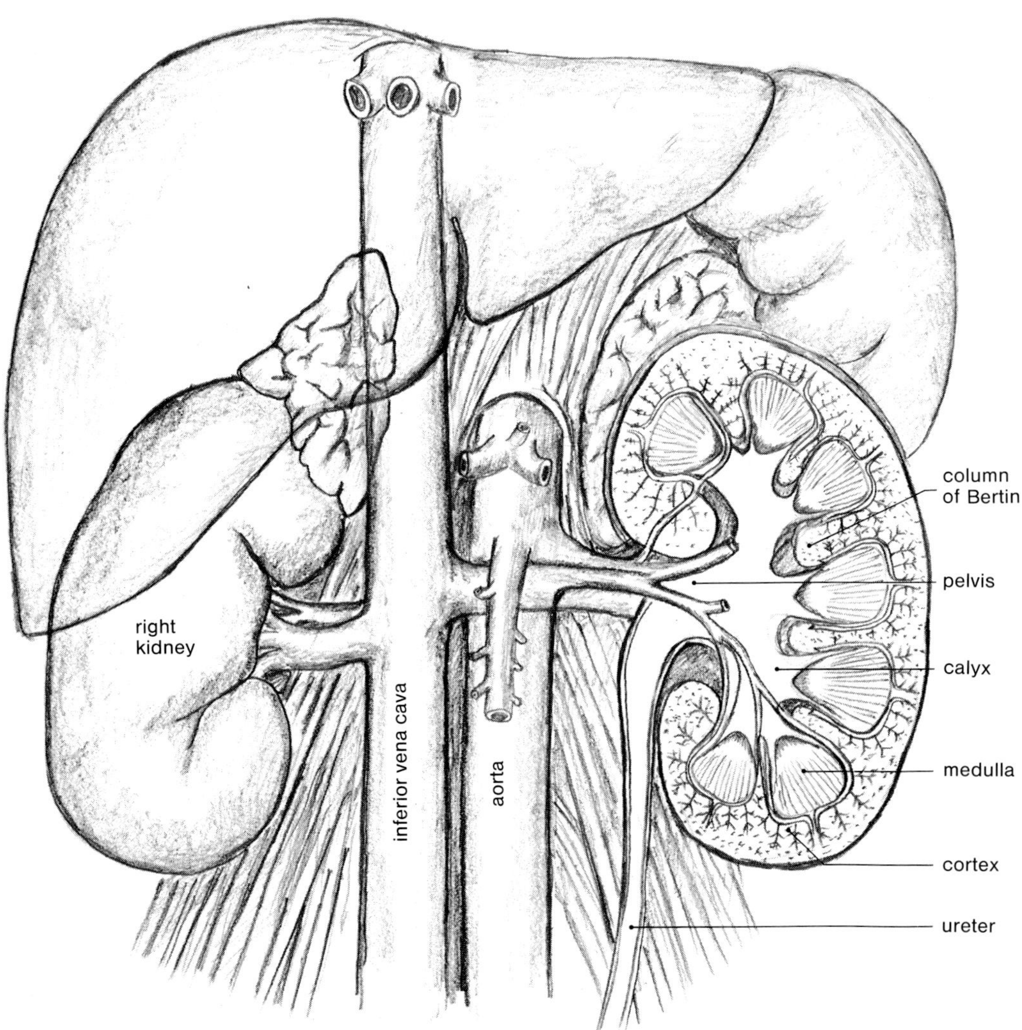

Fig. 7.1. Renal anatomy

The renal parenchyma is further subdivided into the cortex and the medulla. The medullary substance forms the renal pyramids. The tips of the pyramids, called the renal papillae, abut the calices. The renal sinus includes the calices, pelvis, renal artery, renal vein, adipose tissue, and connective tissue.

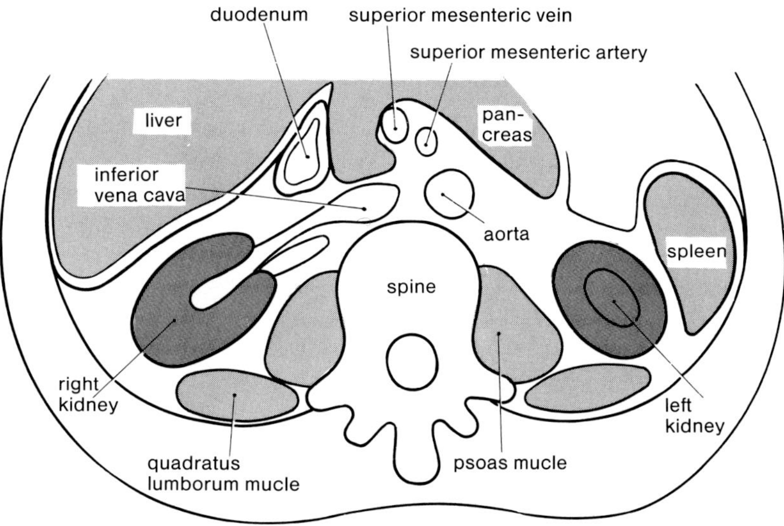

Fig. 7.2. Transverse section of the kidney and surrounding organs

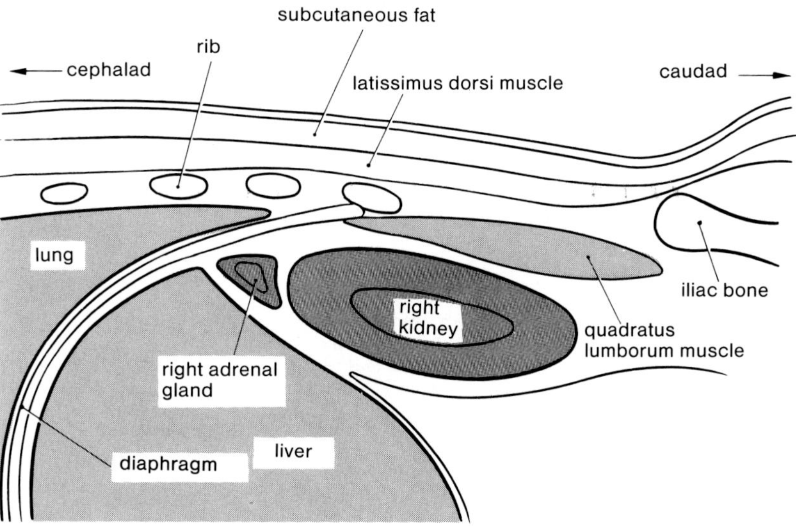

Fig. 7.3. Longitudinal section of the kidney and surrounding organs

Scanning Techniques

The kidneys can be visualized from the surface of the back in the prone position, by intercostal scanning in the supine position, from the right anterior abdominal wall through the right lobe of the liver, and by right subcostal scanning. The intercostal scan usually provides better visualization of the kidneys compared to the posterior approach with the patient in the prone position. This is because there is a thinner muscular layer on the abdomen compared to the back. A coronal section of the kidneys can be obtained by intercostal scanning; this can be easier to interpret because the images are similar to intravenous pyelogram images. In a patient with a longer right lobe of the liver, or in a patient with hepatic enlargement, imaging the kidneys via longitudinal sections through the right anterior abdominal wall is effective. The left kidney cannot be visualized from the left anterior abdominal wall because of intestinal gas. Right subcostal scanning is similar to that used to study the gallbladder; the right kidney can be well visualized by this method.

Ultrasonographic Appearance of a Normal Kidney

The kidney is visualized as an ovoid structure with a normal length of 95–110 mm on ultrasonography, slightly smaller than on excretory urography. The renal parenchyma and the renal sinus are clearly distinguished. Normal ureters are not visualized.

Renal Parenchyma

The renal cortex has a solid homogeneous echo pattern which is slightly hypoechoic relative to liver. The medulla, also referred to as the renal pyramids, is visualized as round areas of lower echogenicity than the cortex. The arcuate arteries may be visual-

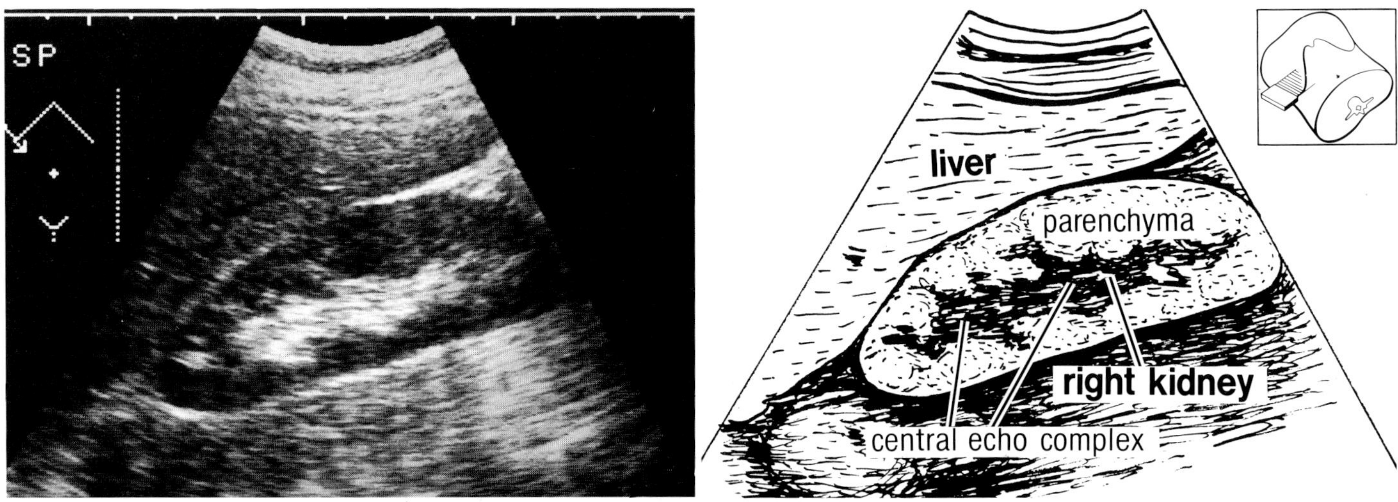

Fig. 7.4. *Case 1.* Normal right kidney

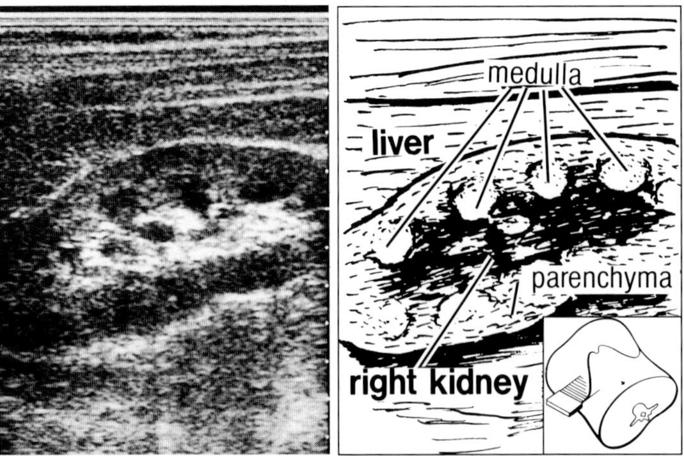

Fig. 7.5. *Case 2.* Normal kidney is slightly longer than standard 8-cm transducer head

ized as punctate hyperechoic areas at the corticomedullary junction. A well-developed portion of the renal cortex protruding toward the renal sinus is called a column of Bertin.

Renal Sinus

The renal sinus contains many complex structures such as the renal pelvis, renal calices, renal artery, renal vein, fat, and connective tissue. It is visualized as a hyperechoic area, referred to as the central echo complex, pyelocalyceal system, or simply the central echo. The renal pelvis and individual renal calices are not separable from the central echo complex unless they are dilated.

Ultrasonographic Appearance of Normal Pararenal Areas

Renal Artery and Vein

The renal veins, especially the right renal vein, are visualized more easily than the renal arteries because of their larger size and more anterior location. The left renal vein is prominent to the left of where it crosses the aorta and is clearly visualized. The right renal artery runs parallel and posterior to the right renal vein. A longitudinal section of the inferior vena cava shows the right renal artery in cross-section, passing posterior to the inferior vena cava (see Fig. 9.8 on p. 178).

Renal Fascia

The fatty tissue around the kidney is separated by the renal fascia into perirenal (inside the fascia) and pararenal (outside the fascia) fat. The renal fascia is usually visualized as a thin linear layer parallel to the renal contour, except in thin patients who have little perirenal fat.

Muscles

The quadratus lumborum muscle is visualized immediately posterior to the kidney. The sacrospinous muscle is seen more posteriorly and the latissimus dorsalis muscle more laterally. The quadratus muscle has a lower echo level than other posterior muscles.

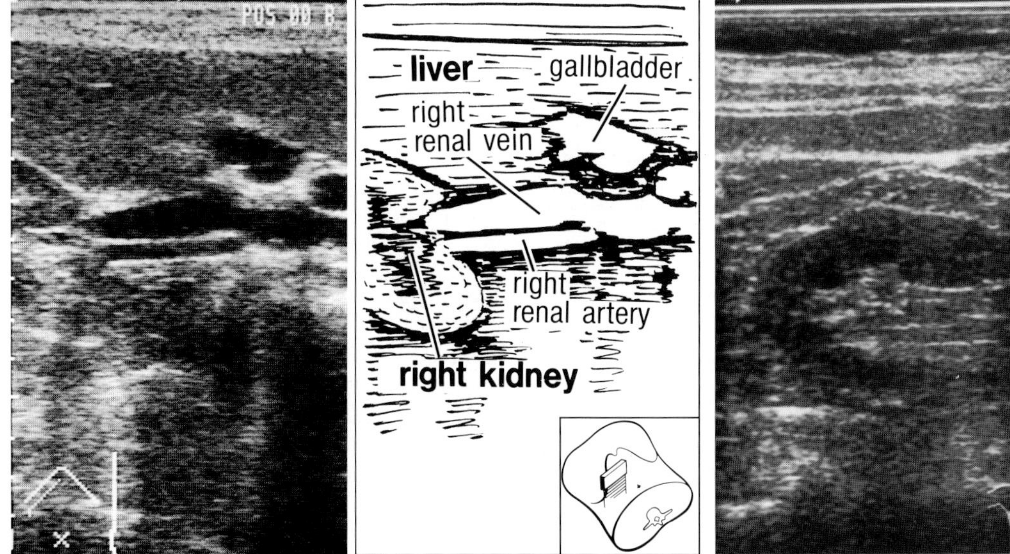

Fig. 7.6. *Case 1.* Right renal vein and right renal artery

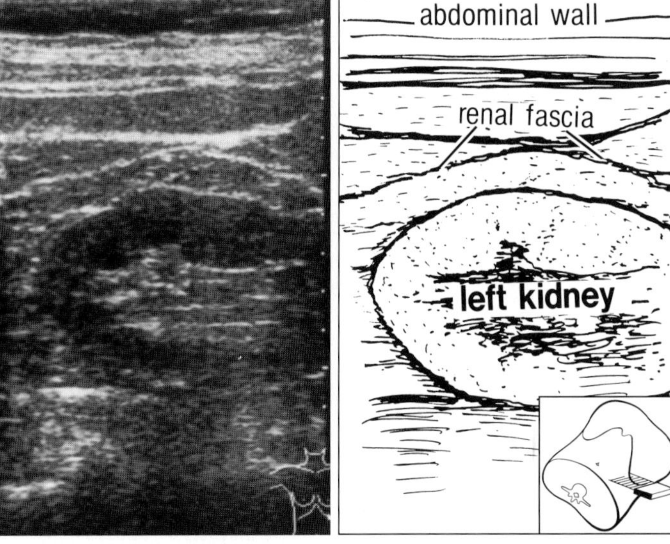

Fig. 7.7. *Case 2.* Renal fascia

Liver and Spleen

The liver and the gallbladder are visualized anterior to the right kidney. Anterolateral to the upper pole of the left kidney is the spleen.

Ribs

In the prone position, the upper poles of the kidneys are frequently difficult to visualize because of the overlapping 11th and 12th ribs.

Renal Cysts

Ultrasonography is sensitive in detecting cystic masses in the kidneys. Even small cysts of 5 mm in size can be visualized with high-resolution equipment in a thin patient. When a cyst is small, a rounded anechoic space is visualized, but there is no posterior echo enhancement. Using current equipment with gray scale display, weak echoes are often visualized within cysts, and differentiation from solid tumors may be difficult. These faint echoes are either due to weak reflection of the beam from the contents of the cyst, or, more likely, secondary to various types of artifacts (side lobe, reverberation) or noise from the equipment itself. When a cyst is primarily anterior or posterior in location, a longitudinal section from the side of the abdomen (coronal section) may not be able to demonstrate these cysts. In these cases, transverse or longitudinal sections with the patient in a prone position should be obtained. The renal pyramids are hypoechoic and should not be mistaken for renal cysts.

Simple Cysts

Cortical cysts can be divided into simple cysts and multilocular cysts. The simple cyst can be further divided, according to the number present, into solitary and multiple cysts. With the recent advent of ultrasonography and CT, simple cysts are frequently diagnosed.

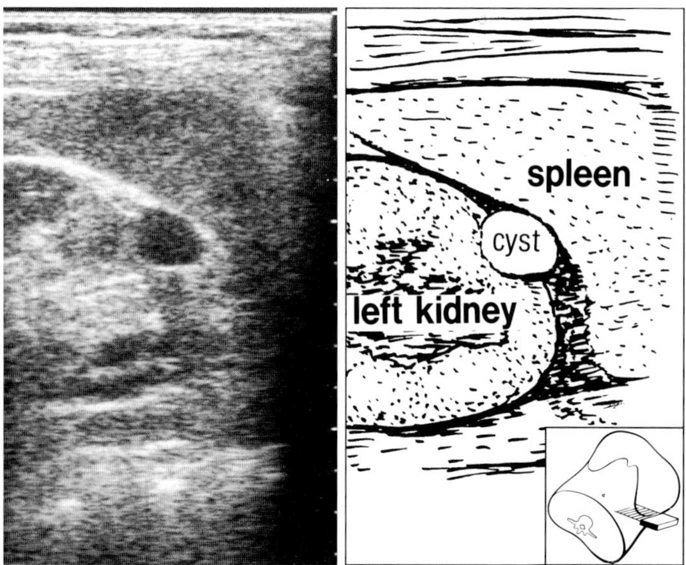

Fig. 7.8. *Case 1.* There is a 17-mm cyst arising from the upper pole of the left kidney and extending toward the spleen

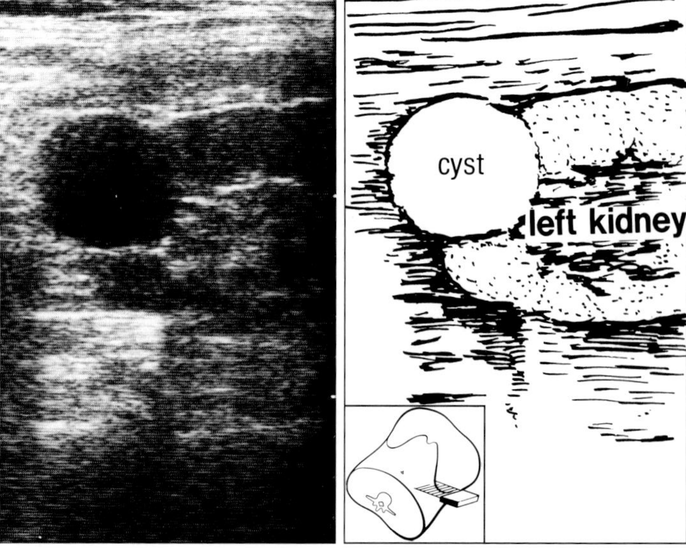

Fig. 7.9. *Case 2.* A 35-mm cyst arising from the lower pole of the kidney. Half of the cyst is extrinsic to the kidney

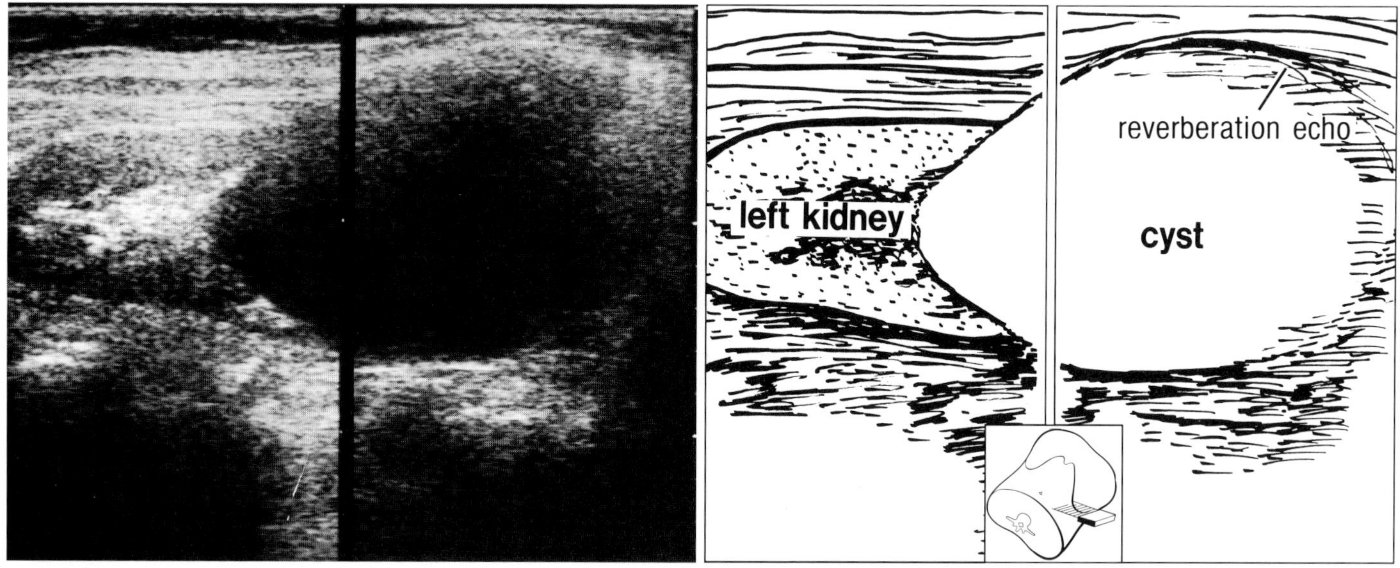

Fig. 7.10. *Case 3*. There is a giant cyst, measuring 10 × 8 cm, arising from the lower pole of the left kidney. Because of reverberation artifacts, the anterior wall is not distinctly visualized

Parapelvic Cysts

A renal cyst arising from a location other than the renal parenchyma is called a parapelvic cyst. Differentiation from hydronephrosis confined to one calix is important.

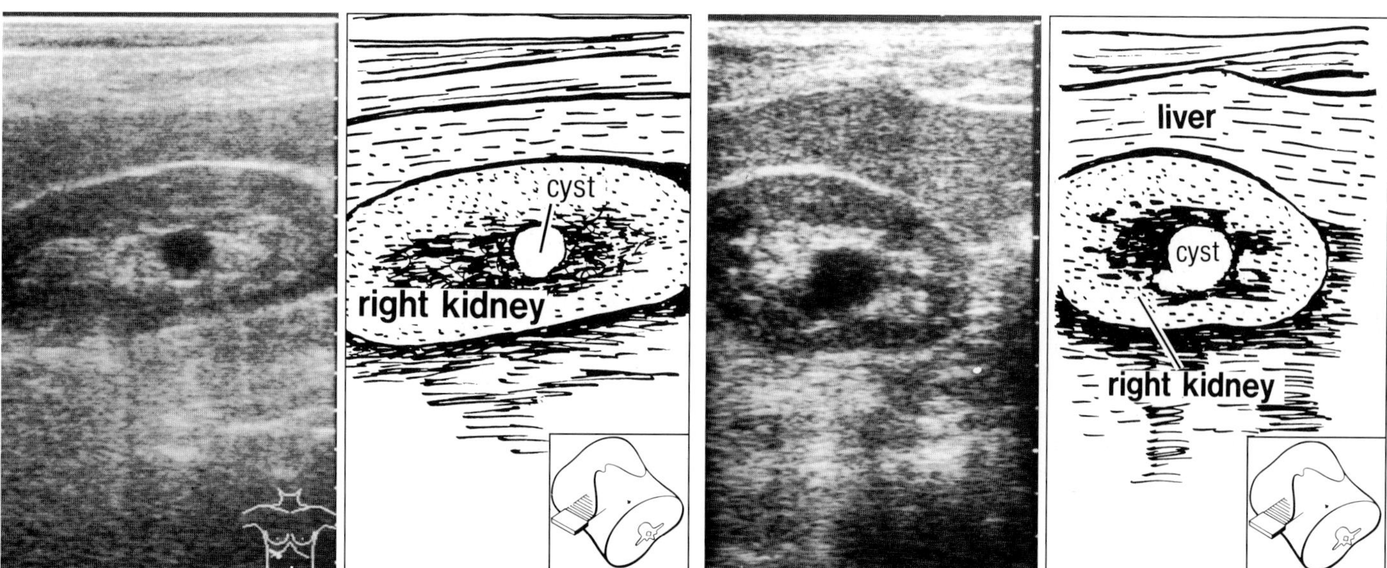

Fig. 7.11. *Case 1*. A 13-mm typical parapelvic cyst in the renal sinus   **Fig. 7.12.** *Case 2*. A 15-mm parapelvic cyst

Polycystic Kidney Disease

Polycystic kidney disease manifests as multiple cysts in bilaterally enlarged kidneys with indeterminate margins. The central strong echo complex, which is characteristic of the renal sinus, is not visualized. In some cases, cysts are seen in the liver and, rarely, in the pancreas and the spleen. There are two inheritance patterns of polycystic kidney disease: autosomal dominant and autosomal recessive. Patients with the autosomal dominant form (also known as the adult type) usually become symptomatic at the age of 30–50 with abdominal masses or high blood pressure. This disease is frequently complicated by renal stones, renal abscesses, and hematuria, and finally the patient develops chronic renal failure. Patients with the autosomal recessive form (also known as the infantile type) usually die several days to several weeks after birth.

A

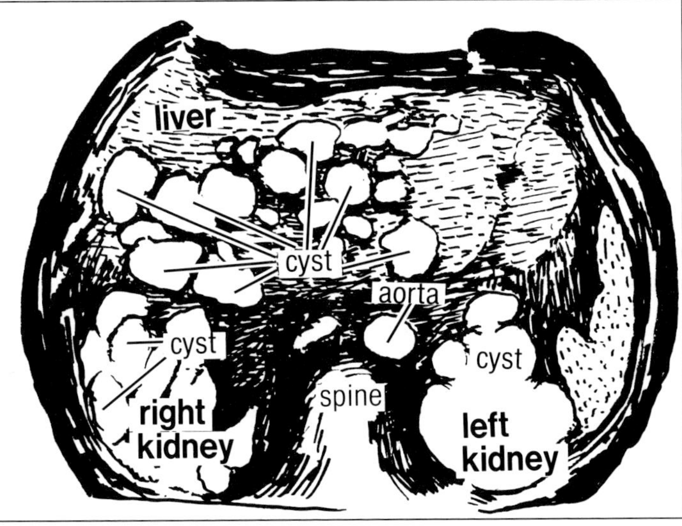

B

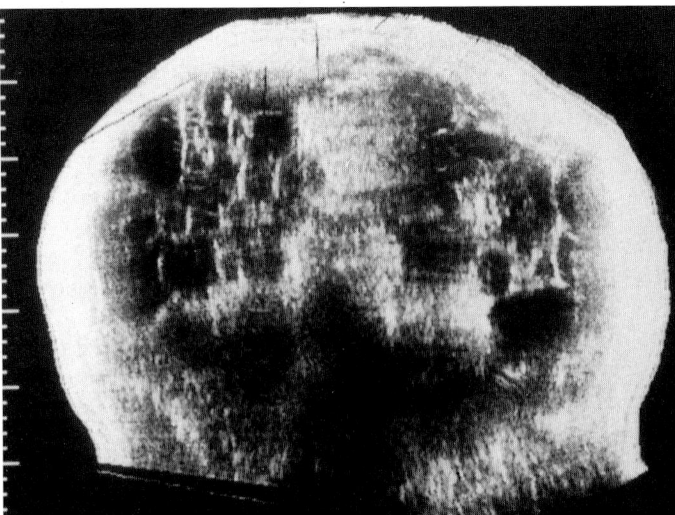

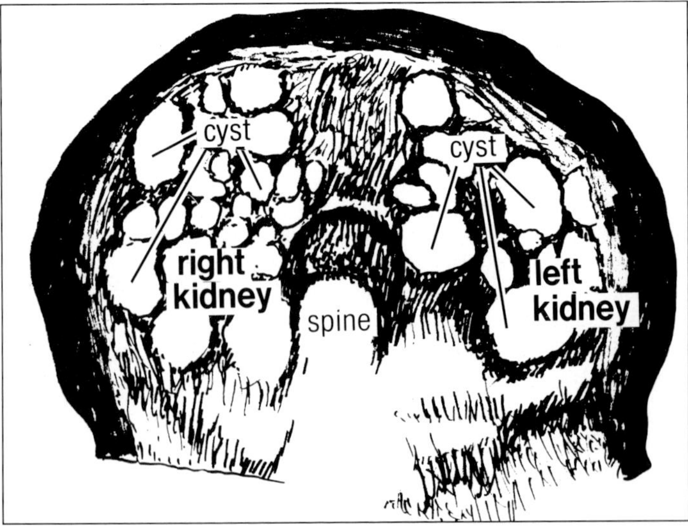

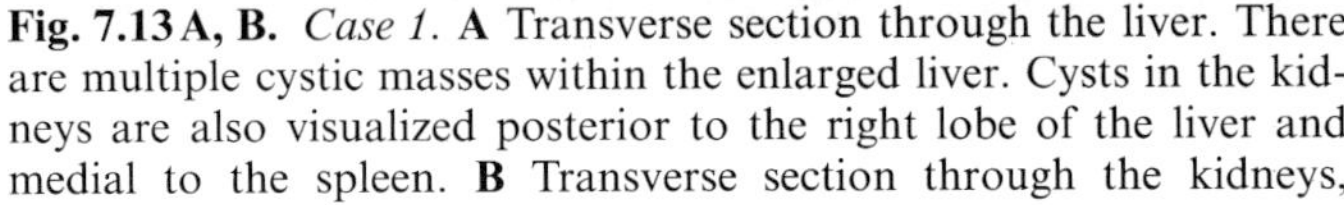

Fig. 7.13 A, B. *Case 1.* **A** Transverse section through the liver. There are multiple cystic masses within the enlarged liver. Cysts in the kidneys are also visualized posterior to the right lobe of the liver and medial to the spleen. **B** Transverse section through the kidneys, demonstrating bilaterally enlarged kidneys approaching the anterior abdominal wall. The kidneys have a honeycomb appearance, and the contours are indistinct

Table 7.1. Cystic diseases of the kidney

Cortex
    Simple cyst(s) — Solitary / Multiple
    Multilocular cyst
	Extraparenchymal
	    Parapelvic cyst
	    Perirenal pseudocyst

Medulla
    Medullary sponge kidney
    Medullary cystic kidney
	Congenital
	    Polycystic disease — Adult / Infantile
	    Multicystic dysplastic kidney

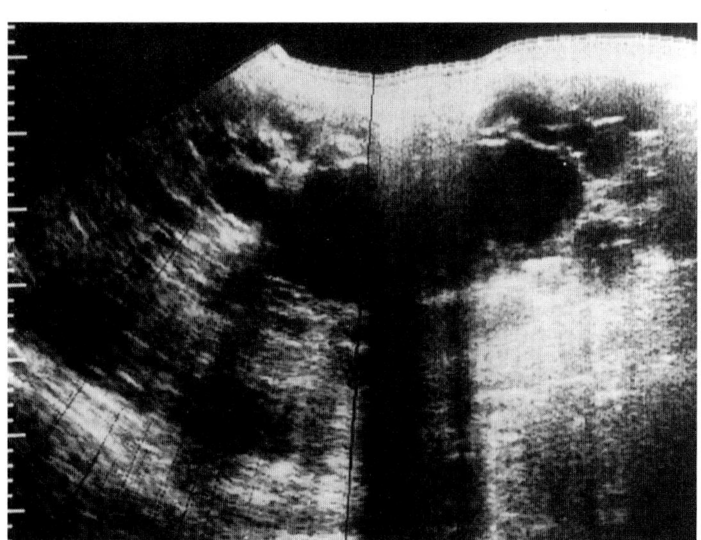

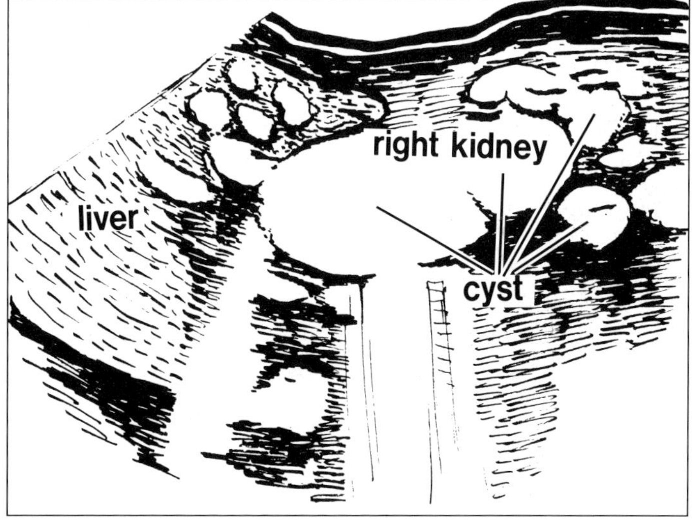

Fig. 7.14. *Case 1.* Longitudinal sections through the right lobe of the liver. There are multiple cysts in the liver and right kidney. The demarcation between these two organs is not clear because multiple cysts arising from both organs are interdigitated

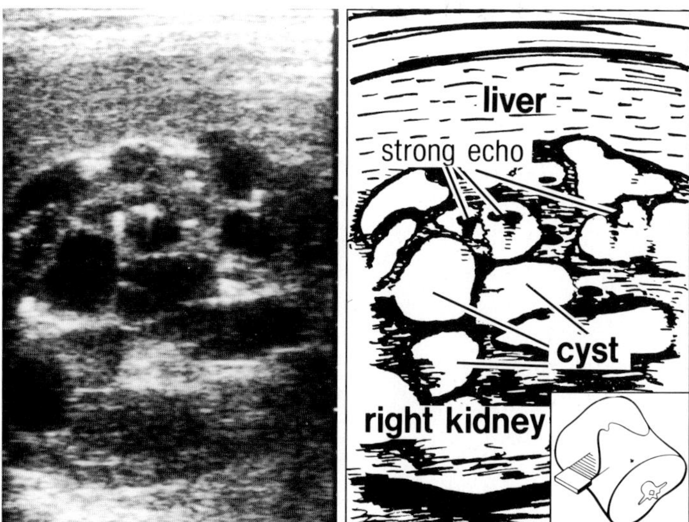

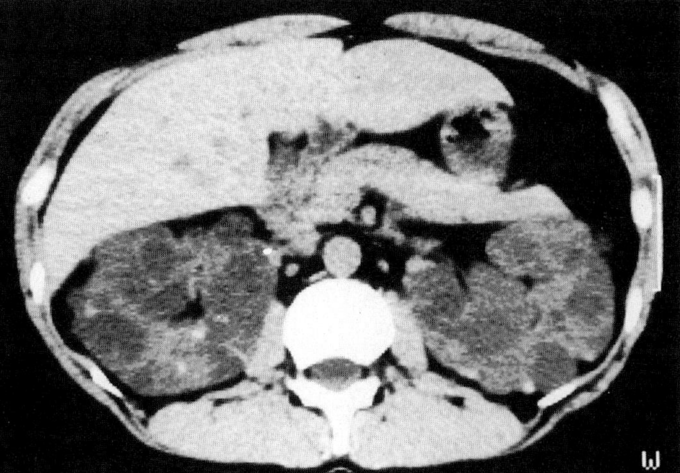

Fig. 7.15. *Case 2.* There is enlargement of the right kidney, and there are multiple cysts measuring 1–3 cm. There is a 2–3-mm strong echo on the cyst wall with comet-like echoes

Fig. 7.16. *Case 2, CT scan.* The kidneys are enlarged bilaterally, and there are multiple renal cysts. There are a few high-density areas on the walls of the cysts, suggesting calcification

Hydronephrosis

Ultrasonographic examination is sensitive in diagnosing hydronephrosis because of the characteristic cystic pattern seen in the region of the renal sinus. Advanced hydronephrosis, which is not visualized on the intravenous pyelogram, can be easily detected with ultrasonography. In normal kidneys, renal pelves and renal calices are not visualized on the ultrasonographic examination, but in the case of hydronephrosis, these are visualized as anechoic structures because of dilatation. These structures can be differentiated from renal cysts because of communcation with each other. In massive hydronephrosis, it becomes more difficult to diagnose the abnormality as renal disease because of total distortion of the echo pattern of the renal parenchyma. The fact that no normal kidney is visualized is important in making this diagnosis.

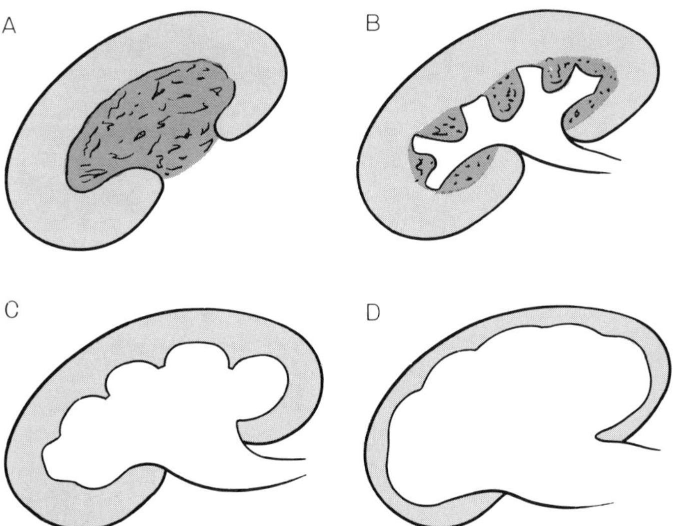

Fig. 7.17 A–D. *Spectrum of hydronephrosis.* **A** None; **B** mild; **C** moderate; **D** marked

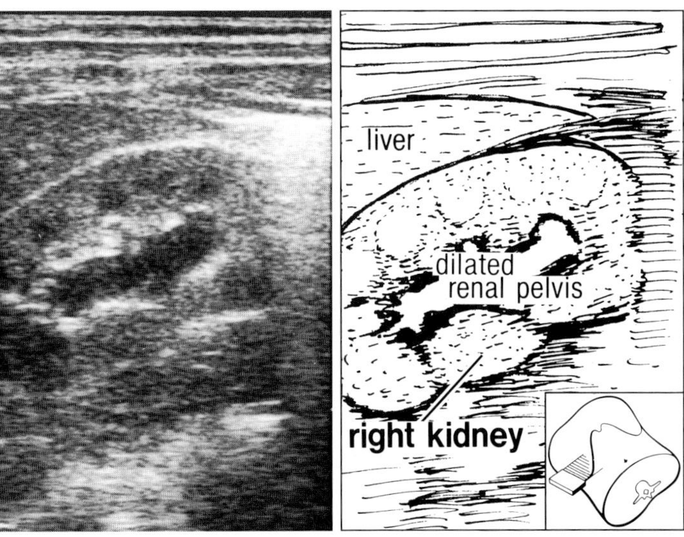

Fig. 7.18. *Case 1.* Minimal hydronephrosis. The central portion of the renal sinus is anechoic, and there is a thin layer of the central echo pattern around the anechoic space

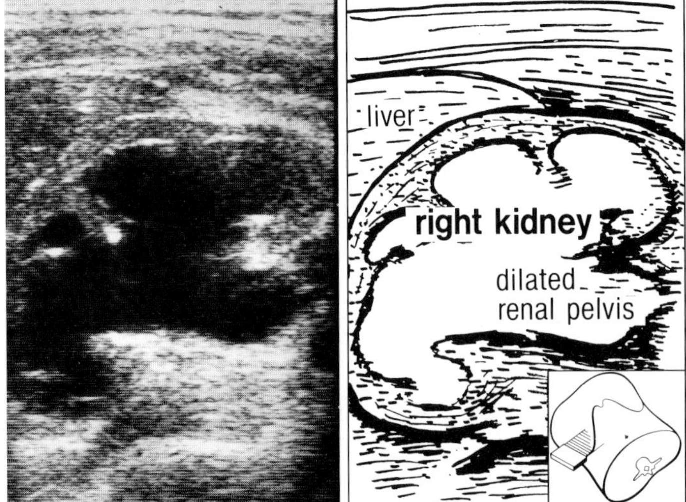

Fig. 7.19. *Case 2.* Moderate hydronephrosis. The renal pelvis and calices are markedly dilated. The dilatation of the renal pelvis extends to the ureteropelvic junction. There is thinning of the renal parenchyma

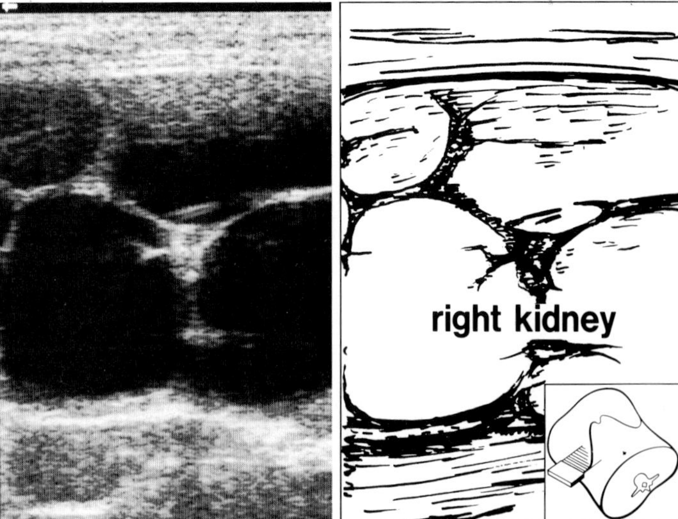

Fig. 7.20. *Case 3.* Marked hydronephrosis. Advanced hydronephrosis with the appearance of a multiloculated cyst. The renal parenchyma is barely visualized

Nephrolithiasis

Renal stones are visualized as hyperechoic areas associated with acoustic shadowing. However, these findings are not as distinct as is seen with cholelithiasis. Since the central echo complex of the renal sinus normally contains multiple strong echoes, strong echoes caused by stones can be quite difficult to identify, and only the acoustic shadowing suggests the presence of stones. Consequently, only relatively large stones can be diagnosed on the ultrasonographic examination. When the stone is within the renal parenchyma, relatively small stones can also be identified.

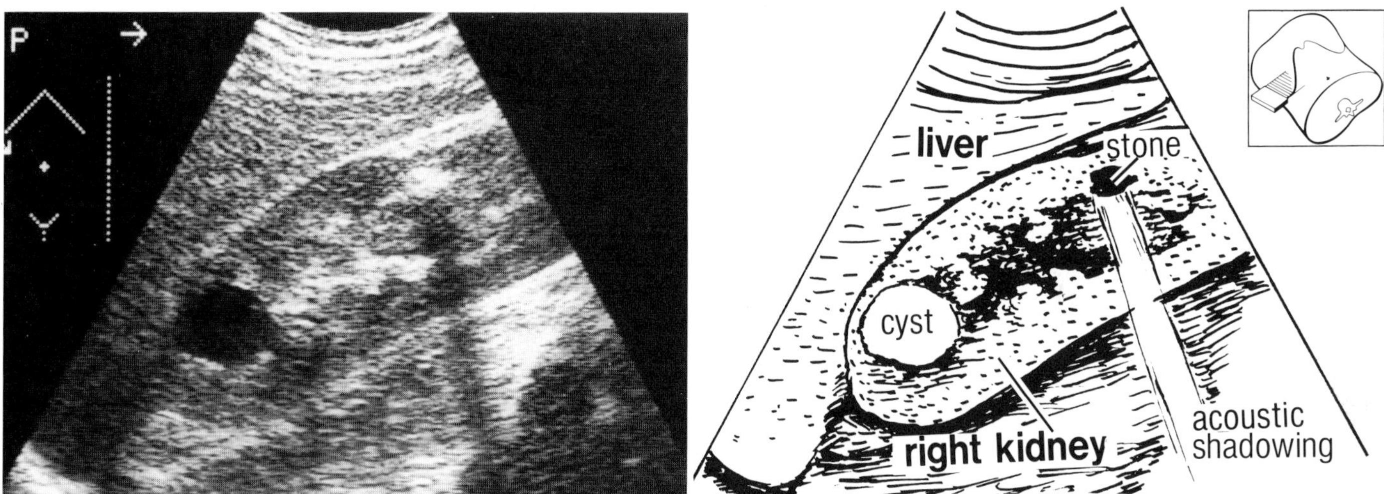

Fig. 7.21. *Case 1.* There is a 10-mm hyperechoic area near the lower pole of the right kidney associated with distinct acoustic shadowing. There is a 25-mm cyst in the upper pole of the right kidney

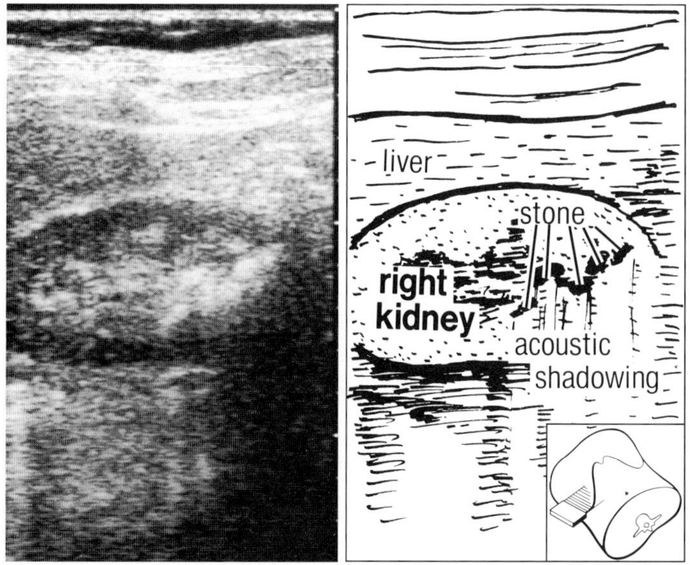

Fig. 7.22. *Case 2.* There are multiple hyperechoic areas associated with acoustic shadowing in the lower pole of the right kidney. These findings represent small stones

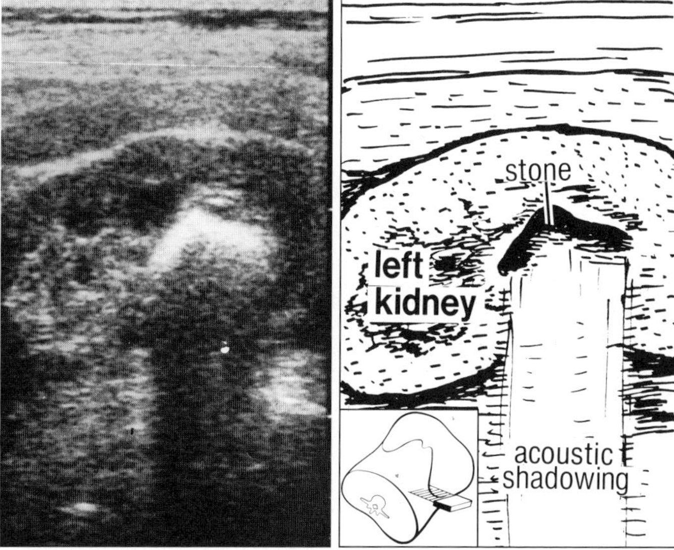

Fig. 7.23. *Case 3.* There is a 25-mm crescent-shaped hyperechoic area in the renal sinus of the left kidney, associated with posterior acoustic shadowing. Because of the large size of the stone, only the anterior surface of the stone is visualized

Renal Cancer

Renal Cell Carcinoma   Renal cell carcinoma is frequently visualized as a solid mass with relatively weak internal echoes, but it can be hyperechoic or partially cystic. There will be focal enlargement of the kidney and distortion of the central echo complex in that portion of the kidney. It is important to look for tumor thrombus within the inferior vena cava or renal vein in cases of renal cell carcinoma.

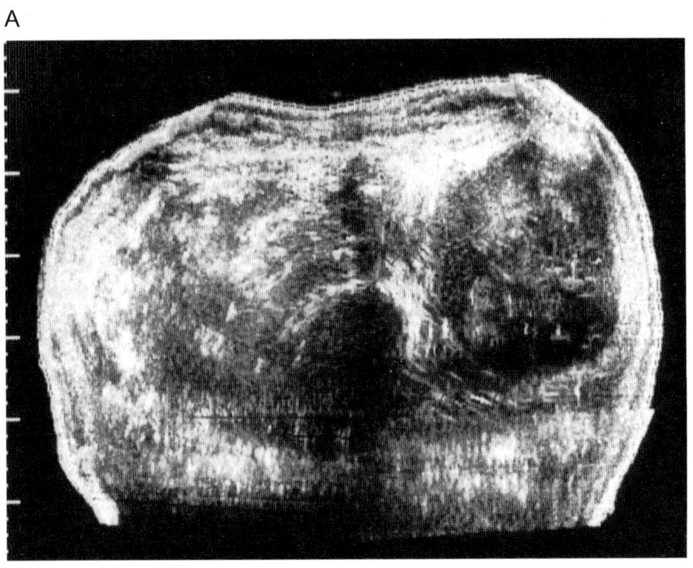

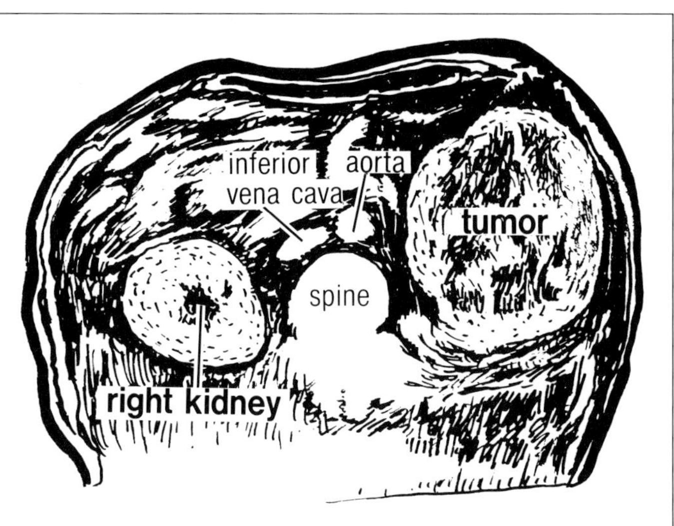

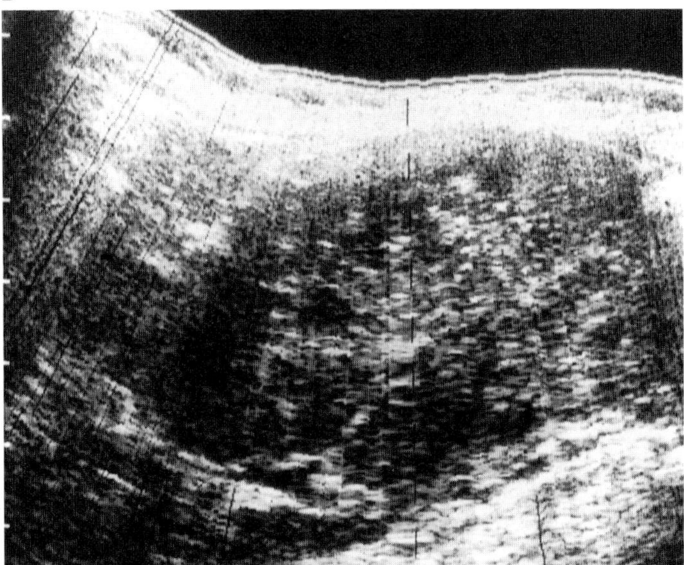

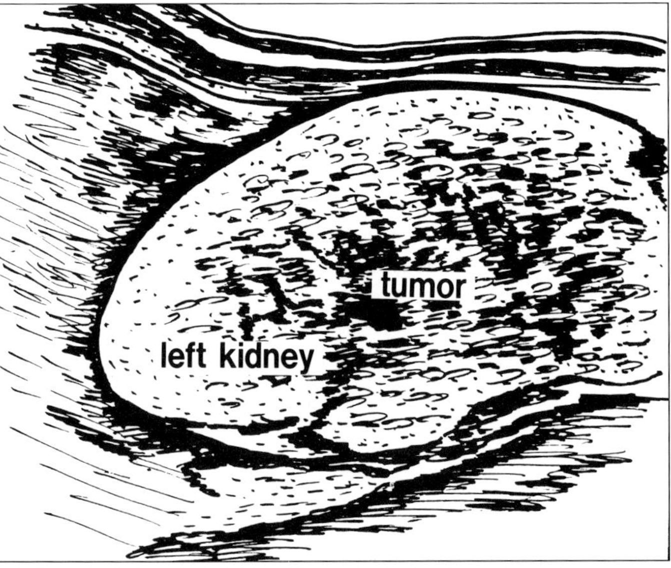

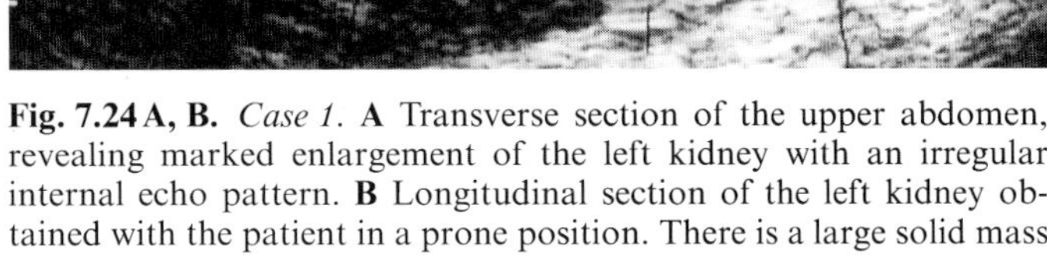

Fig. 7.24 A, B. *Case 1.* **A** Transverse section of the upper abdomen, revealing marked enlargement of the left kidney with an irregular internal echo pattern. **B** Longitudinal section of the left kidney obtained with the patient in a prone position. There is a large solid mass involving the mid and lower portions of the left kidney. The internal echo pattern is heterogeneous. A normal renal echo pattern is seen in the upper pole

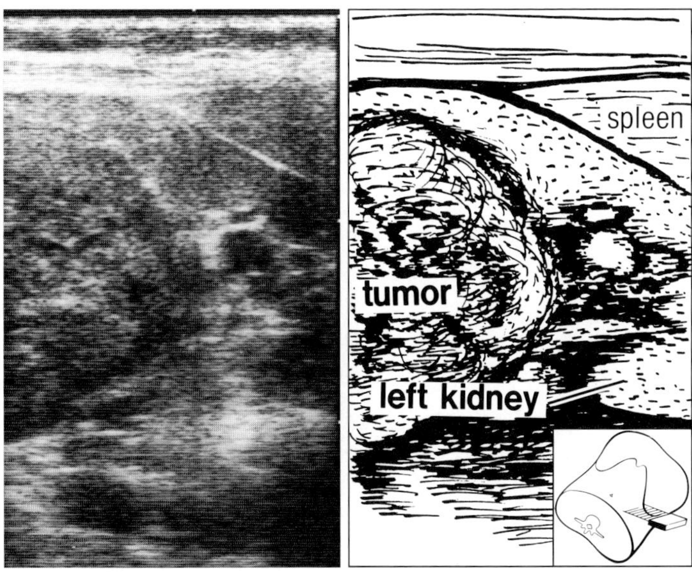

Fig. 7.25. *Case 1.* Intercostal scan on the left side of the abdomen shows a large solid tumor in the lower half of the left kidney

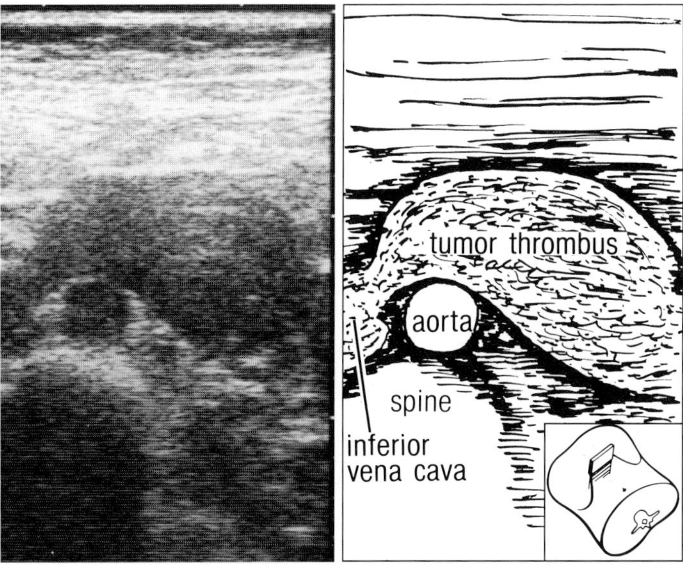

Fig. 7.26. *Case 1.* There is abnormal dilatation of the left renal vein, the lumen of which is filled by solid tumor, representing tumor thrombus

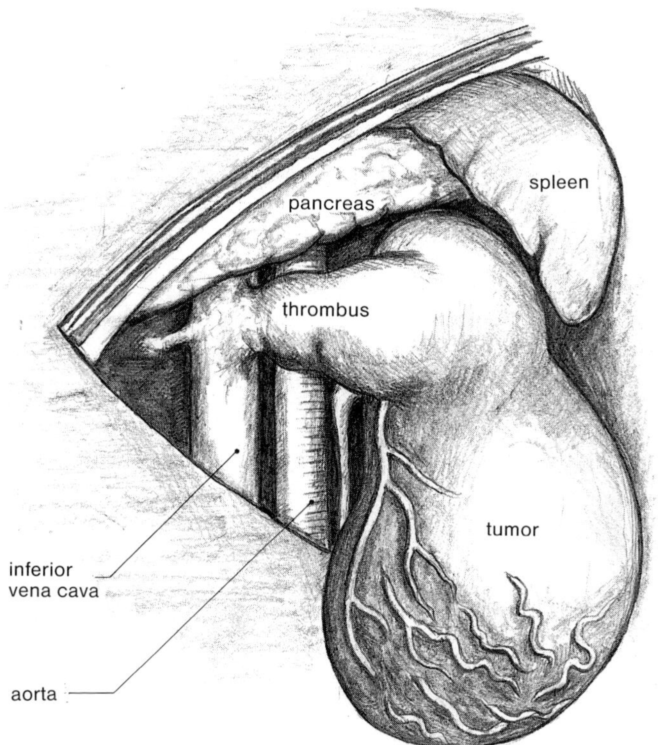

Fig. 7.27. *Case 1.* Surgical findings as revealed by transverse incision of the left upper abdomen. There was a huge tumor involving the lower pole of the left kidney with multiple dilated venous structures on its surface. The left renal vein was markedly dilated by tumor thrombus

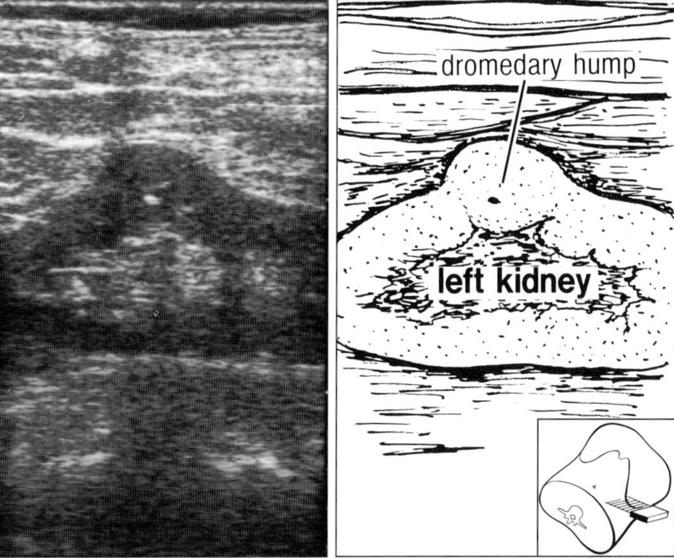

Fig. 7.28. *A case for comparison.* Lateral portion of the left renal parenchyma appears to be tumor like. This is called a dromedary hump and is a normal variant. This finding is seen only in the lateral portion of the left kidney, as in this case

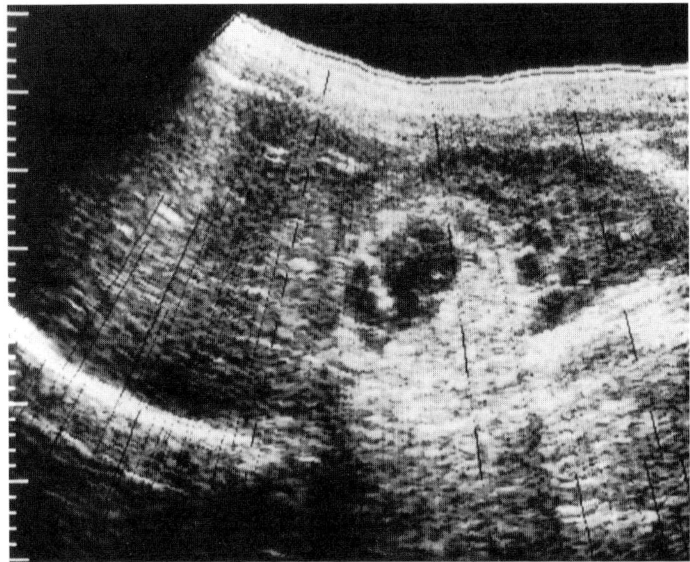

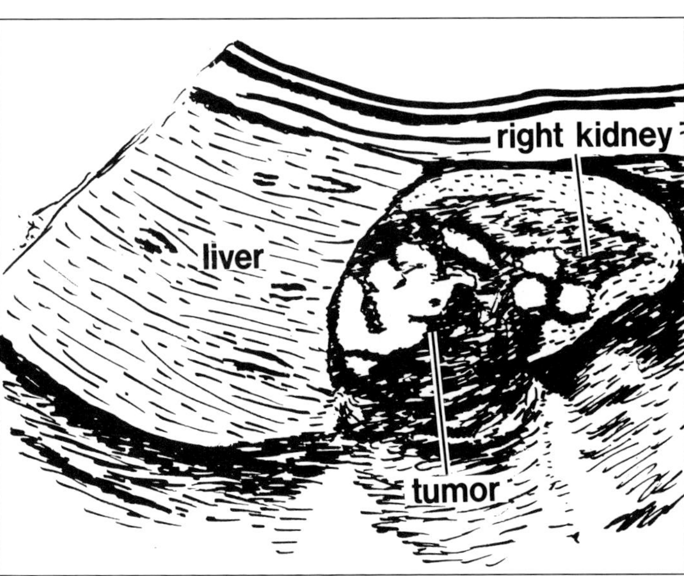

Fig. 7.29. *Case 2*. Longitudinal section of the right kidney obtained with a contact compound scanner in the supine position in a 26-year-old female patient. There is a 65-mm tumor in the upper pole of the right kidney. The central portion of the tumor shows a multiloculated cystic pattern. The peripheral portion of the tumor is abnormally echogenic

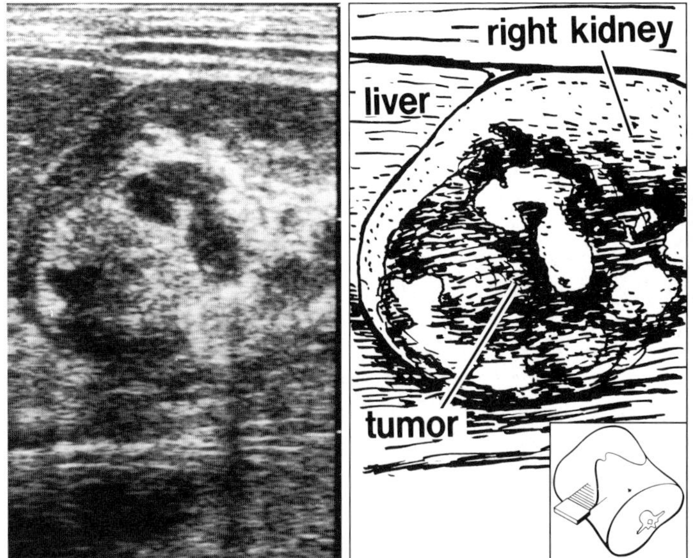

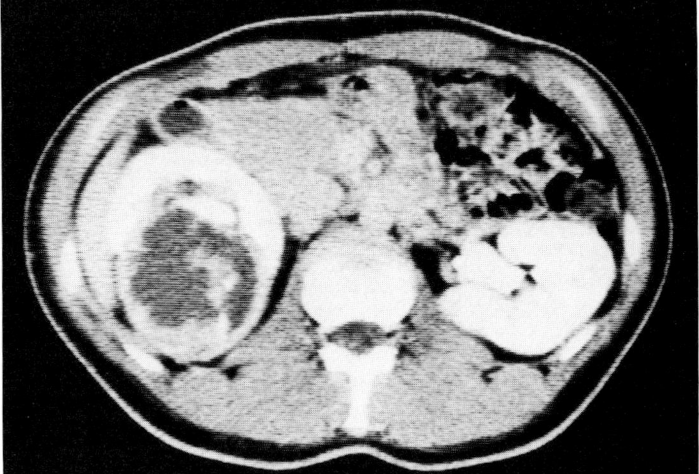

Fig. 7.30. *Case 2*. On the image obtained with a linear scanner, findings similar to those in Fig. 7.29 are seen. This was proven to be renal cell carcinoma with hemorrhage and necrosis within the tumor

Fig. 7.31. *Case 2, CT scan*. This demonstrates a large mass in the posterior portion of the right kidney with an irregular central area of hypodensity with contrast enhancement, suggesting necrosis

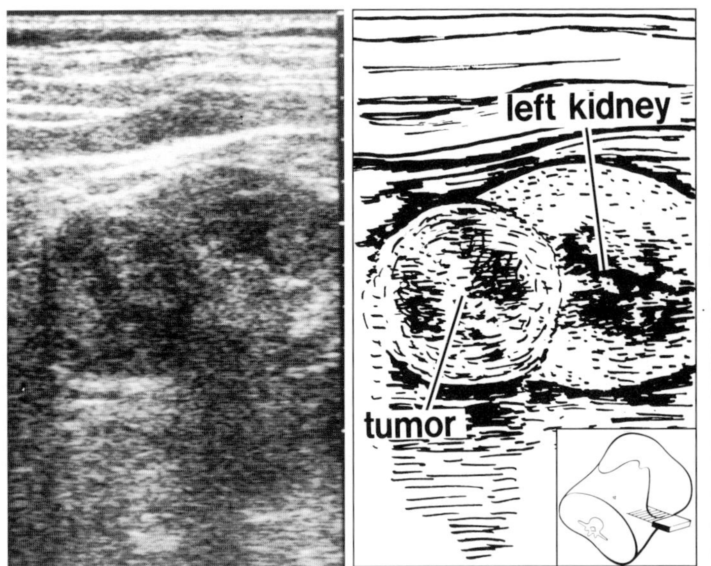

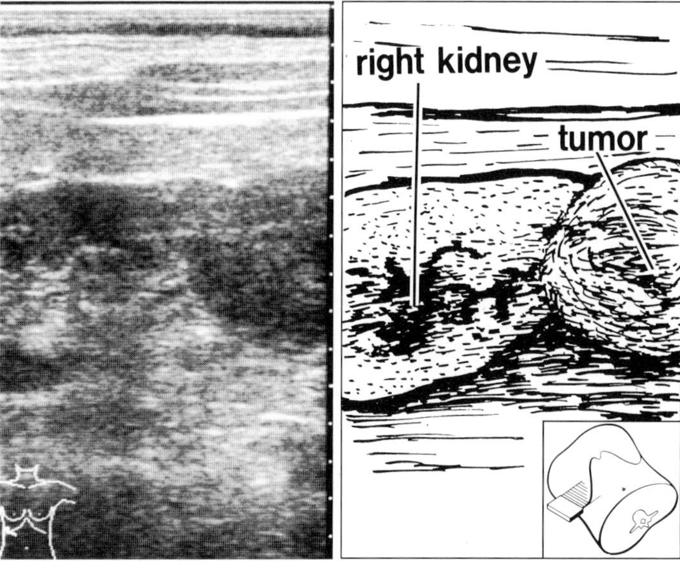

Fig. 7.32. *Case 3.* Longitudinal section of the left kidney, obtained from the left side of the abdomen, demonstrates a 4-cm solid tumor in the lower pole with partial exophytic growth. This proven case of renal cell carcinoma was incidentally found on a screening ultrasonographic examination of the abdomen

Fig. 7.33. *Case 4.* There is a 5-cm solid tumor arising from the lower pole of the right kidney with partial exophytic growth. The internal echo pattern is relatively homogeneous

Transitional Cell Carcinoma of the Kidneys

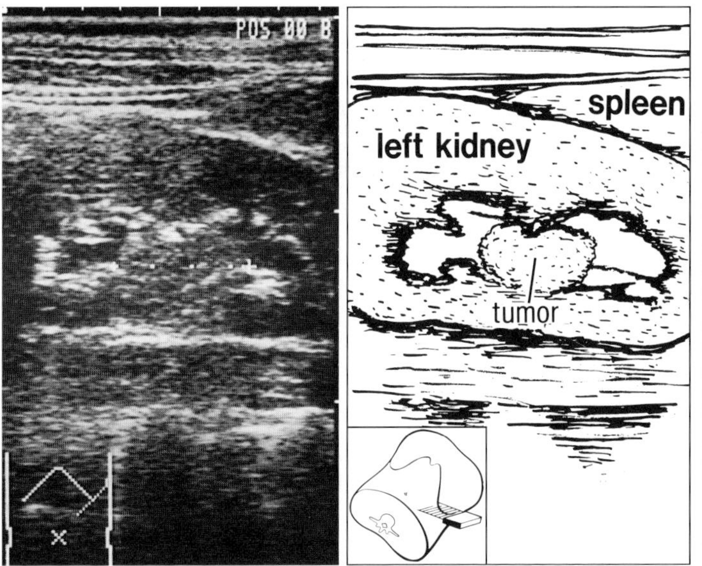

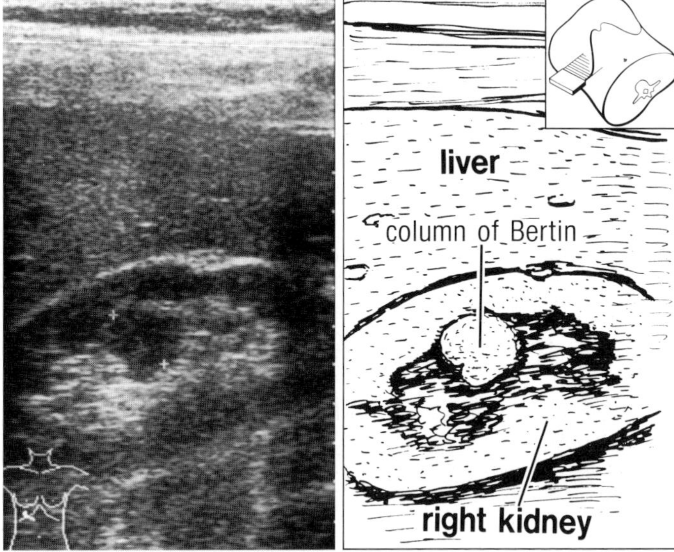

Fig. 7.34. *Case 1.* The patient is a 33-year-old with hematuria. There is a 3.5-cm solid mass within the left renal pelvis. On this image alone, differentiation from a blood clot is difficult

Fig. 7.35. *A case for comparison.* There is a 19-mm solid mass in the renal sinus. This is a column of Bertin, which is partial hypertrophy of the renal cortex protruding into the renal sinus

**Metastatic Tumor
to the Kidneys**

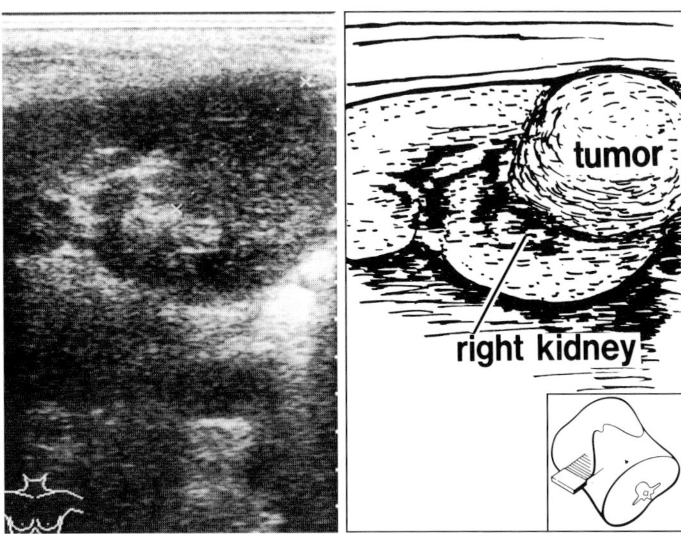

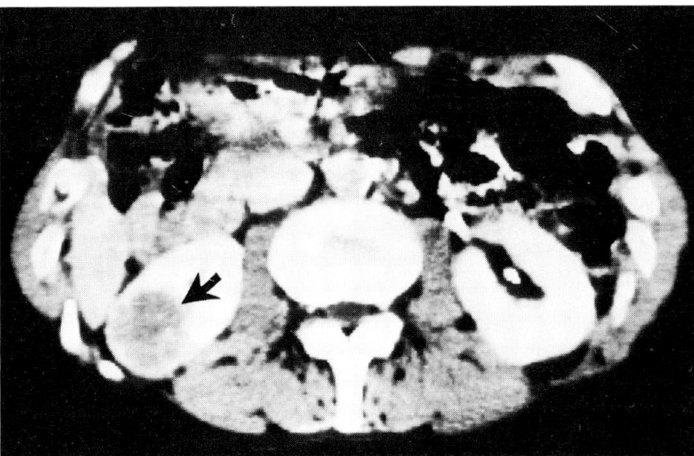

Fig. 7.36. *Case 1.* There is a 5-cm solid tumor in the lower pole of the right kidney. This patient had had surgery for carcinoma of the lung, and recent CT and ultrasonographic examination showed metastases to the liver and kidneys

Fig. 7.37. *Case 1, CT scan.* This showed a 5-cm low-density mass in the lower pole of the right kidney

Renal Hamartoma

Renal hamartoma is a benign tumor containing fat, smooth muscle, and blood vessels. It is also called angiomyolipoma and is often seen in patients with tuberous sclerosis. The ultrasonographic findings are variable, depending on the predominant component of the tumor. The portion of the tumor within which adipose tissue is visualized is markedly hyperechoic.

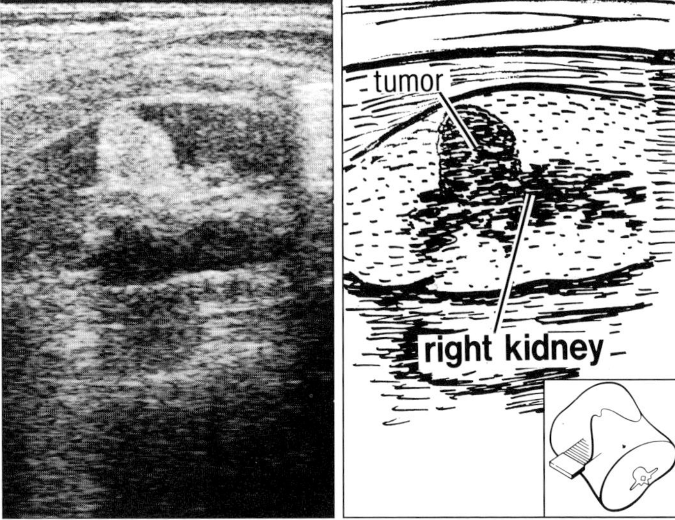

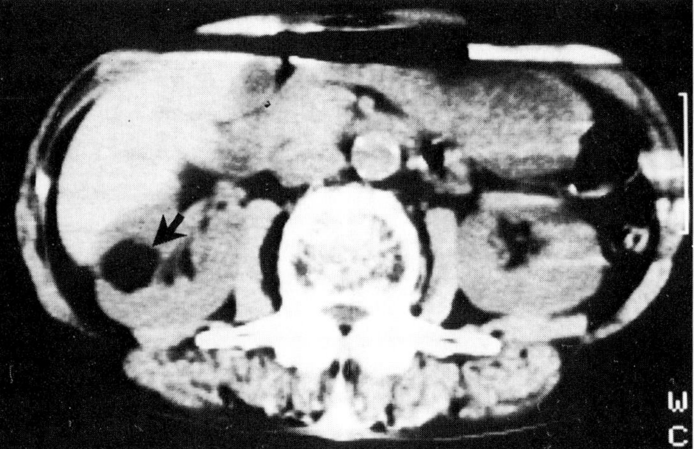

Fig. 7.38. *Case 1.* There is a 2-cm hyperechoic mass in the lateral portion of the right kidney

Fig. 7.39. *Case 1, CT scan.* This shows a 2-cm low-density mass in the lateral portion of the right kidney (−67 HU). This density is consistent with fatty tissue

Chronic Renal Failure

Ultrasonographic changes are seen only in cases of severe nephritis with deformity. In acute renal failure, there is swelling of the kidney, and the renal parenchyma becomes hypoechoic. Pyonephrosis may exhibit hypoechoic areas suggesting abscess or necrosis within the renal substance. In advanced renal failure, the kidneys become decreased in

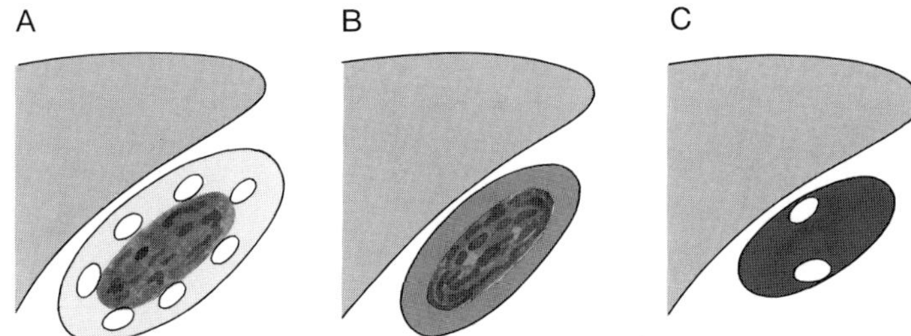

Fig. 7.40 A–C. *Ultrasonographic pattern of chronic renal failure.* In renal failure, the kidney becomes small in size and the echo level of the renal parenchyma is increased. In severe cases of renal failure, the kidneys become diffusely hyperechoic. **A** Normal kidney; **B** minimal renal failure; **C** severe renal failure

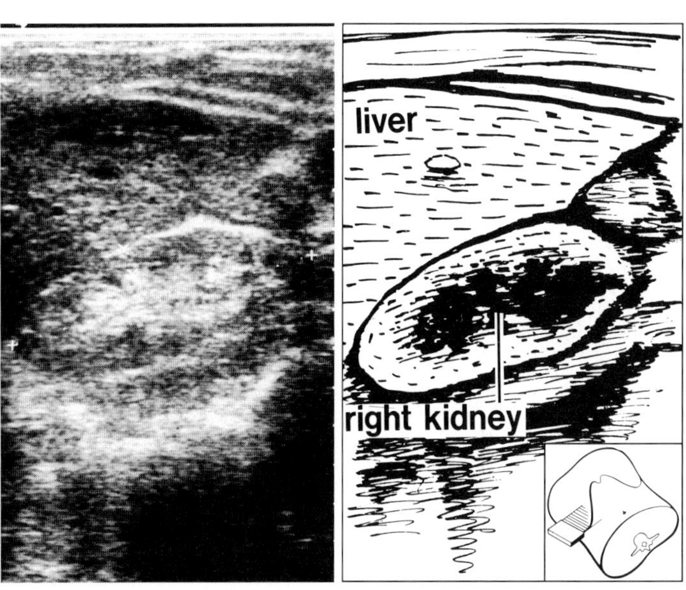

Fig. 7.41. *Case 1.* The length of the right kidney is decreased to 75 mm, and there is decreased thickness of the renal parenchyma. The echo level of the renal parenchyma is increased and slightly higher than that of the liver (blood urea nitrogen 69 mg/dl, creatinine 6.9 mg/dl)

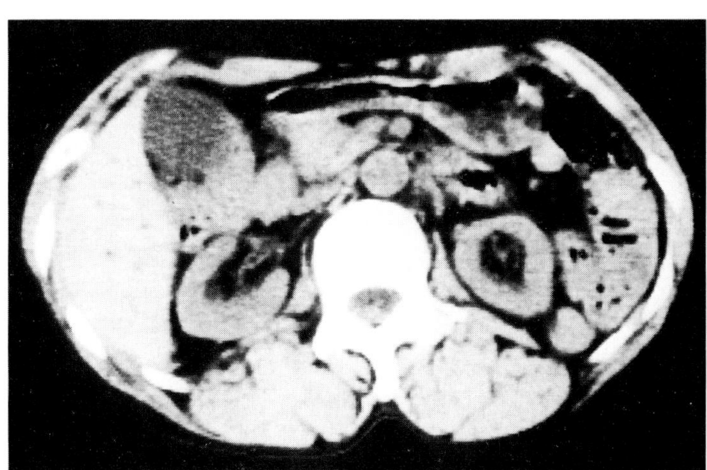

Fig. 7.42. *Case 1, CT scan.* Both kidneys are generally decreased in size

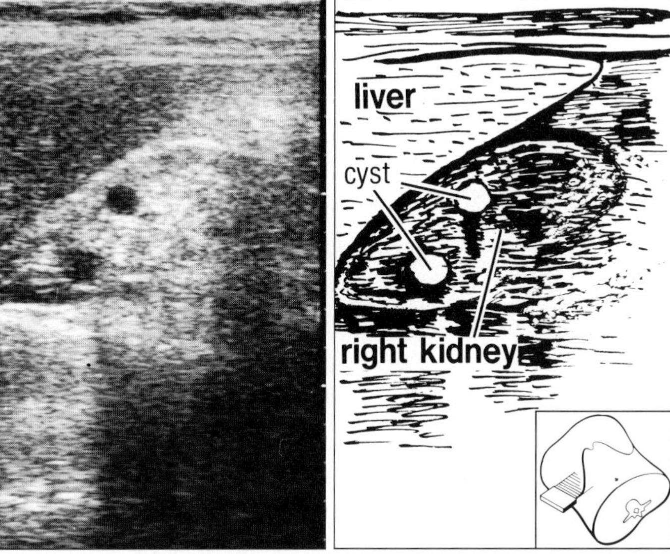

Fig. 7.43. *Case 2.* There is marked atrophy of the kidney. The overall echogenicity of the kidney is increased, and there is no differentiation between the renal parenchyma and the renal sinus. There are two small cysts. This is a typical appearance of chronic renal failure (creatinine 5.7 mg/dl)

size. Secondary to fibrosis, the echogenicity of the renal cortex becomes increased relative to normal. Consequently, the entire kidney appears rather homogeneous with poor corticomedullary distinction. Owing to their small size and change in overall echogenicity, the kidneys tend to blend into the surrounding structures, and thus the kidneys become more difficult to localize. Small renal cysts are often seen.

Complications of Renal Transplantation

Ultrasonography is now an important modality in the evaluation of renal transplants. In acute rejection, ultrasonographic findings include globular enlargement of the kidney, swelling and hypoechogenicity of the medullary pyramids, an indistinct corticomedullary junction, and foci in the renal cortex. A Doppler study may show decreased diastolic flow of the renal arteries (increased pulsatility index). Note should be made, however, that rejection may be present in the absence of significant ultrasonographic findings. The clinical features of acute tubular necrosis may be similar to acute rejection, but ultrasonographically the transplanted kidney with acute tubular necrosis is usually normal.

Ultrasonography can easily detect hydronephrosis of the transplanted kidney. The proximal ureter may be visualized when dilated, but the distal ureter is usually difficult to visualize because of overlapping intestinal gas. Obstruction may be caused by ureteral stricture, extrinsic compression by mass or fluid collection, or a blood clot or stone in the collecting system.

Perinephric fluid collections are also easily visualized by ultrasonography. These include lymphoceles, urinomas, hematomas, abscesses, and seromas. The ultrasonographic appearance is nonspecific, and the exact nature of the fluid can be determined only by aspiration.

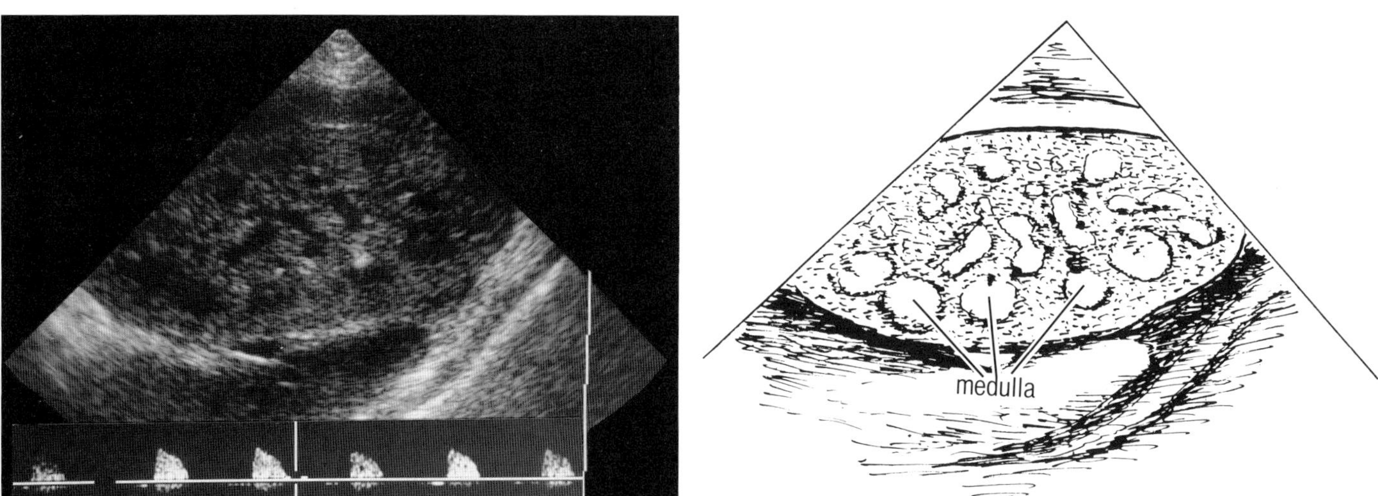

Fig. 7.44. *Case 1.* Acute transplant rejection. There is globular enlargement of the kidney. The medullary pyramids are swollen and decreased in echogenicity. The central echo complex is also hypoechoic. The Doppler study shows complete loss of diastolic flow (pulsatility index is 1.0)

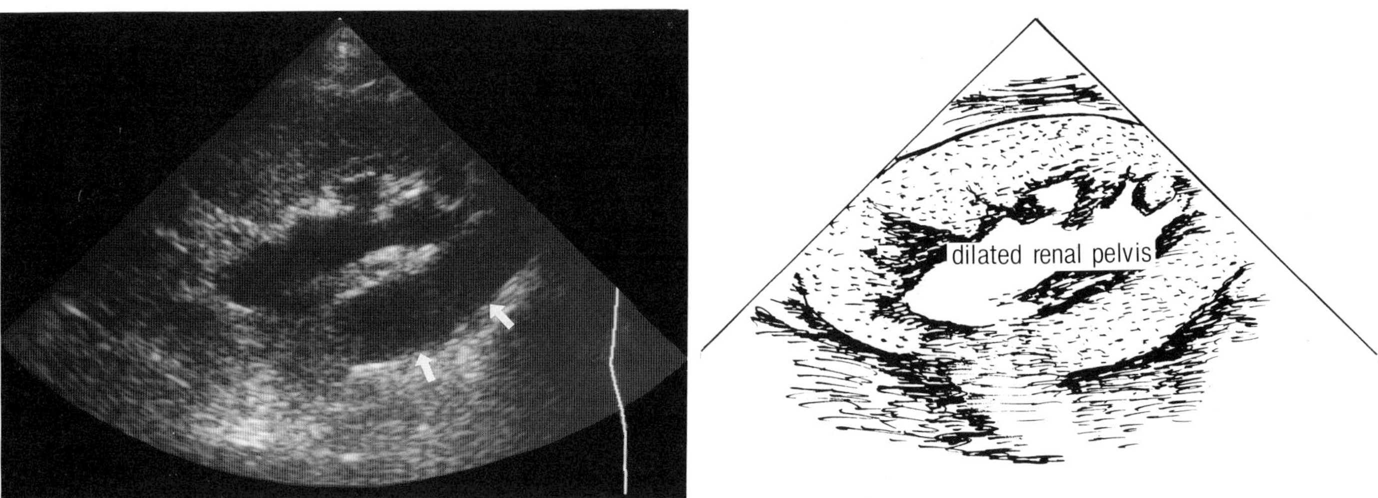

Fig. 7.45. *Case 2*. Obstruction. There is moderate dilatation of the collecting system. Nephrostogram showed severe stricture of the ureter

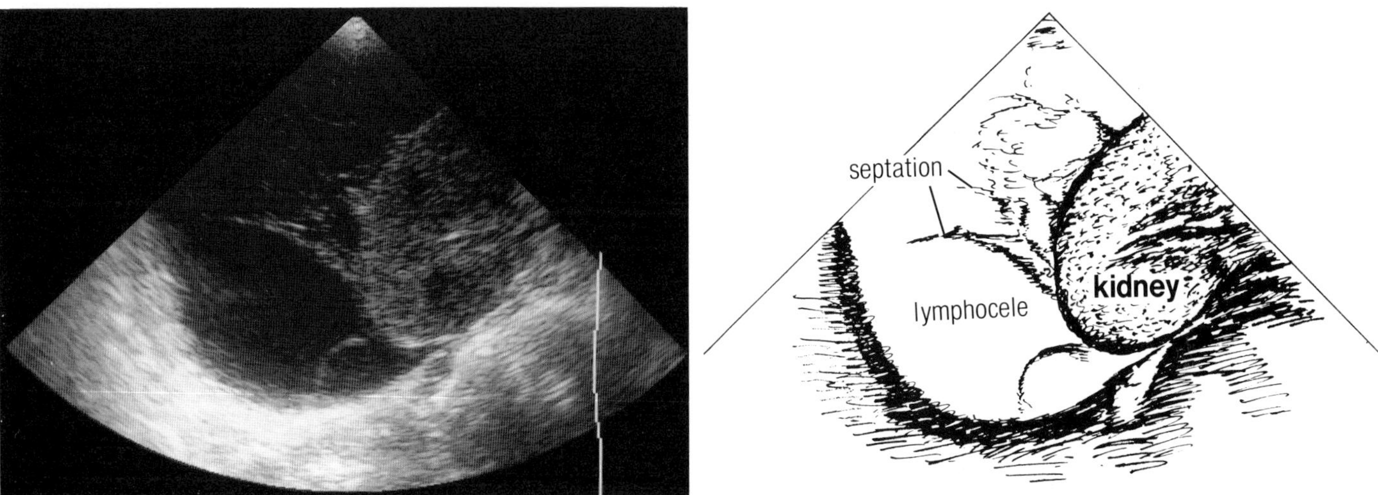

Fig. 7.46. *Case 3*. Lymphocele. An extrarenal fluid collection is seen 3 weeks after transplantation. Fine septations are seen, which is not uncommon in lymphoceles

Perirenal Hematoma

Perirenal hematoma can be caused by trauma or renal biopsy. Iatrogenic hematoma secondary to renal biopsy seldom forms within the kidney, forming more often in the perirenal space around the needle puncture site. When there is a large hematoma, the kidney is displaced anteriorly. Scanning from the back in the area of the skin puncture with the patient in the prone position usually reveals a thin, solid mass posterior to the kidney. The hematoma is more easily recognized when a comparison is made with opposite kidney.

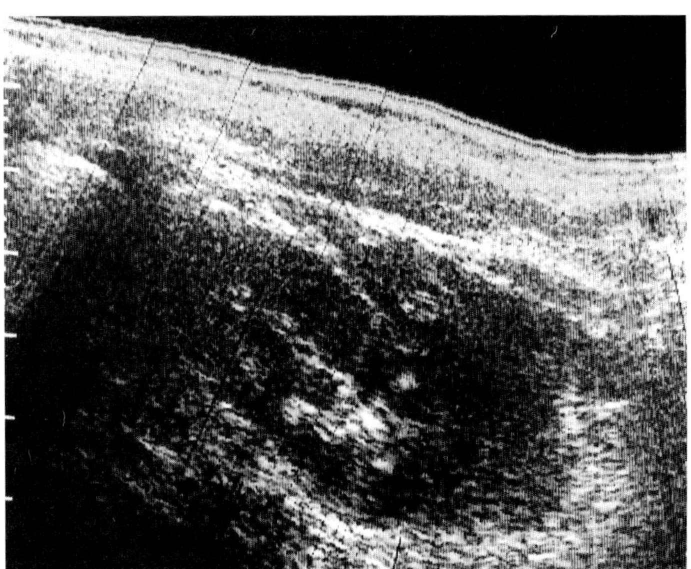

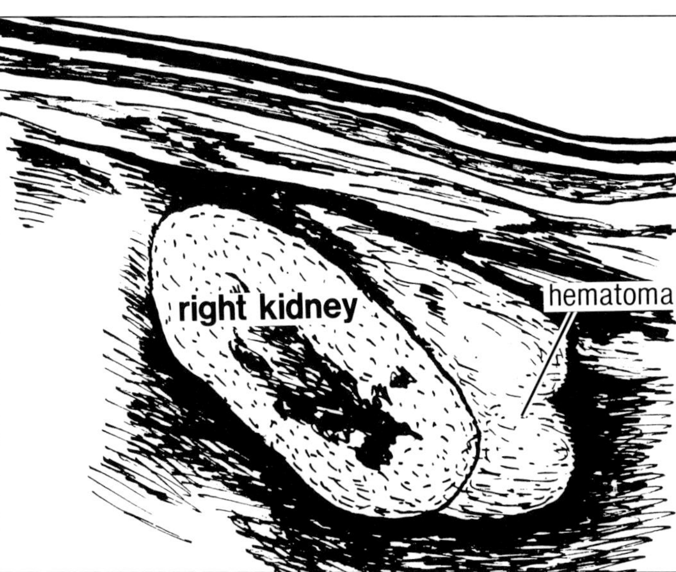

Fig. 7.47. *Case 1.* Contact compound scanner image obtained from the back in a patient who had had blunt right flank trauma in a motor vehicle accident 10 days earlier. There is a hypoechoic mass around the lower pole of the right kidney, suggesting hematoma. The lower pole of the right kidney is significantly anteriorly displaced

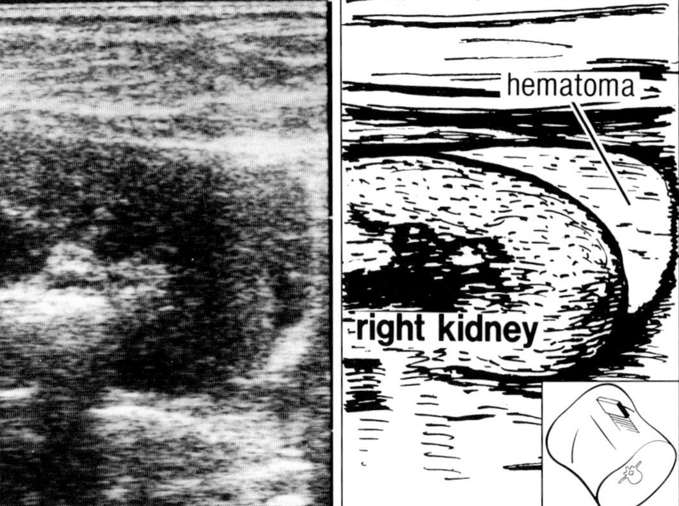

Fig. 7.48. *Case 2.* There is a crescent-shaped hematoma, approximately isoechoic to the renal parenchyma, dorsal to the lower pole of the right kidney. This mass was secondary to a renal biopsy

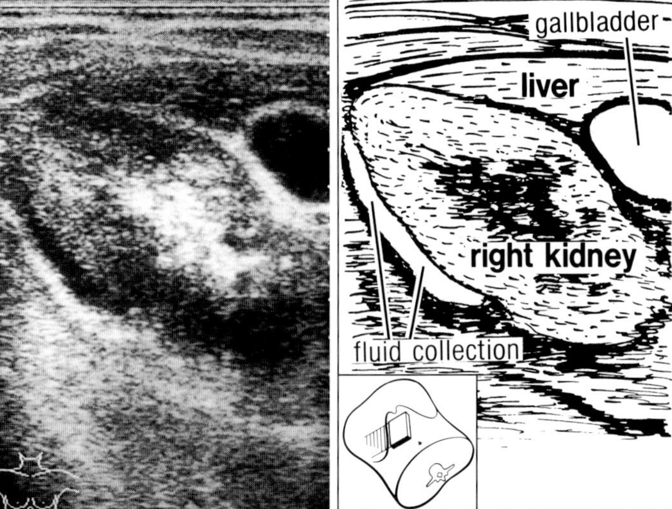

Fig. 7.49. *Case 3.* There is an anechoic space posterior to the right kidney representing a postbiopsy hematoma

Perirenal Pseudocyst

A collection of urine in the perirenal space, which has extravasated from a small rent in a renal calix, the renal pelvis, or the ureter, is called a perirenal pseudocyst, urinoma, or hydrocele renalis. Urinary tract extravasation can be caused by intrinsic obstruction (for example calculus or blood clot) or extrinsic compression of the ureter. This entity is differentiated from a true cyst as the collection of urine is not surrounded by epithelial cells.

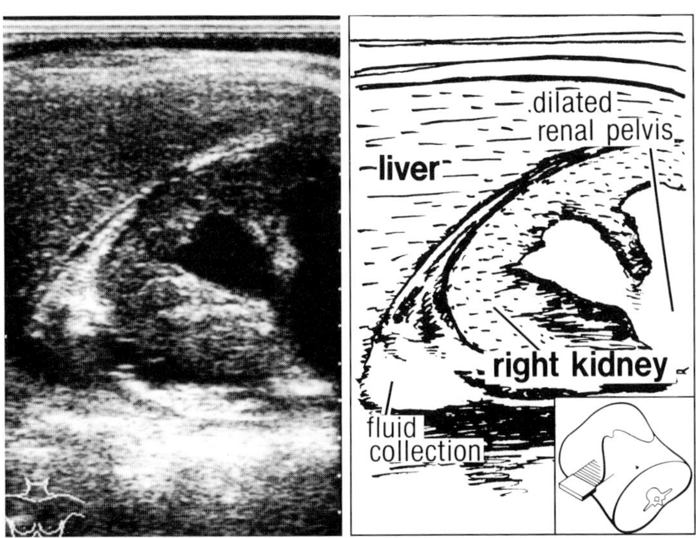

Fig. 7.50. *Case 1.* There is an anechoic space around the upper pole of the right kidney. There is also a thin anechoic space in Morison's pouch, suggesting ascites. The renal pelvis and renal calices are dilated and appear anechoic, indicating hydronephrosis

Fig. 7.51. *Case 1, intravenous pyelogram.* The right kidney shows moderate hydronephrosis. There is an abnormal collection of contrast outside the renal collecting system, indicating contrast extravasation

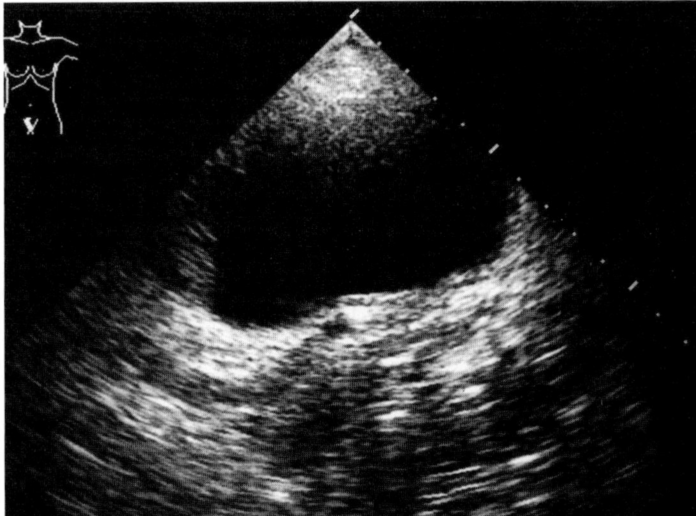

Fig. 7.52. *Case 1.* Oblique transverse section of the urinary bladder. There is a hyperechoic area measuring approximately 1 cm at the orifice of the right ureter and associated with acoustic shadowing.

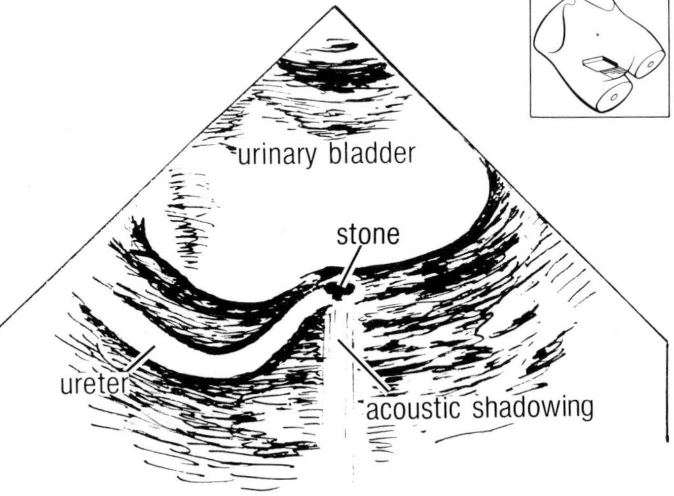

There is mild dilatation of the ureter. Normally, the ureter is not visualized in this location. This case represents a pararenal pseudocyst secondary to obstruction of the right ureter by a stone

Horseshoe Kidney

A horseshoe kidney is a congenital abnormality which occurs secondary to fusion of the lower poles of the kidneys. The ultrasonographic examination should be performed in the supine position, as the isthmus of the horseshoe kidney cannot be visualized in the prone position due to obscuration by the spine. When the isthmus of the kidneys is visualized, diagnosis of horseshoe kidney can be confirmed. However, it is often difficult to visualize the connective tissue which connects the kidneys. Ultrasonographic diagnosis of horseshoe kidney is usually made only when there is a very small amount of intestinal gas or when the patient is thin.

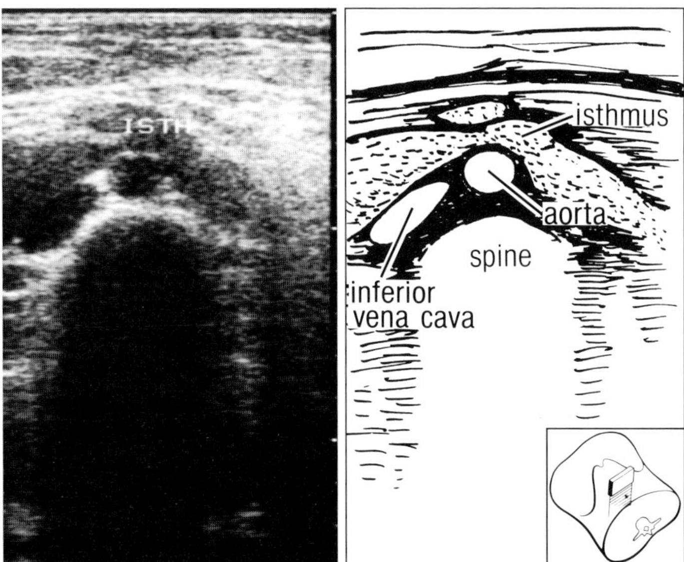

Fig. 7.53. *Case 1.* Transverse section through the isthmus of a horseshoe kidney. The isthmus connecting the lower poles of the kidneys is visualized anterior to the abdominal aorta and inferior vena cava

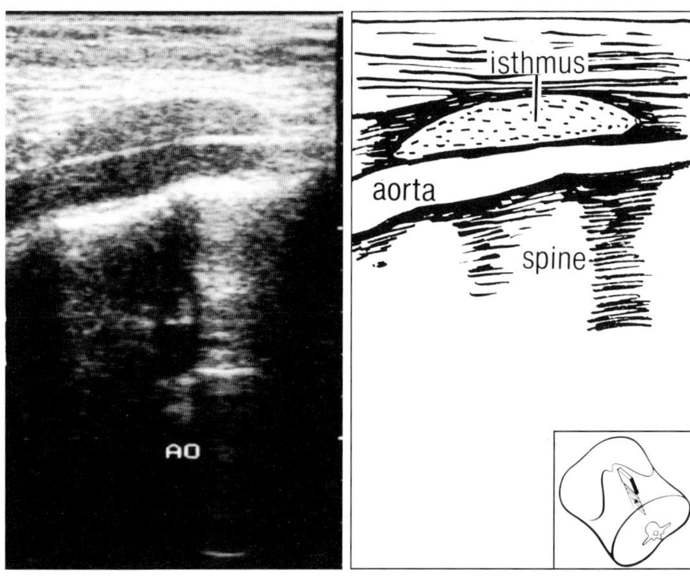

Fig. 7.54. *Case 1.* Longitudinal section of the abdominal aorta. Discoid tissue anterior to the abdominal aorta represents the isthmus of the horseshoe kidney

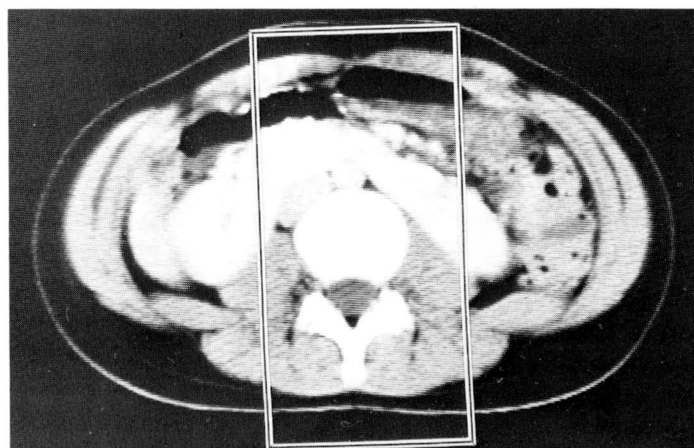

Fig. 7.55. *Case 1, CT scan.* This shows contrast enhancement of the lower poles of the kidneys and the isthmus

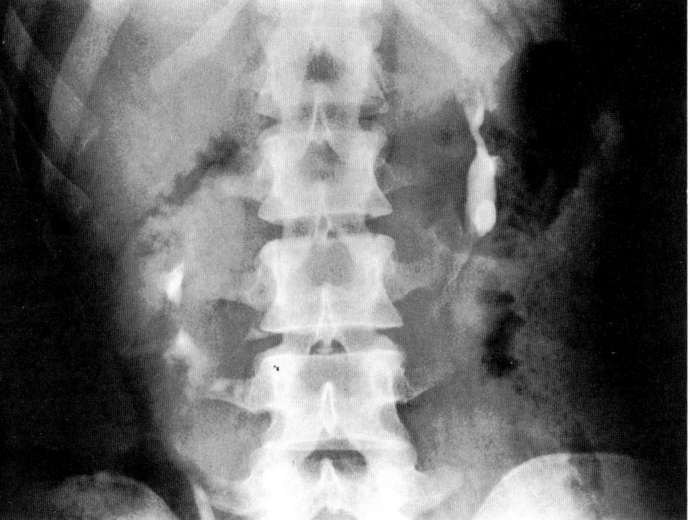

Fig. 7.56. *Case 1, intravenous pyelogram.* Judging from the distribution of the renal calices, the long axis of the kidneys is reversed (converging inferiorly), and the renal pelves are directed anteriorly. This is a typical intravenous pyelogram image of a horseshoe kidney with fusion of both kidneys inferiorly

Duplex Renal Pelvis and Double Ureters

The duplex renal pelvis is a relatively frequent congenital anomaly of the urinary tract. The ureter may show complete duplication, or double ureters may join to form a single ureter distally. Ultrasonographic examination of the kidneys will demonstrate a central echo complex which is separated into two discrete regions. Note that the central echo complex can appear to be separated in a normal kidney with certain angulations of the transducer head.

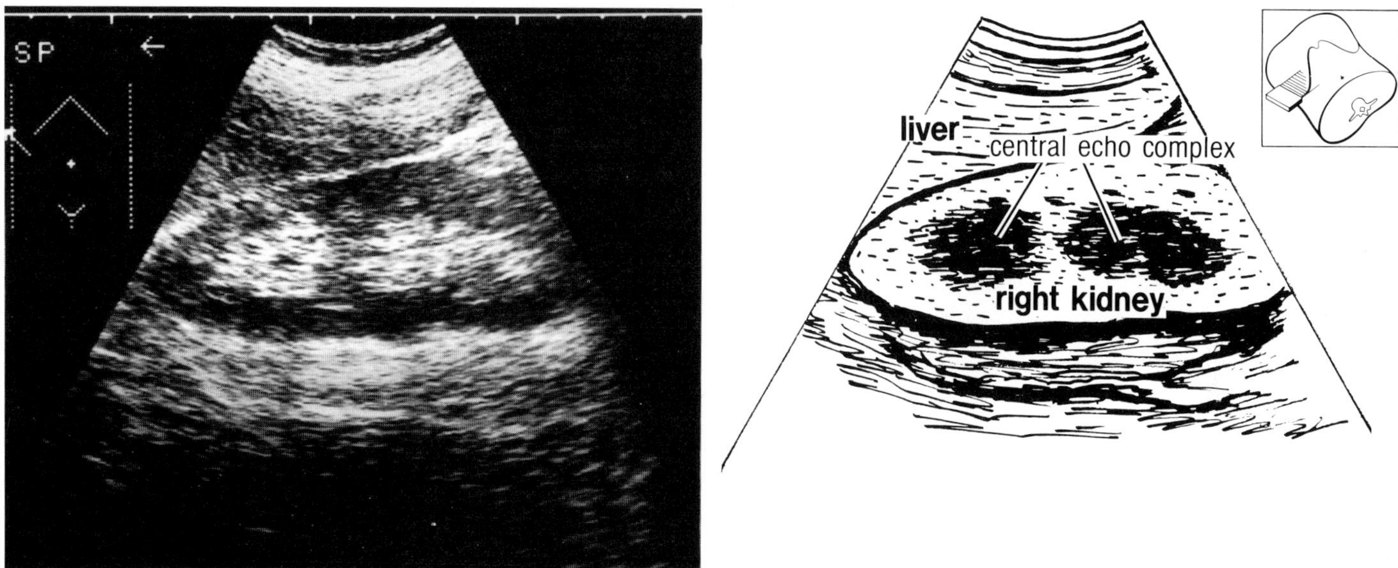

Fig. 7.57. *Case 1.* Coronal section of the right kidney, obtained from the right side of the abdomen. The central echo complex is divided into two portions. The superior portion is slightly smaller than the inferior portion. Frequently, these have a ratio of 1 : 2

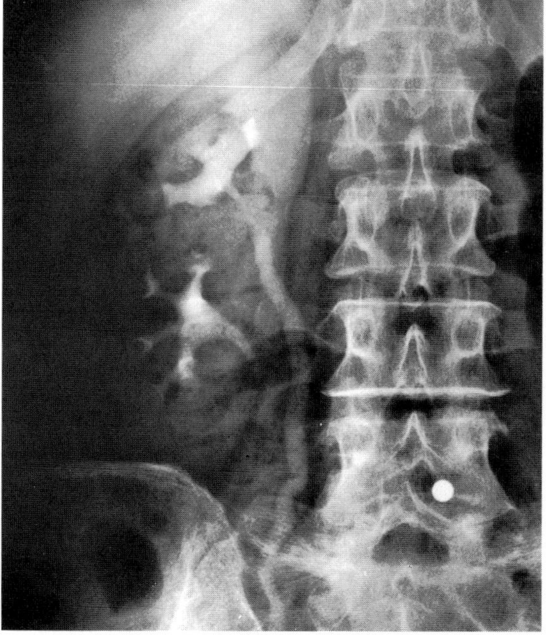

Fig. 7.58. *Case 1, intravenous pyelogram.* There is a duplication of the right renal pelvis and ureter. The ureters join to form a single lower ureter distally (duplex renal pelvis with incomplete double ureter)

Complete Duplication of the Renal Pelvis and Ureter, with Associated Ureterocele

Ureterocele is an anomaly of the urinary tract manifested by cystic dilatation of the distal ureter immediately above the ureteral orifice of the bladder. Ectopic ureterocele is seen in children and is always associated with ureteral duplication.

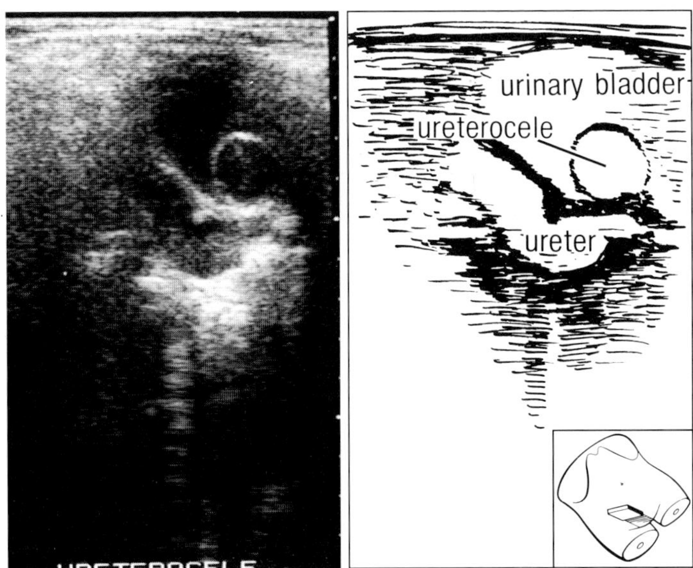

Fig. 7.59. *Case 1.* The lower segment of the right ureter, located behind the bladder, is dilated. A ureterocele is visualized as a balloon-like cystic orifice of the right ureter. The size of the ureterocele is different on ultrasonography when compared to the intravenous pyleogram of the same case (Fig. 7.60). As in this case, the size of a ureterocele changes with time

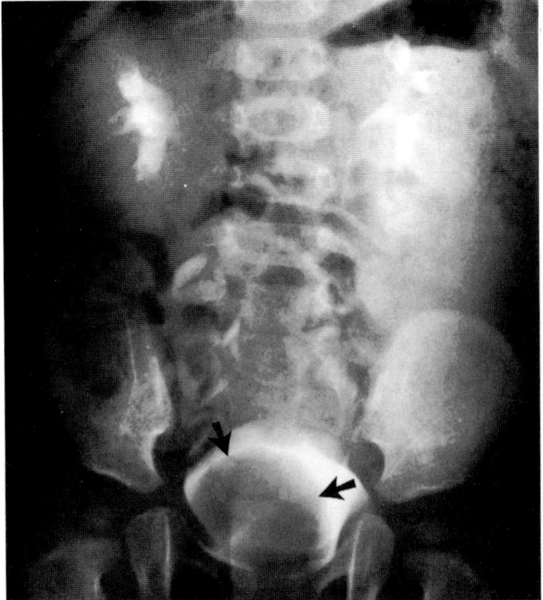

Fig. 7.60. *Case 1, Intravenous pyelogram.* Only the mid and lower portions of the right kidney are visualized. The large filling defect in the urinary bladder represents a ureterocele

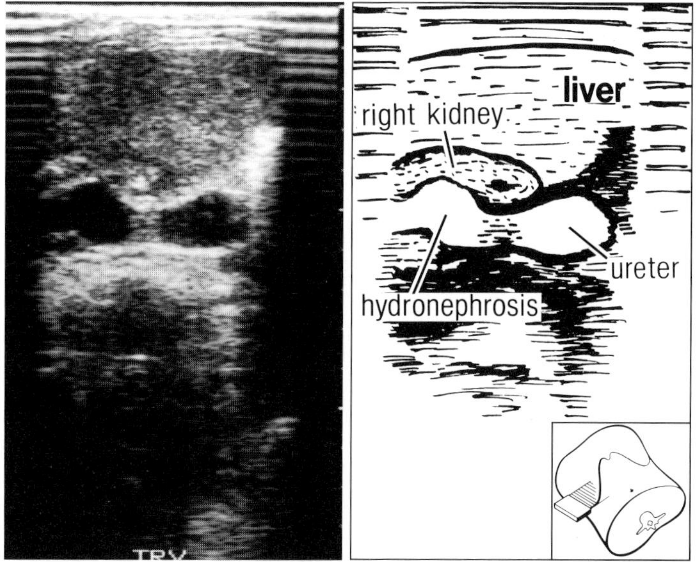

Fig. 7.61. *Case 1.* The renal pelvis in the upper pole of the right kidney and the ureter are dilated and appear anechoic

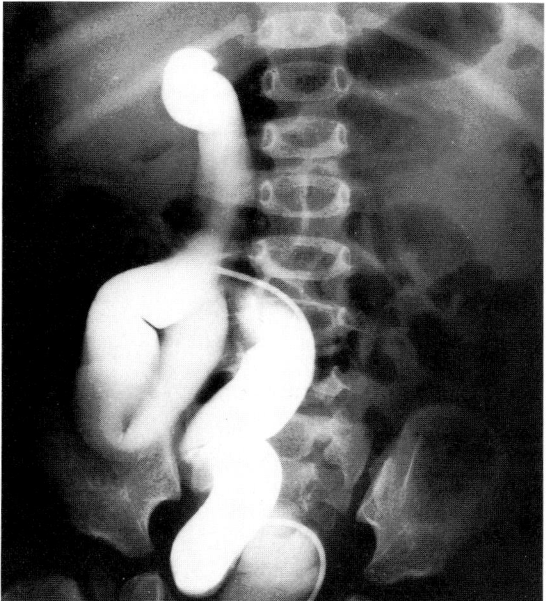

Fig. 7.62. *Case 1, retrograde pyelogram.* The catheter is inserted into the right ureter through the ureterocele. The renal pelvis of the right upper pole and ureter are markedly dilated

8 Adrenal Glands

**Anatomy
of the Adrenal Glands**

The adrenal glands are small, yellow, retroperitoneal organs located within the adipose tissue near the upper poles of the kidneys. The right adrenal gland is triangular in shape and appears as a cap over the upper pole of the right kidney. On transverse section, it lies medial to the right lobe of the liver, posterior to the inferior vena cava and adjacent to the right crus of the diaphragm. The left adrenal is half-moon shaped and is located on a line connecting the upper pole of the left kidney and the aorta, adjacent to the left crus of the diaphragm.

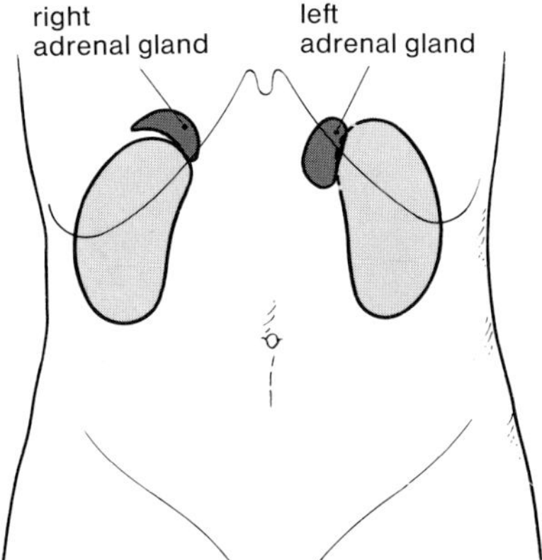

Fig. 8.1. Position of the adrenal glands

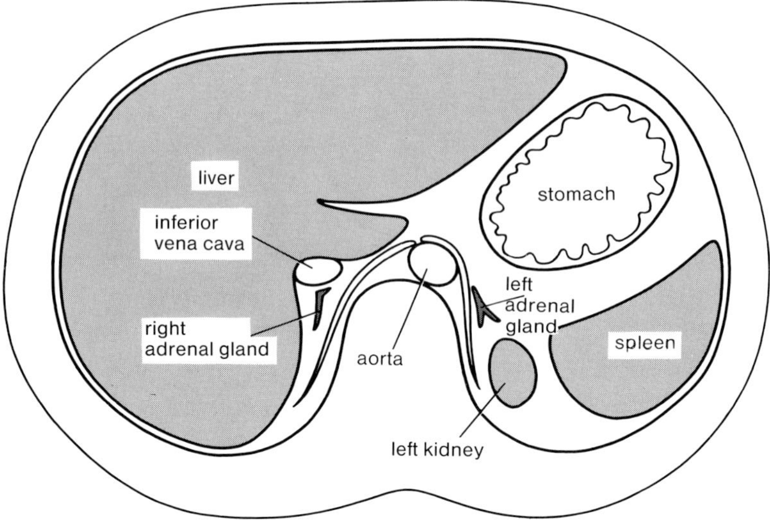

Fig. 8.2. Transverse section of the adrenal glands and surrounding organs

Scanning Techniques

The right adrenal gland is relatively easy to visualize by careful observation in the region between the liver and the upper pole of the right kidney. The liver can function as an acoustic window, and intercostal or subcostal scanning can be useful. Because of intestinal gas, the left adrenal gland cannot be visualized from the abdomen in the supine position, except when there is an enlarged spleen. It can be examined from the posterior abdomen with right lateral decubitus positioning on an image which contains the left kidney and the aorta.

Ultrasonographic Appearance of a Normal Adrenal Gland

A normal adrenal gland is difficult to visualize because of its small size and deep position. Using a contact compound scanner with a sharp focal zone in the deep portion of the abdomen, the normal adrenal gland is occasionally visualized in a thin patient, whereas it is extremely difficult with a linear scanner.

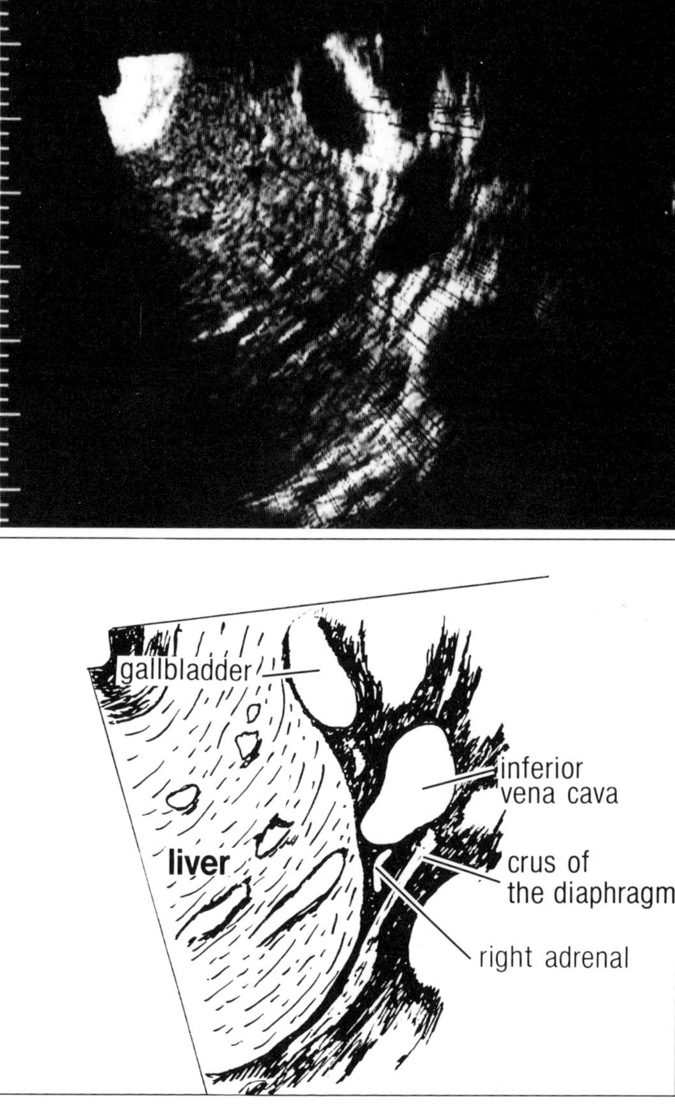

Fig. 8.3. Right adrenal gland imaged from an intercostal space with a contact compound scanner

Metastatic Tumor of the Adrenal Gland

There is a relatively high incidence of adrenal gland metastases from lung cancer. Metastases can also be seen in cases of breast, renal, and hepatocellular carcinomas. These metastatic tumors can be visualized as solid masses with weak internal echoes.

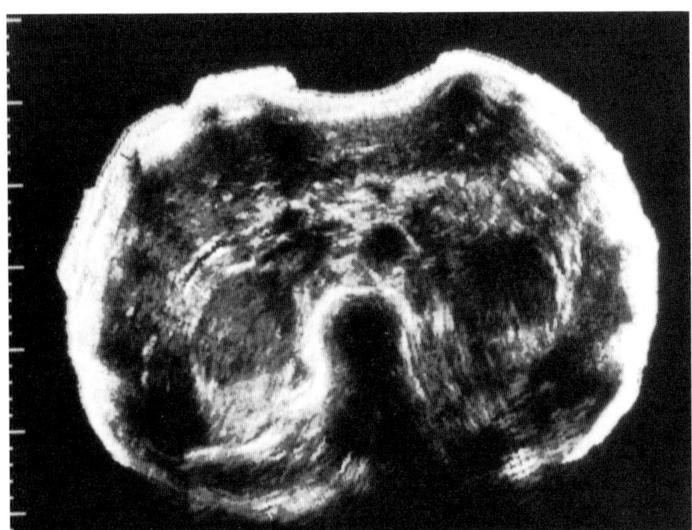

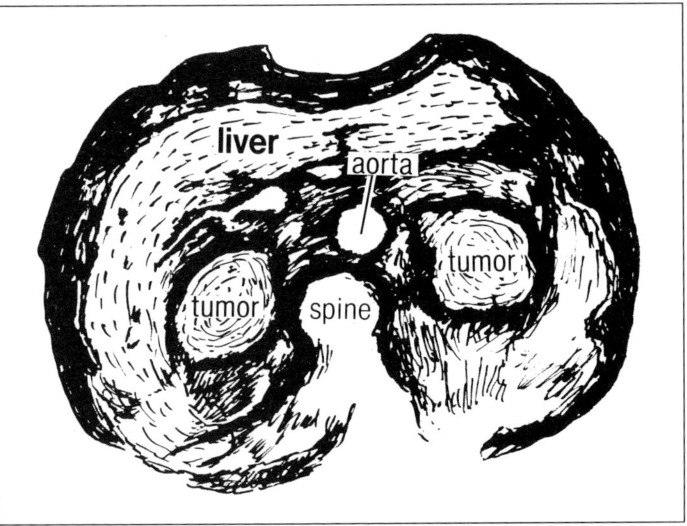

Fig. 8.4. *Case 1.* A patient with lung cancer and cervical lymph node enlargement. Ultrasonographic examination of the liver to rule out metastases showed marked enlargement of the adrenal glands. There was also enlargement of multiple lymph nodes posterior to the inferior vena cava and around the pancreas. There were no significant abnormalities in the liver

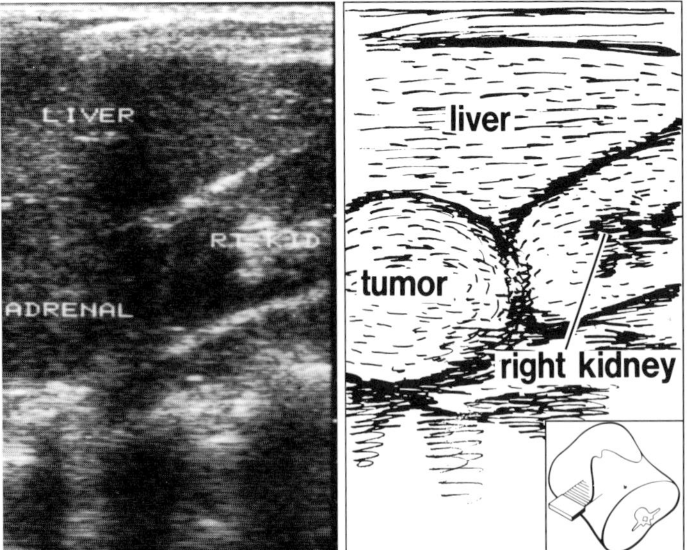

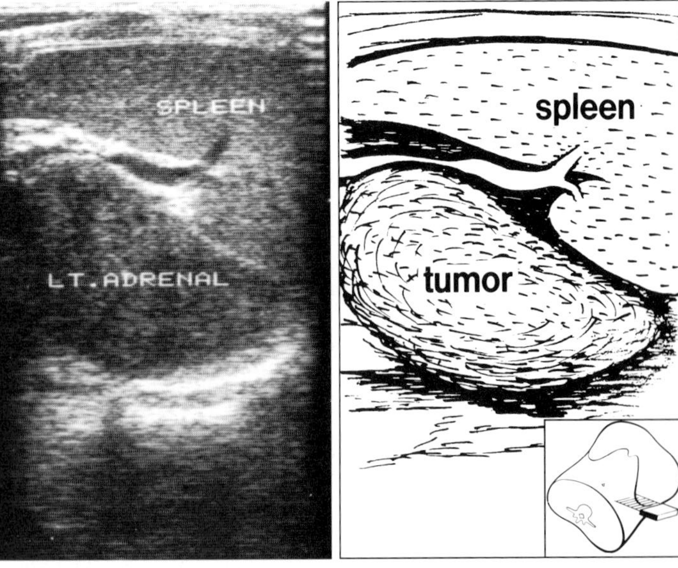

Fig. 8.5. *Case 1, image of the right adrenal gland performed with a linear scanner.* There is a 45-mm solid tumor with a homogeneous echo texture seen adjacent to the upper pole of the right kidney

Fig. 8.6. *Case 1, intercostal image of the left adrenal gland.* There is an ovoid-shaped solid tumor adjacent to the splenic hilum

Pheochromocytoma

When present in the region of the adrenal glands, pheochromocytoma is frequently visualized on ultrasonographic examination. It is usually visualized as a solid tumor of 3–6 cm in size, often with multiple small cystic components inside the tumor. This finding is secondary to degeneration and necrosis of the tumor.

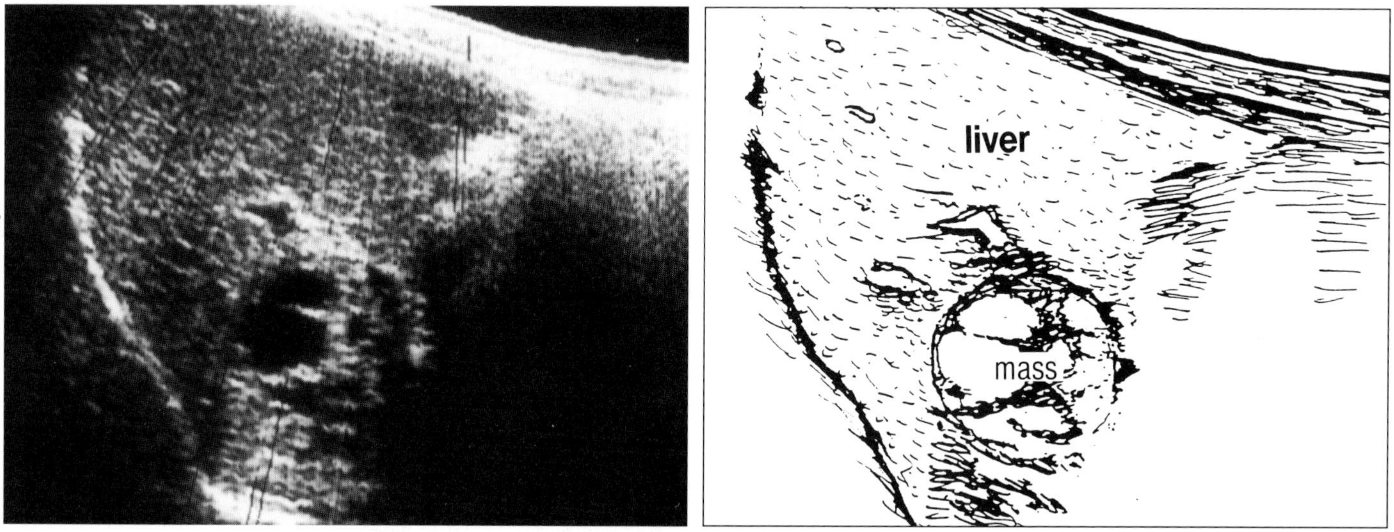

Fig. 8.7 A, B. These images were obtained using a contact compound scanner. The transverse section (**A**) shows a 6 × 4-cm solid mass medial to the right lobe of the liver. There is an irregularly shaped, anechoic space inside the tumor. Tumor arising from the liver can be excluded as this is separated from the liver by a distinct tissue plane. The longitudinal section (**B**) shows a solid mass indenting the lower surface of the liver. Again, cystic components are visualized within the tumor as on the transverse section

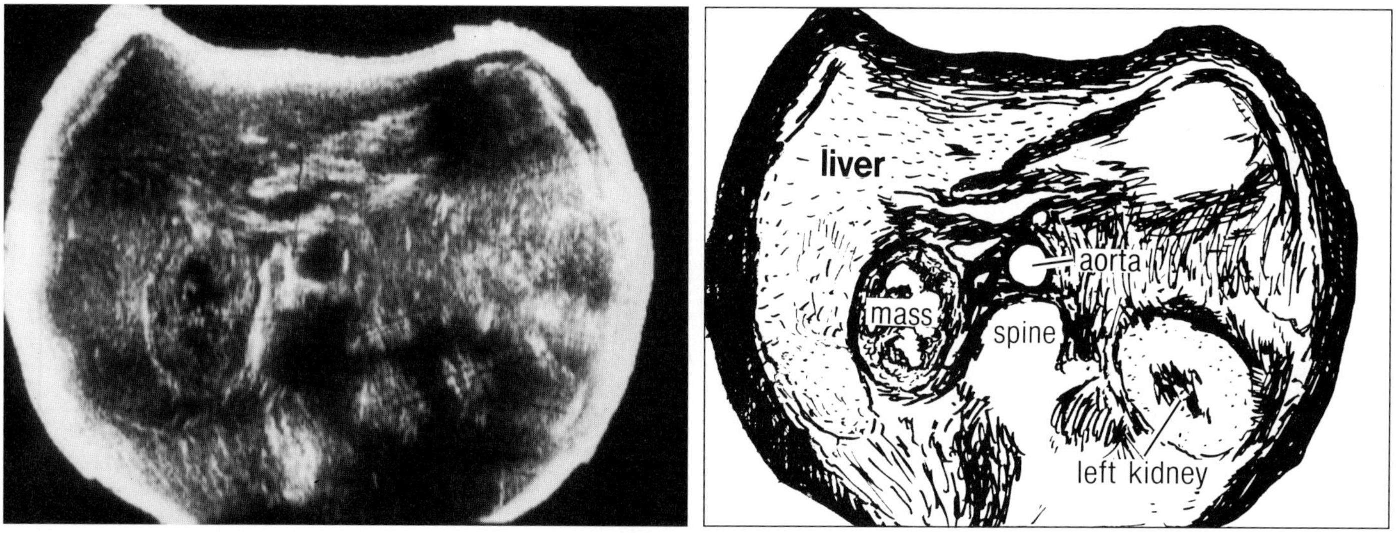

9 Retroperitoneum

**Anatomy
of the Retroperitoneum**

The organs of the retroperitoneum include the kidneys, adrenal glands, pancreas, part of the duodenum, and the ascending and descending colon. However, generally speaking, diseases of the retroperitoneum include diseases of connective tissue, fatty tissue, muscle, fascia, the lymphatic system, the vascular system, and the sympathetic system.

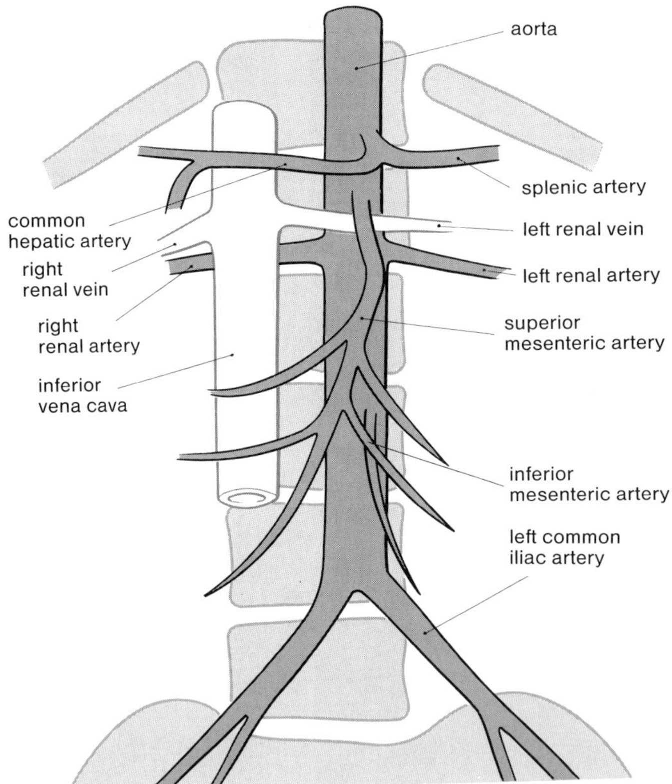

Fig. 9.1. Anatomy of the retroperitoneum

**Ultrasonographic
Appearance
of Normal Blood Vessels
in the Upper Abdomen**

The following are representative ultrasonographic images of the normal upper abdominal vasculature. Interpretation is facilitated by comparison with Fig. 9.1.

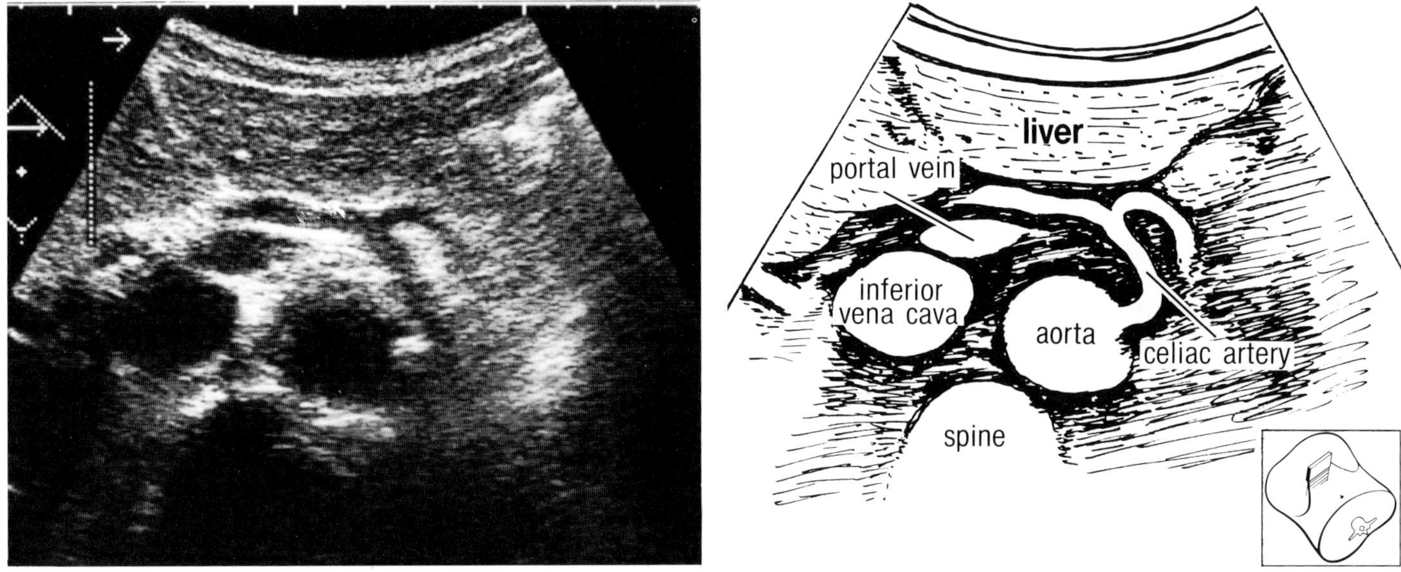

Fig. 9.2. *Case 1.* The celiac artery arising from the abdominal aorta and its branches (common hepatic artery and splenic artery) are visualized

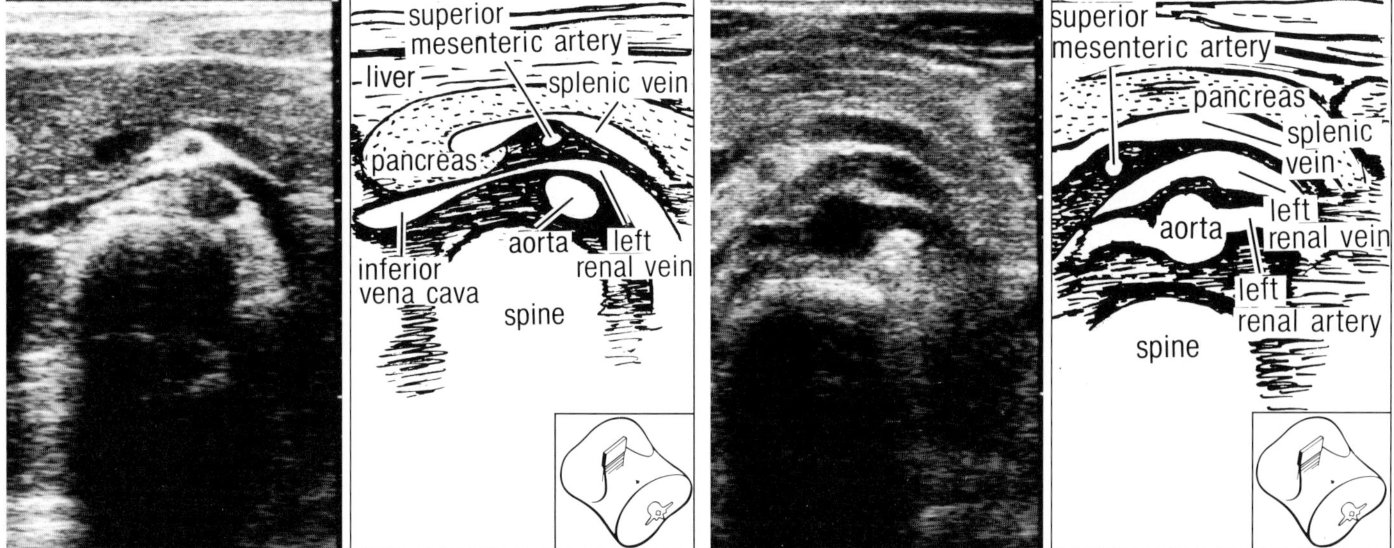

Fig. 9.3. *Case 2.* The splenic vein running transversely in the midline of the upper abdomen and the left renal vein are visualized. While the splenic vein runs anterior to the superior mesenteric artery, the left renal vein courses posterior to the superior mesenteric artery and is on the anterior surface of the abdominal aorta

Fig. 9.4. *Case 3.* The splenic vein, left renal vein, and bilateral renal arteries are clearly visualized. It is rather unusual that the left renal vein is as prominent as in this case

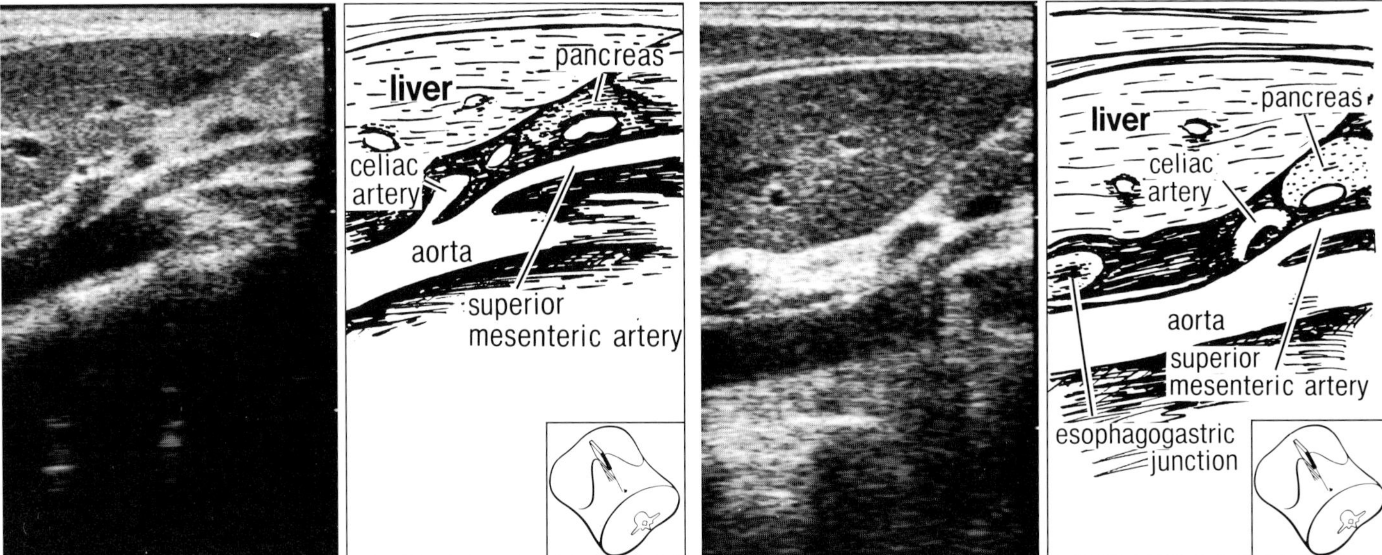

Fig. 9.5. *Case 4.* Longitudinal section of the abdominal aorta demonstrates the origins of the celiac artery and superior mesenteric artery from the abdominal aorta

Fig. 9.6. *Case 5.* The esophagogastric junction and left crus of the diaphragm are visualized between the abdominal aorta and the left lobe of the liver

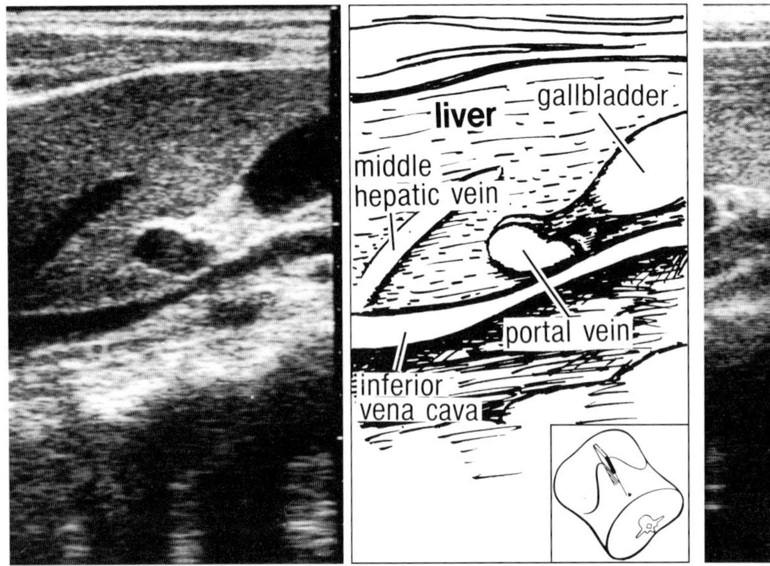

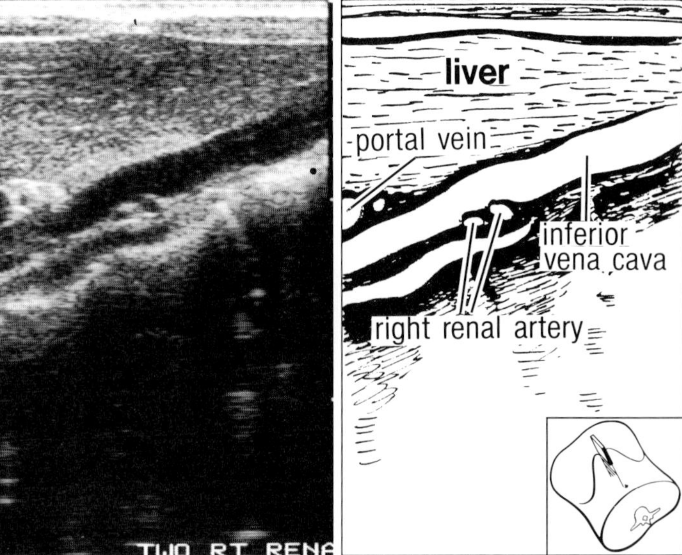

Fig. 9.7. *Case 6.* Longitudinal section of the inferior vena cava shows the middle hepatic vein which drains into the inferior vena cava away from the liver. The main trunk of the portal vein is visualized adjacent to the inferior vena cava near the neck of the gallbladder

Fig. 9.8. *Case 7.* There are two cystic structures adjacent to the posterior wall of the inferior vena cava, representing the right renal arteries in cross-section. In this patient, there are two right renal arteries

Left Inferior Vena Cava   Left inferior vena cava is a congenital anomaly due to anomalous development during fetal life. The left inferior vena cava crosses the abdominal aorta anteriorly, immediately above the level of the renal vein, and is located to the left of the abdominal aorta below this level. This anomaly is found incidentally on abdominal CT or ultrasonographic examination.

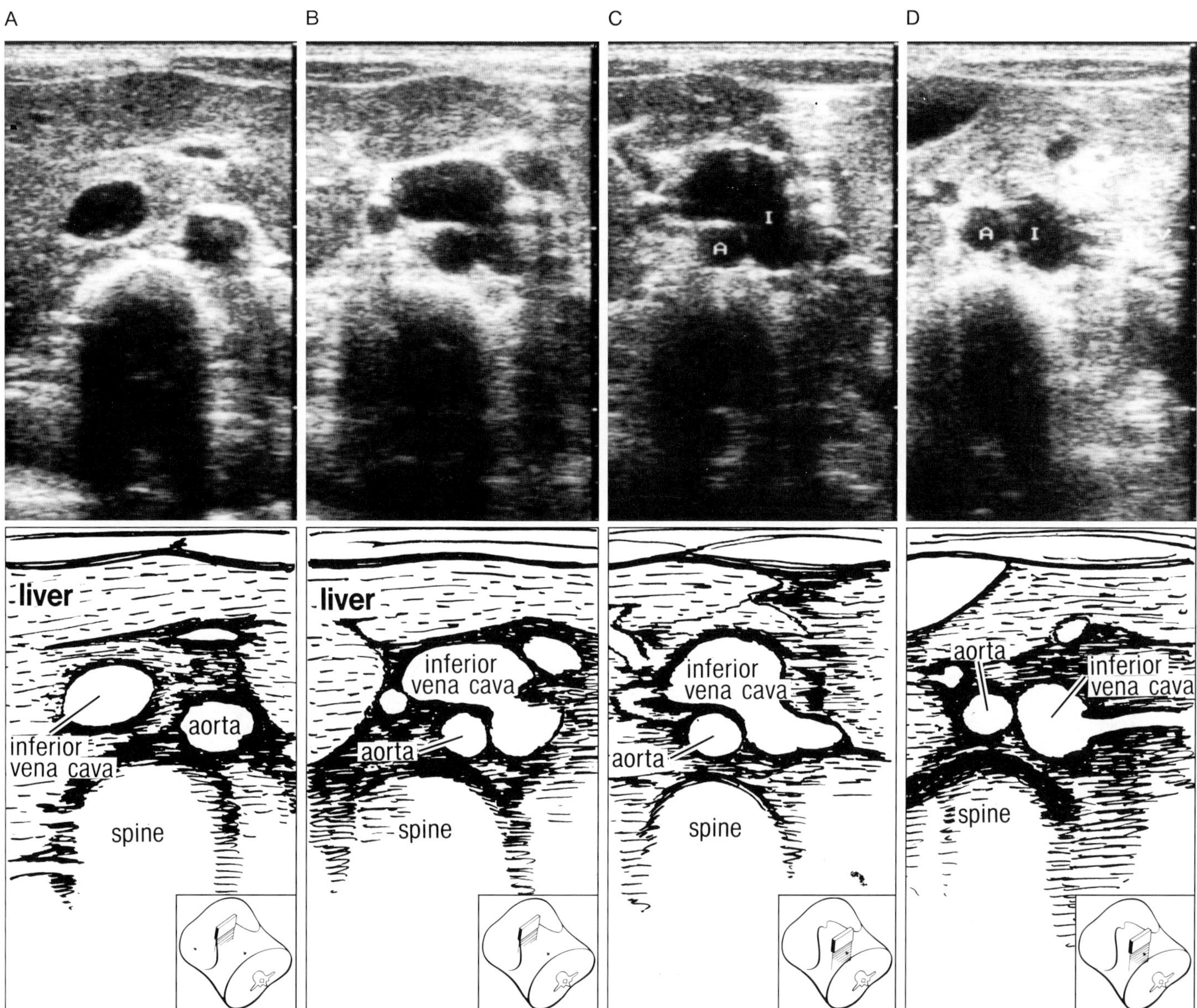

Fig. 9.9 A–D. *Case 1*. Transverse sections in the midline. The scan slice is moving caudally from **A** to **D**. The inferior vena cava which was located to the right of the abdominal aorta crosses the abdominal aorta anteriorly as it descends and is finally situated to the left of the abdominal aorta. In an elderly patient with severe atherosclerosis, the abdominal aorta can be markedly tortuous and located behind the inferior vena cava, but in that case the inferior vena cava courses to the right of the vertebral body. In the case of a left inferior vena cava, the abdominal aorta and its branches are in a normal location, and the inferior vena cava crosses over the aorta and is located on the left side. These two entities can be easily differentiated

Abdominal Aortic Aneurysm

The presence of an abdominal aortic aneurysm can easily be diagnosed by ultrasonographic examination alone. The normal abdominal aorta can always be visualized at the level of the liver and spleen, but can be difficult to visualize in the lower abdomen because of intestinal gas. If there is a large abdominal aneurysm which is in contact with the abdominal wall, displacement of intestinal gas occurs, and consequently the aneurysm is easily visualized on ultrasonographic examination. Thrombus within the lumen of an aneurysm can be clearly visualized on ultrasonographic examination.

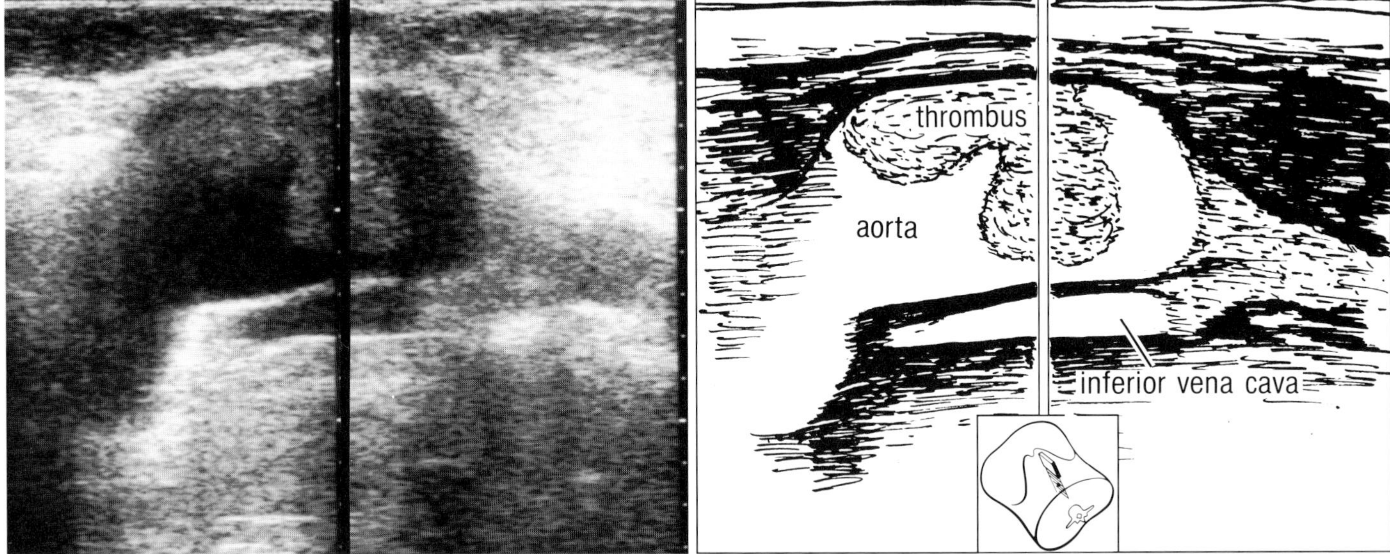

Fig. 9.10. *Case 1.* Longitudinal section of the abdominal aorta. The abdominal aorta is markedly dilated, up to 10 cm in greatest outer dimension, cephalad to the aortic bifurcation. The lumen measures approximately 5 cm. There is organized thrombus on the anterior wall of the aneurysm

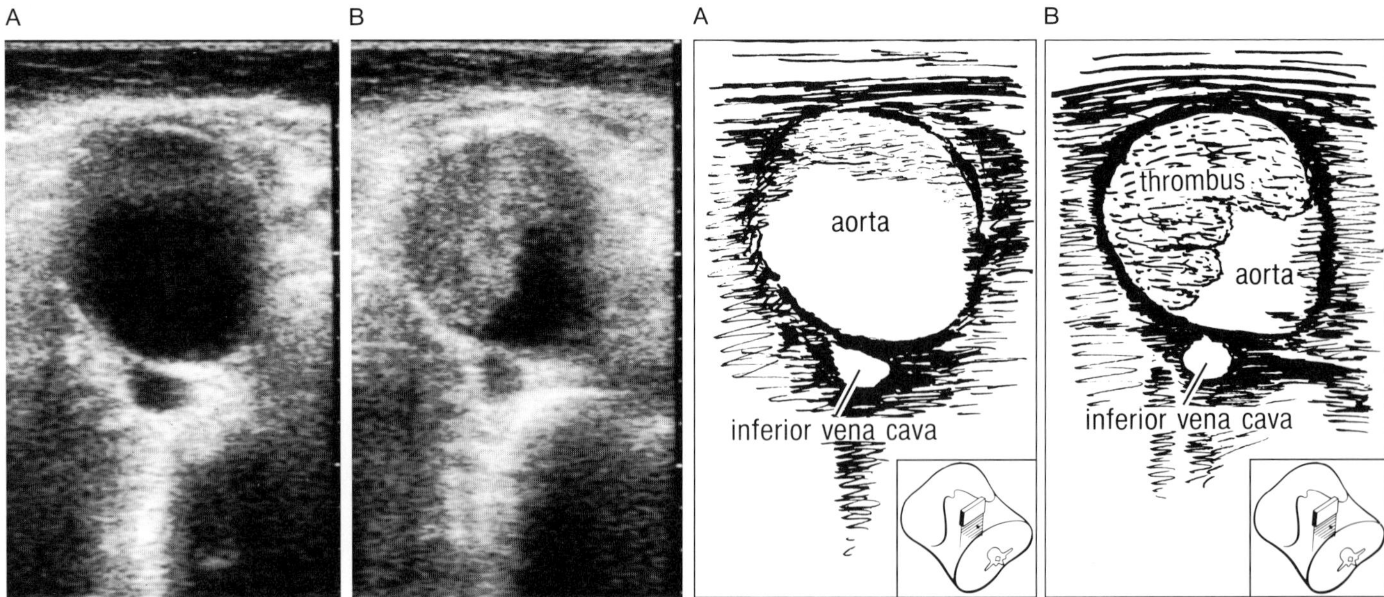

Fig. 9.11 A, B. *Case 1.* Transverse section at different levels of abnormal dilatation of the aorta. **B** shows the thrombus occupying more than half of the lumen. The abdominal aorta is deviated to the right at this level, and the inferior vena cava is seen immediately behind the aneurysm

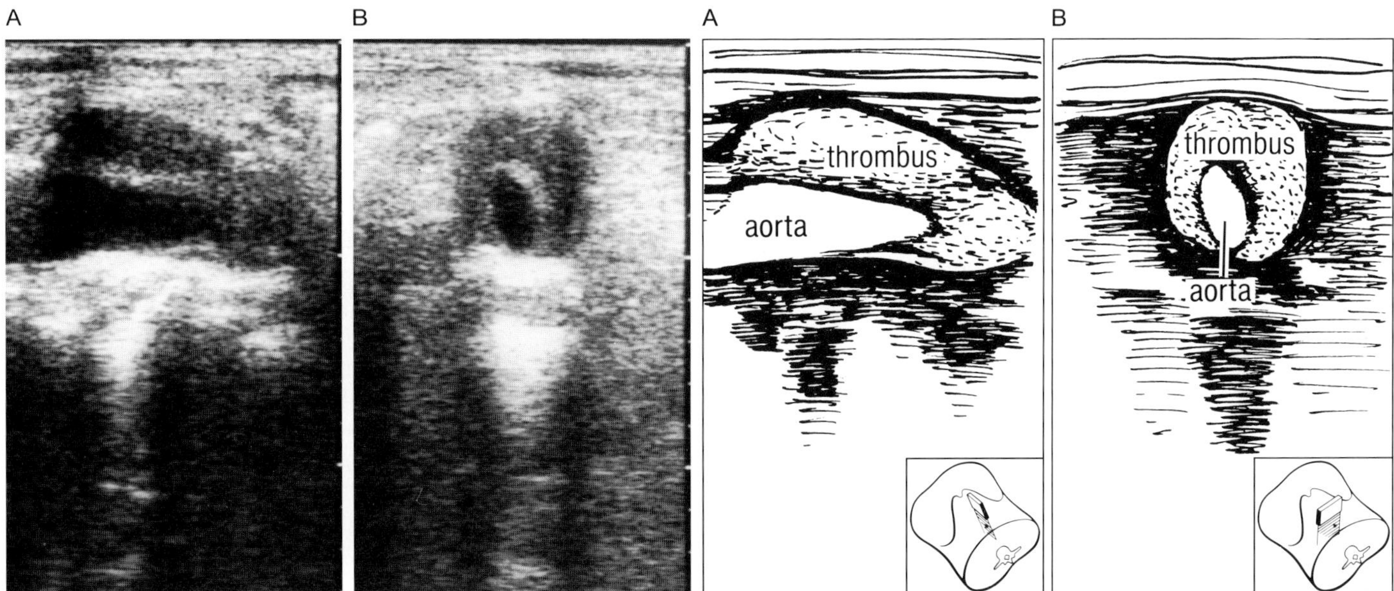

Fig. 9.12 A, B. *Case 2.* **A** Longitudinal section of the abdominal aorta. **B** Transverse section at the same location. There is a hypoechoic layer around the abdominal aorta. This represents organized thrombus within an aneurysm. In this case, the lumen of the aorta is almost normal in caliber

Dissecting Aneurysm of the Abdominal Aorta

Most dissecting aneurysms of the abdominal aorta are contiguous with a dissecting aneurysm of the aortic arch. The intimal flap will be observed to be moving synchronous to the cardiac pulsations on real-time scanning.

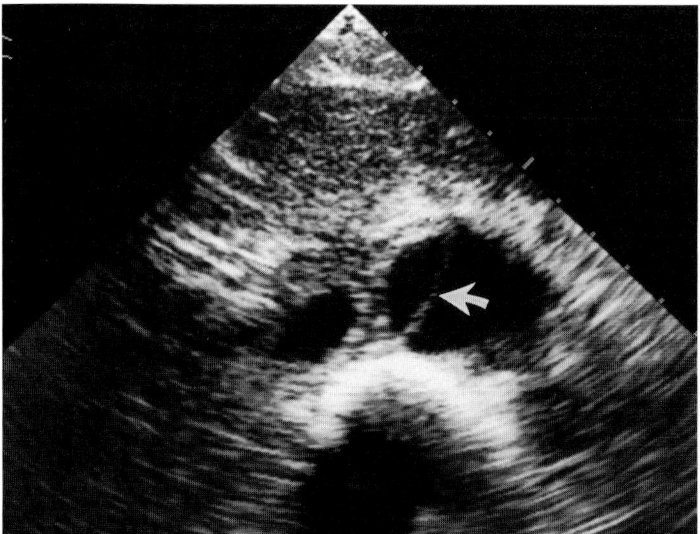

Fig. 9.13. *Case 1.* Transverse section of the upper abdomen demonstrates the abdominal aorta with a diameter of 24 mm, which is enlarged. There is a linear echo within the lumen (*arrow*), which continues in a craniocaudal direction. This was observed to be moving within the lumen of the aorta, synchronous to the arterial pulse

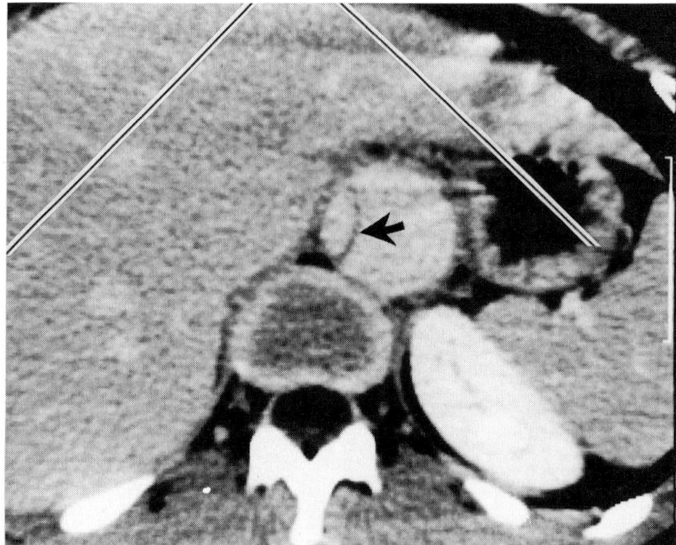

Fig. 9.14. *Case 1, CT scan.* This was obtained with intravenous contrast at approximately the same level as the ultrasonographic examination (Fig. 9.13). The lumen of the abdominal aorta is of high density due to the presence of contrast material. The intimal flap is seen as a filling defect. The triangular area between the *two lines* roughly corresponds to the ultrasonographic field in Fig. 9.13

Lymph Node Enlargement   Enlarged lymph nodes are hypoechoic and may mimic cystic masses. On transverse section, differentiation of enlarged lymph nodes from a cross-section of the abdominal aorta and inferior vena cava is difficult. On longitudinal section, the aorta and the inferior vena cava will be observed to be anteriorly displaced by lymph node enlargement of the retroperitoneum.

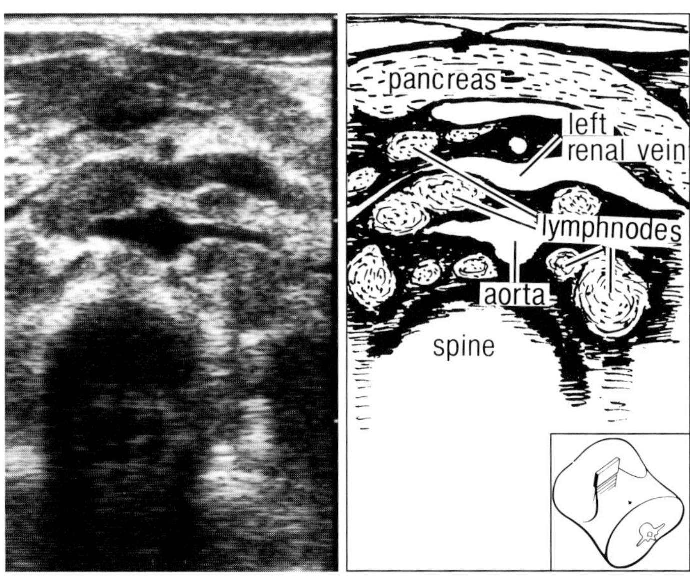

Fig. 9.15. *Case 1.* Metastases to the retroperitoneal lymph nodes from lung carcinoma. There are multiple solid masses, measuring 10–25 mm in size, around the abdominal aorta

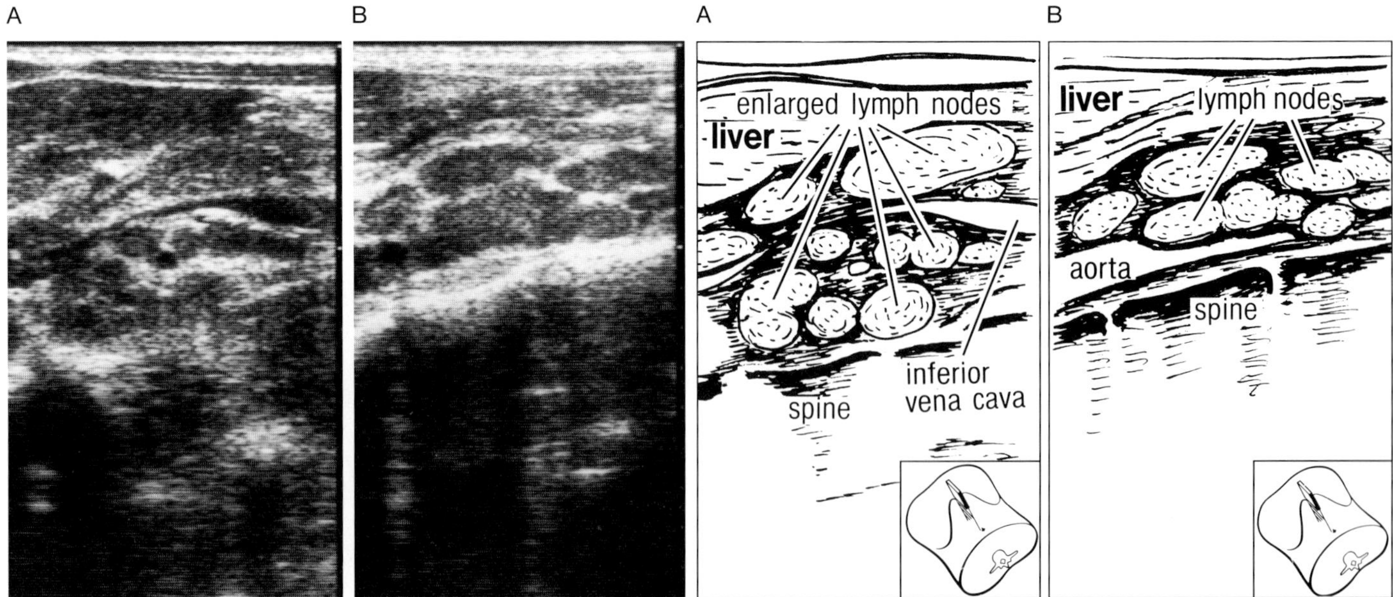

Fig. 9.16 A, B. *Case 1, longitudinal sections.* **A** There is lymph node enlargement posterior to the inferior vena cava, which is anteriorly displaced. **B** Longitudinal section along the abdominal aorta, showing enlargement of mesenteric lymph nodes. Similar findings can be seen in cases of malignant lymphoma

Peritoneal Carcinomatosis   In advanced peritoneal carcinomatosis, the abdominal organs appear amorphous, forming a single large mass. The abdominal aorta and inferior vena cava are clearly visualized throughout their length because of decreased intestinal gas from stenosis of the gastrointestinal tract. In cases of massive ascites, such as with cirrhosis of the liver, the intestine will be floating in the ascites, and peristaltic motion can be visualized. In contrast, in cases of peritoneal carcinomatosis, peristaltic motion is not visualized.

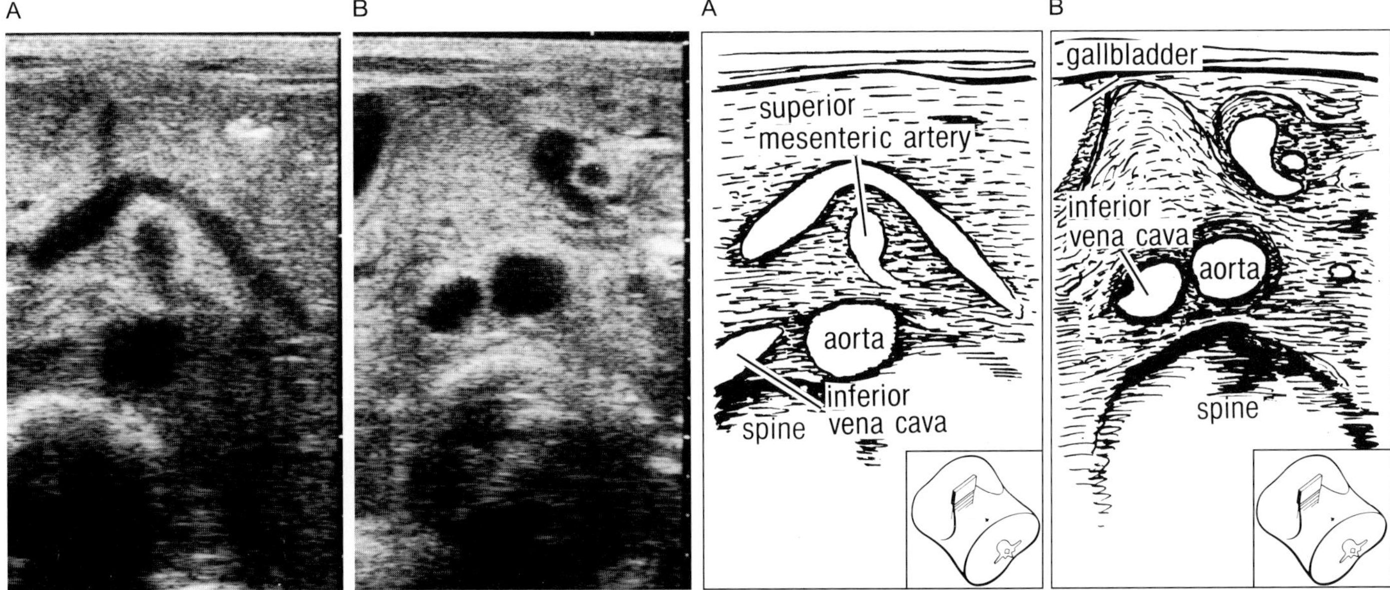

Fig. 9.17 A, B. *Case 1.* **A** Amorphous appearance of the abdominal contents, except for the abdominal aorta, superior mesenteric artery, and splenic vein. **B** The abdominal vasculature and the gallbladder are abnormally well visualized. In normal patients, blood vessels are difficult to evaluate at this level because of intestinal gas

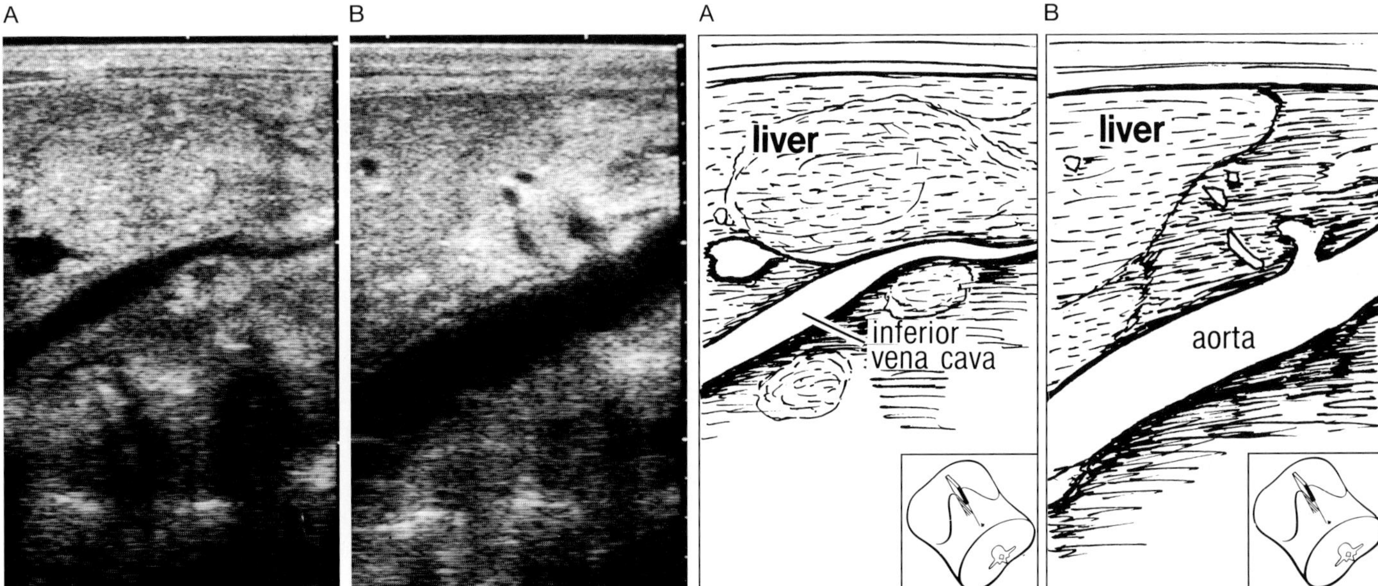

Fig. 9.18 A, B. *Case 1.* **A** Longitudinal section through the inferior vena cava. **B** Longitudinal section of the abdominal aorta. Except for the vessels, the structures in the peritoneal cavity appear homogeneous. No intestinal gas is visualized on these sections

Gastrointestinal Tract

Normal Ultrasonographic Image of the Stomach

The normal wall of the stomach is 3–5 mm in thickness on ultrasonographic examination. Using a high-resolution transducer head, five separate layers of the stomach can be visualized in a thin patient. Beginning from the luminal side, the first layer is hyperechoic, the second layer hypoechoic, the third layer hyperechoic, the fourth layer hypoechoic, and the fifth layer is hyperechoic. The hypoechoic fourth layer represents the muscular layer of the stomach and is the thickest of all the layers. On a typical examination, only this fourth layer, measuring 2–3 mm in thickness, is visualized as hypoechoic. The gastric angle and the antrum are visualized in all fasting patients. When there is a large amount of air within the lumen of the stomach, the wall of the stomach is not well seen, and in this situation the examination should be done in the erect position following oral administration of a large amount of water.

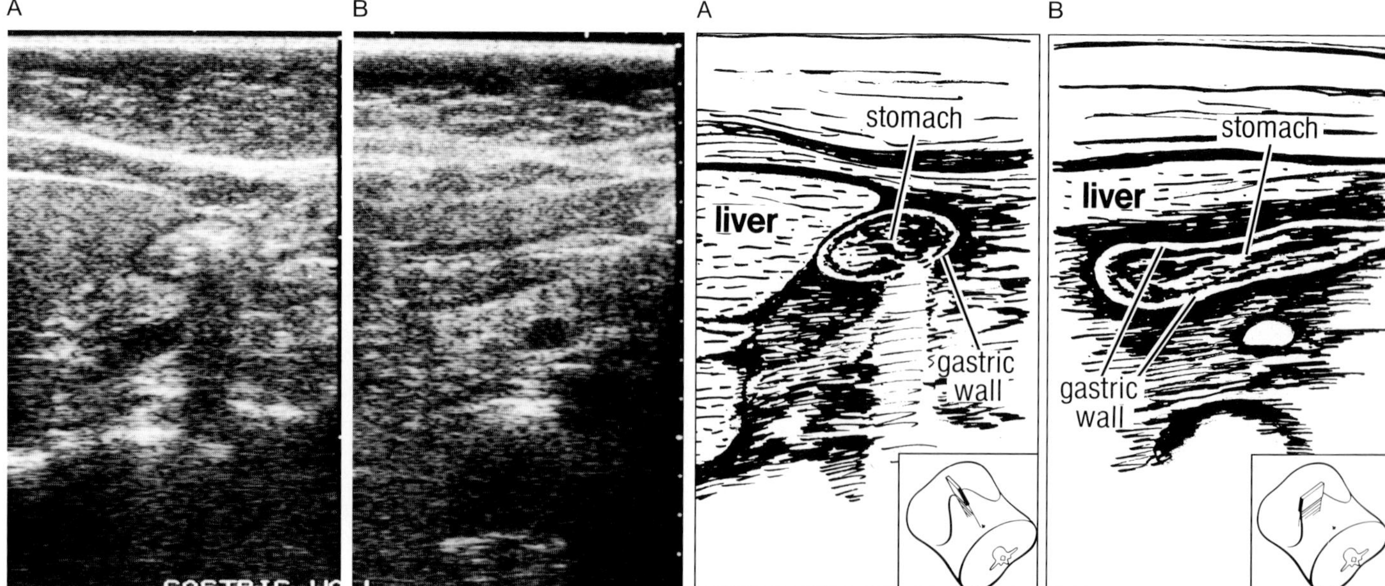

Fig. 10.1 A, B. *Case 1.* Longitudinal (**A**) and transverse (**B**) sections of the stomach. The gastric angle and the gastric antrum are visualized as ring-shaped (**A**) or as two parallel lines (**B**)

**Detecting Lesions
of the Gastrointestinal Tract**

Since sound is reflected by air, air-containing portions of the gastrointestinal tract are difficult to visualize on ultrasonographic studies. However, when there is marked wall thickening by either a mass or inflammatory disease, these abnormalities can be visualized. On X-ray or endoscopic examination, only the lumen of the gastrointestinal tract is visualized, whereas a thickened wall can be visualized by an ultrasonographic examination.

Acute Gastritis

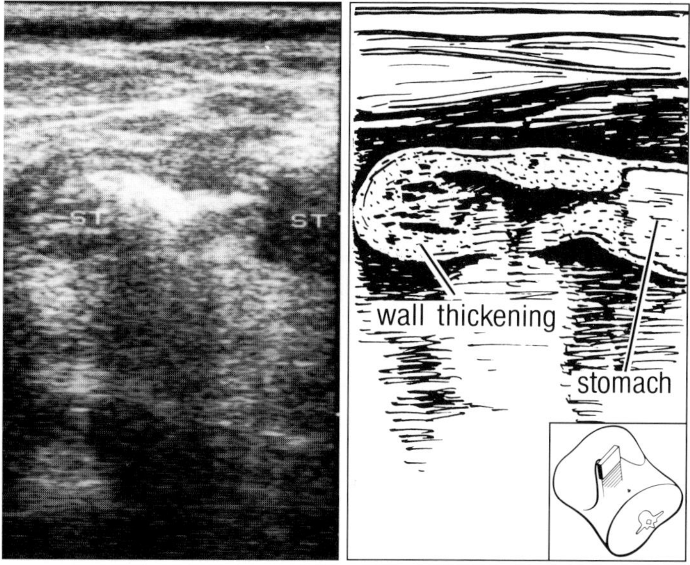

Fig. 10.2. There is marked thickening of the stomach wall from the gastric angle, gastric antrum, and duodenal bulb. The upper portion of the stomach, proximal to the gastric angle, shows abnormal dilatation with a large amount of retained fluid. This case demonstrates edema of the gastric wall in a case of acute gastritis caused by ingesting large quantities of alcohol

**Congenital Hypertrophic
Pyrolic Stenosis**

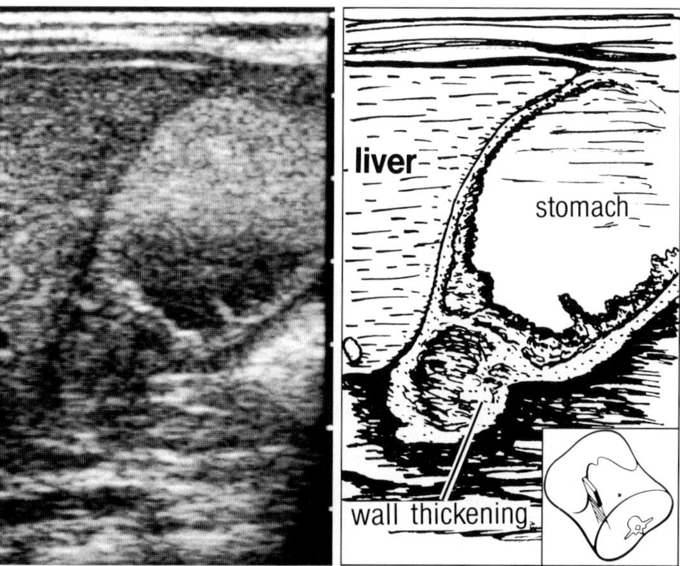

Fig. 10.3. Near the hepatic hilum, there is a structure which mimics a gallbladder. This is the stomach filled with food. The wall of the pyloris is markedly thickened, and there is no visualized lumen in this area

Intestinal Obstruction

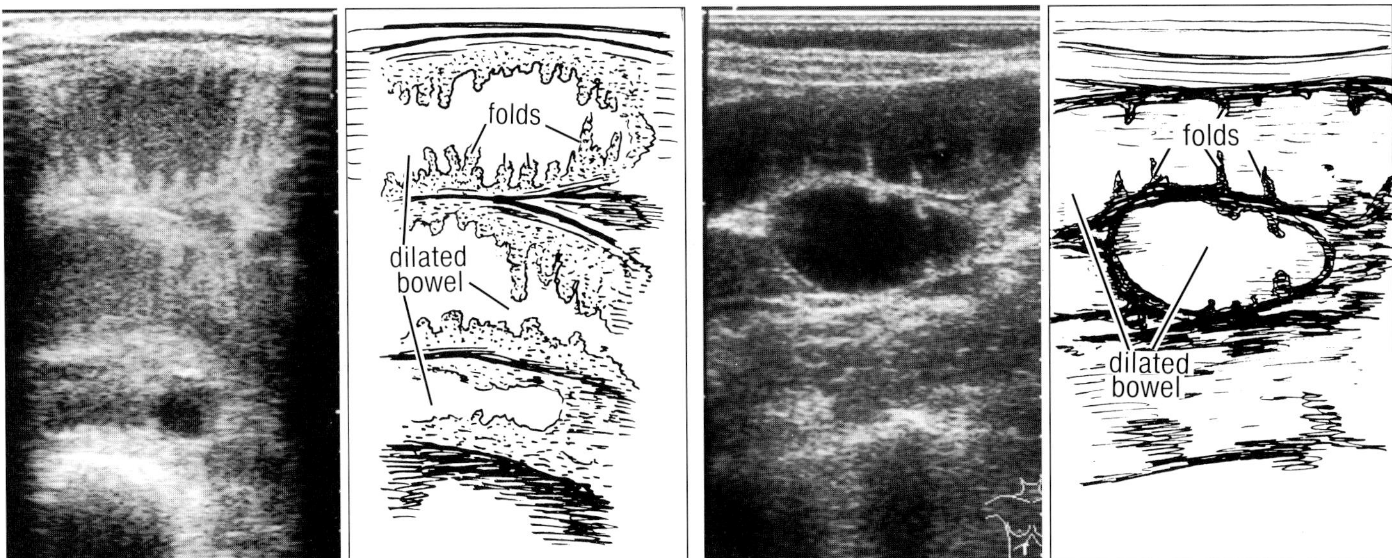

Fig. 10.4. *Case 1.* There is dilatation of the small intestine with multiple fine echoes, suggesting residual food particles. The valvulae conniventes are clearly visualized. During the examination, no peristaltic motion of the small intestine was detected

Fig. 10.5. *Case 2.* There is dilatation of the small intestine. The valvulae conniventes are visualized. The lumen of the dilated small intestine is relatively anechoic in this case

Gastric Cancer

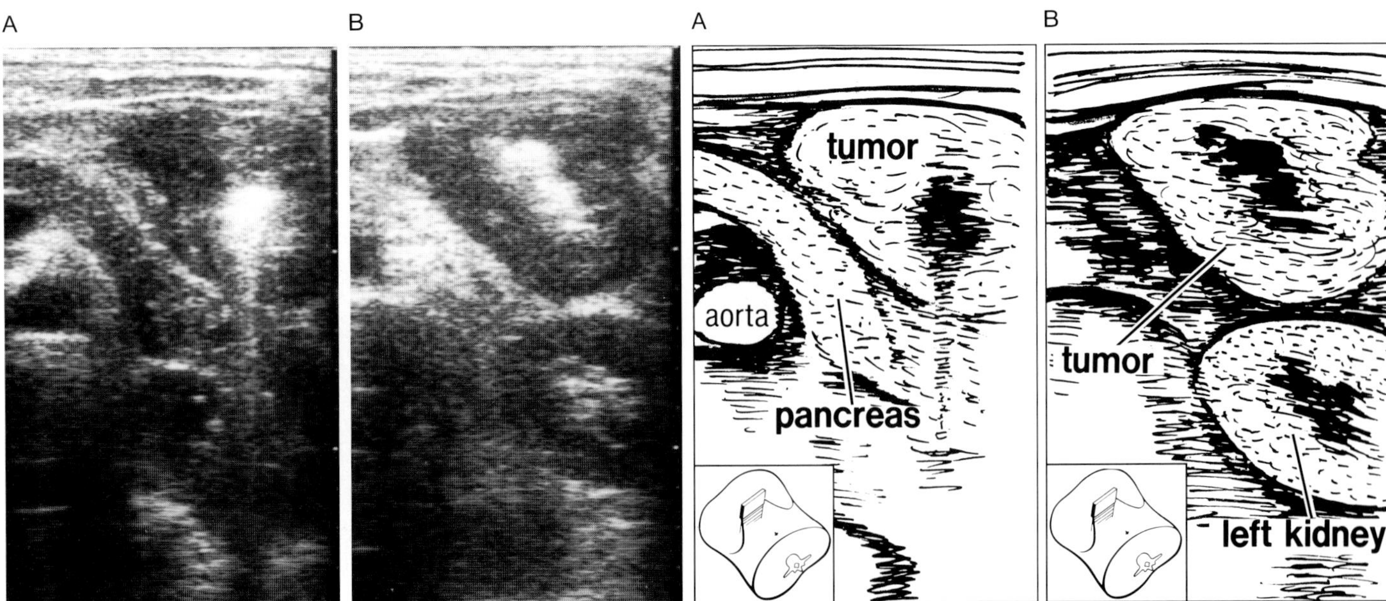

Fig. 10.6 A, B. *Case 1.* **A** Donut-shaped mass anterior to the tail of the pancreas. There is a strong echo in the central portion, suggesting the presence of gas. **B** The same mass is visualized anterior to the left kidney. Since the echo pattern of gastric cancer is similar to the echo pattern of the kidney, this is called the pseudokidney sign. This is a case of advanced gastric carcinoma

Colon Carcinoma

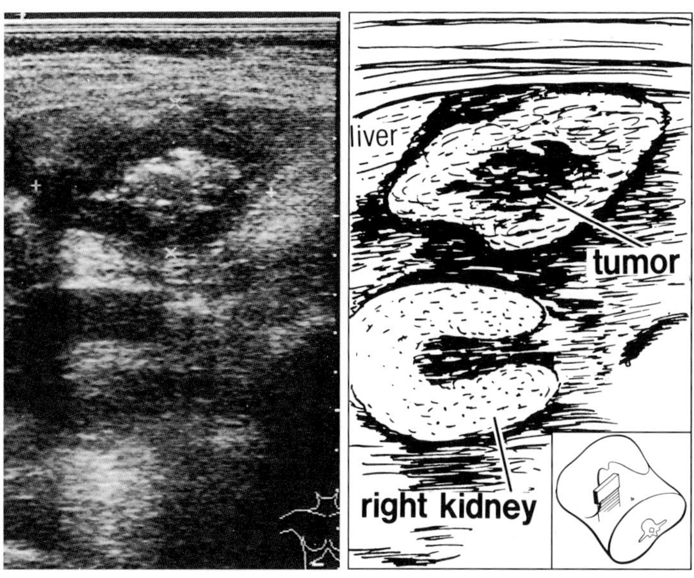

Fig. 10.7. *Case 1.* There is a 6–7-cm solid mass in the right upper quadrant with central hyperechoic areas (pseudokidney sign). This image demonstrates a mass-forming lesion of the gastrointestinal tract

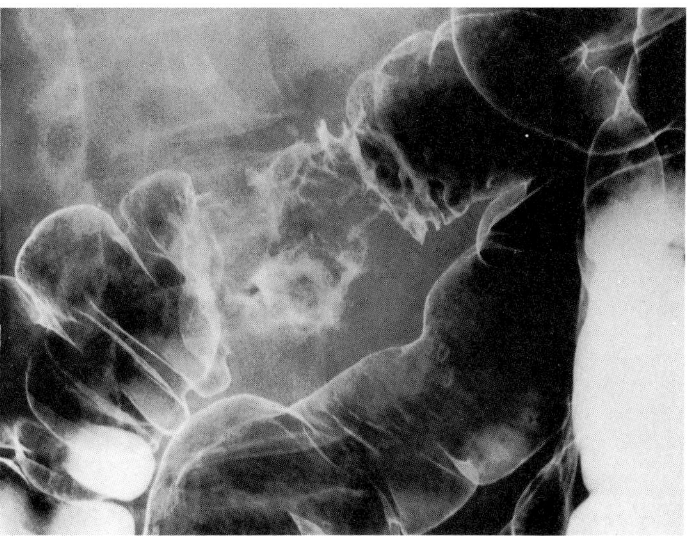

Fig. 10.8. *Case 1, barium enema.* This is a carcinoma of the transverse colon

Rectal Cancer

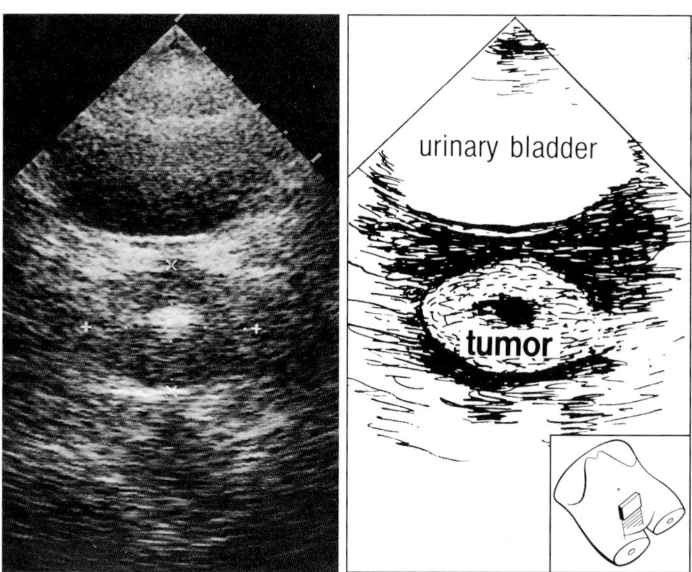

Fig. 10.9. *Case 1.* A transverse section in the midline of the lower abdomen demonstrates a 3 × 4-cm solid mass posterior to the urinary bladder. Central hyperechoic areas suggest a mass lesion of the intestinal tract

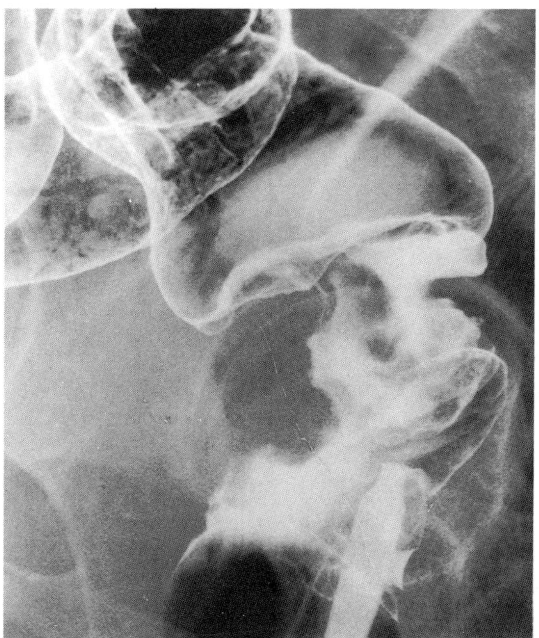

Fig. 10.10. *Case 1, barium enema.* There is a circumferential mass in the rectum

Abdominal Wall and Peritoneum

Some tumor-forming processes of the abdominal wall and the peritoneum are illustrated below. An adequate image cannot be obtained using a conventional transducer head because the lesions are too superficial relative to the focal length of the transducer head. It is necessary to use a polymer gel or water bath between the patient and the transducer head in these situations.

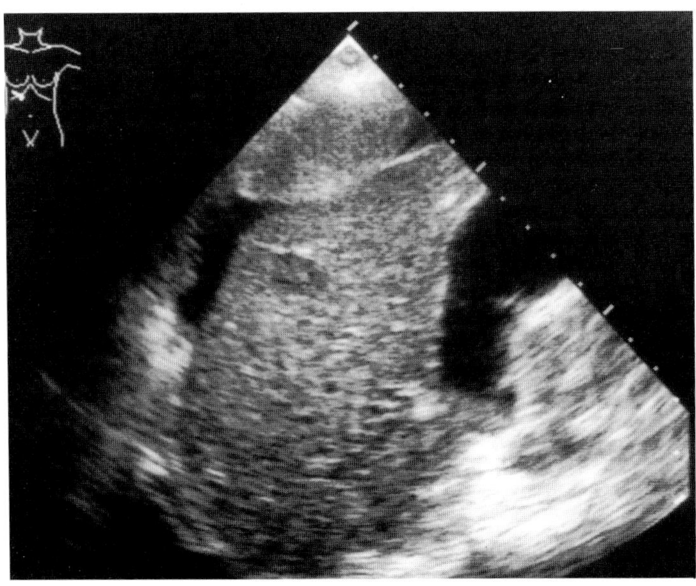

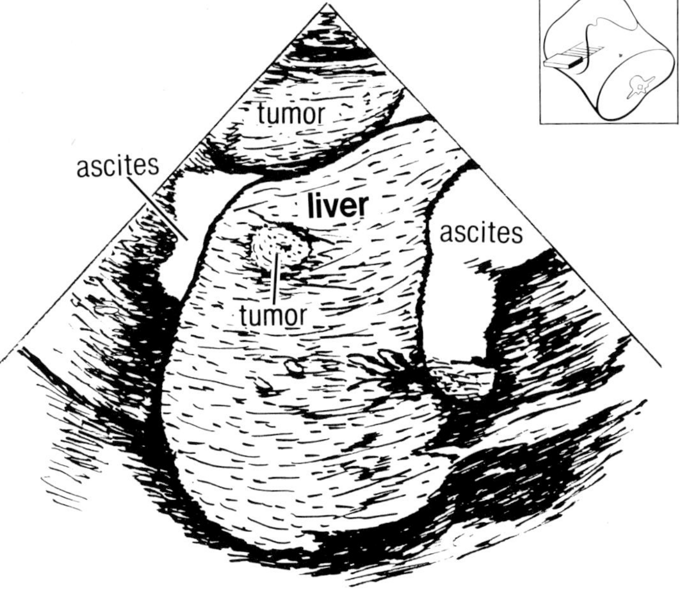

Fig. 10.11. Peritoneal metastases from gastric carcinoma. This patient has had gastrectomy for gastric carcinoma. Metastatic tumor arising from the peritoneum is compressing the liver. Tumors are also seen on the diaphragm. There is a 12-mm metastatic focus in the liver. A moderate amount of ascites is present

Metastatic Tumor Seeding the Abdominal Wall from Gastric Carcinoma

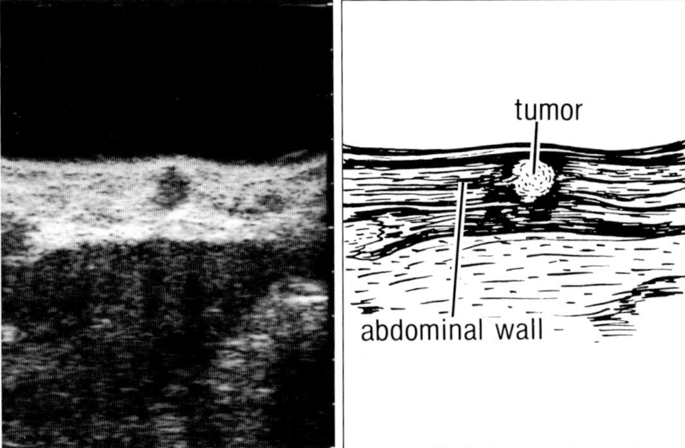

Fig. 10.12. Same case as in Fig. 10.11. Three solid nodules were palpated in the region of the skin incision site. Ultrasonography shows a 1-cm solid tumor within the abdominal wall

Abdominal Herniation

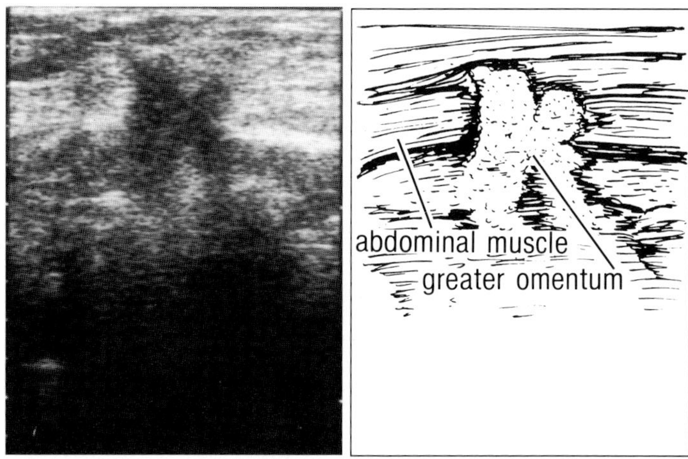

Fig. 10.13. This patient had had previous surgery for appendicitis. There is a rent in the abdominal musculature with interposition of fatty tissue from the greater omentum. This herniation does not contain intestine

Ascites

Ultrasonographic examination is sensitive to the presence of ascites. When there is a small amount of ascites, there is an anechoic space between the right kidney and the liver (hepatorenal fossa, Morison's pouch). This anechoic space varies in size according to the respiratory cycle. As the amount of ascites increases, an anechoic space appears between the liver and the abdominal wall. When there is a small amount of ascites, an anechoic space may only be seen in the pouch of Douglas. When ascites is clinically suspected, the pouch of Douglas should be examined through the urinary bladder, even if there is no evidence of ascites in the upper abdomen.

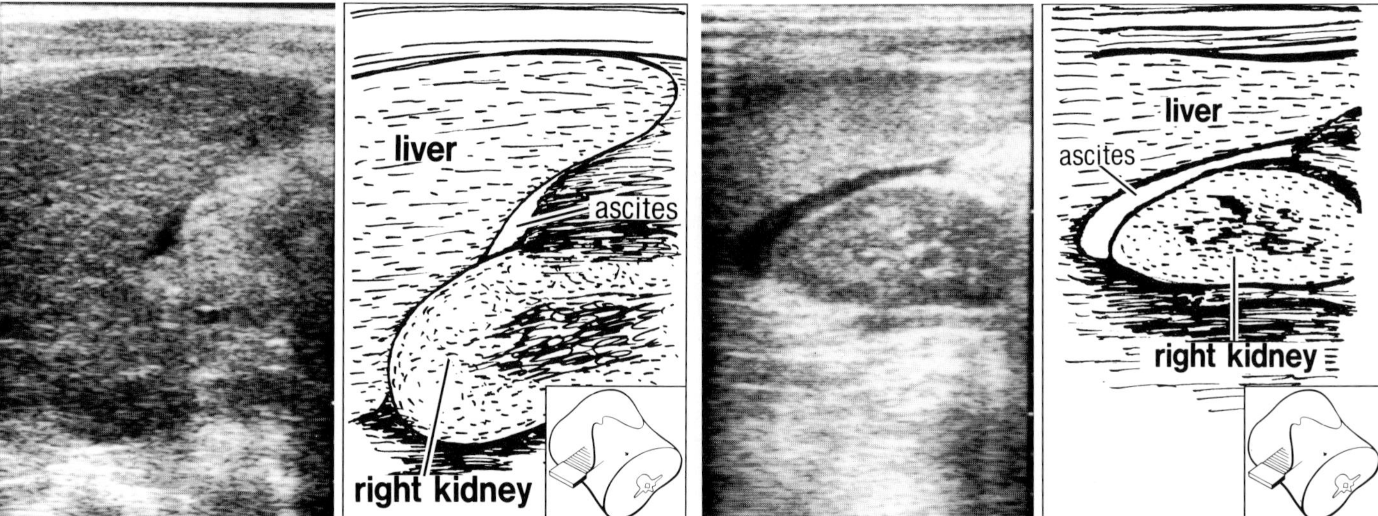

Fig. 10.14. *Case 1*. There is a thin anechoic space along the inferior surface of the liver suggesting a small amount of ascites

Fig. 10.15. *Case 2*. There is a long thin anechoic space between the liver and the right kidney (Morison's pouch)

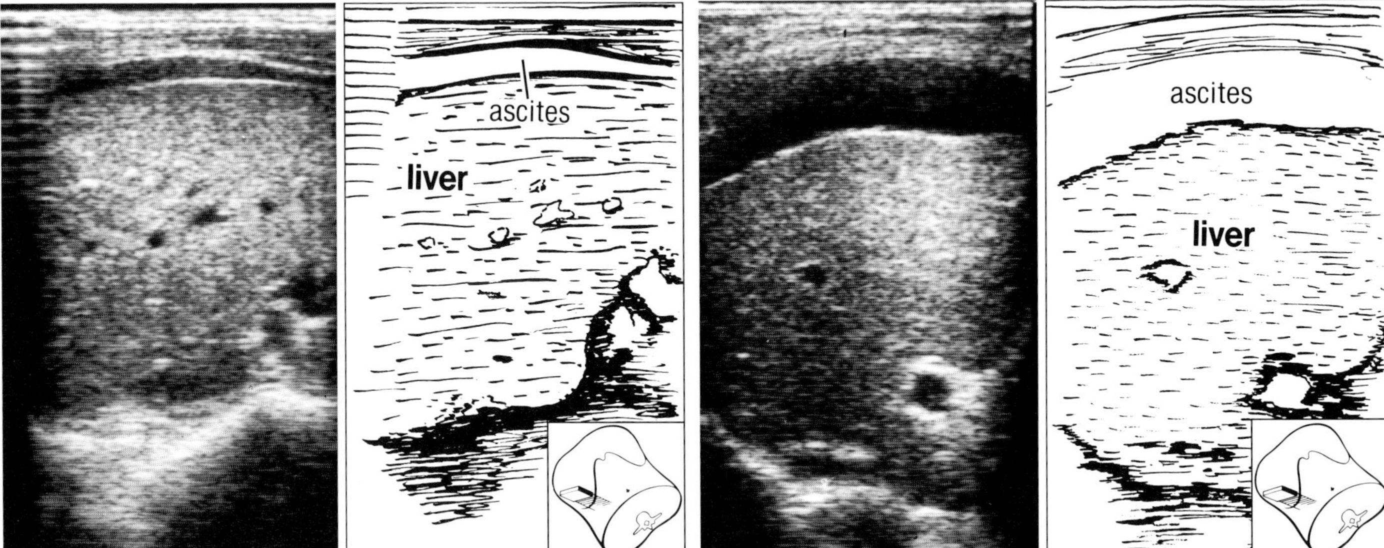

Fig. 10.16. *Case 3.* There is an anechoic space, 5 mm in thickness, between the right lobe of the liver and the abdominal wall

Fig. 10.17. *Case 4.* There is separation of the liver from the abdominal wall, secondary to a large amount of ascites

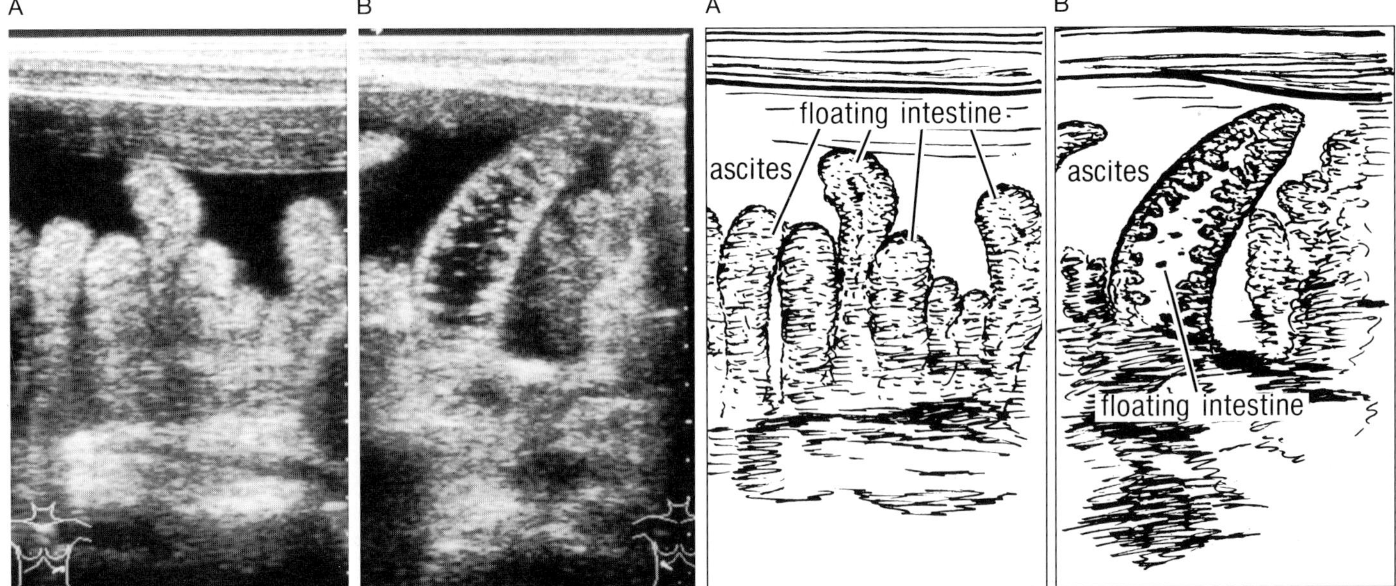

Fig. 10.18 A, B. *Case 5.* There is a large amount of ascites in this patient. The intestinal tract appears to be suspended within the ascites and resembles seaweed on the seabed. Part of the intestinal lumen is filled with fluid and food particles, and the valvulae conniventes are clearly visualized (**B**)

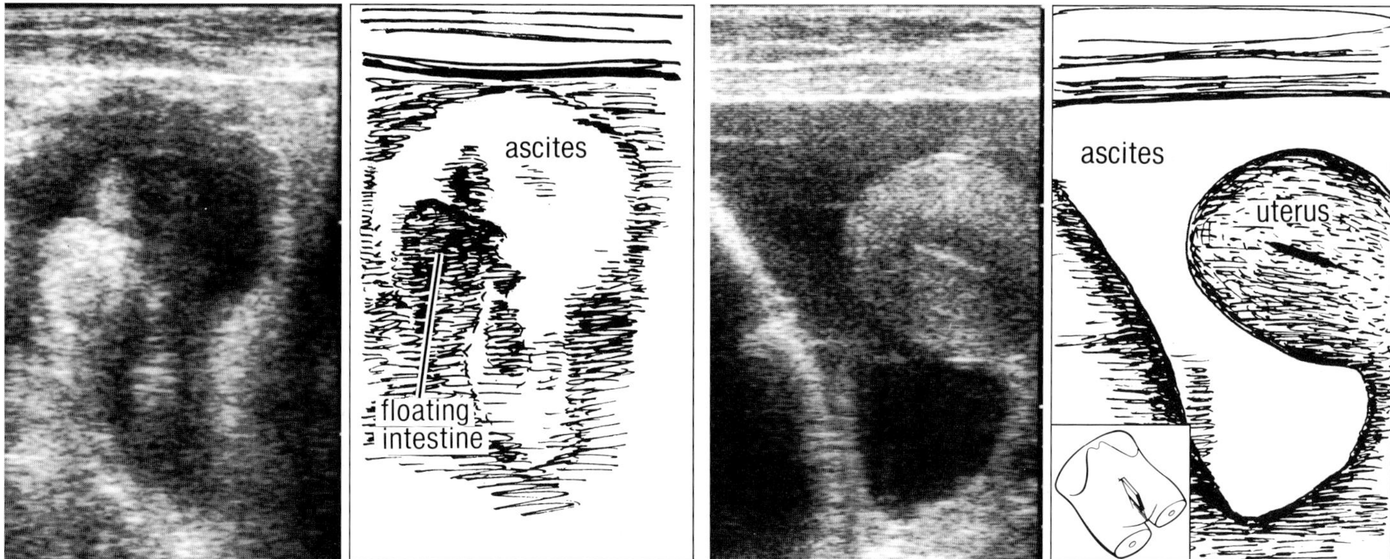

Fig. 10.19. *Case 6.* Ascites is visualized as an anechoic space between loops of the intestinal tract

Fig. 10.20. *Case 7.* There is a large amount of ascites in the pelvis. The anechoic space posterior to the uterus is fluid in the pouch of Douglas

Pleural Effusion

During ultrasonographic examination of the abdomen, pleural effusion, if present, may be visualized through the liver or spleen.

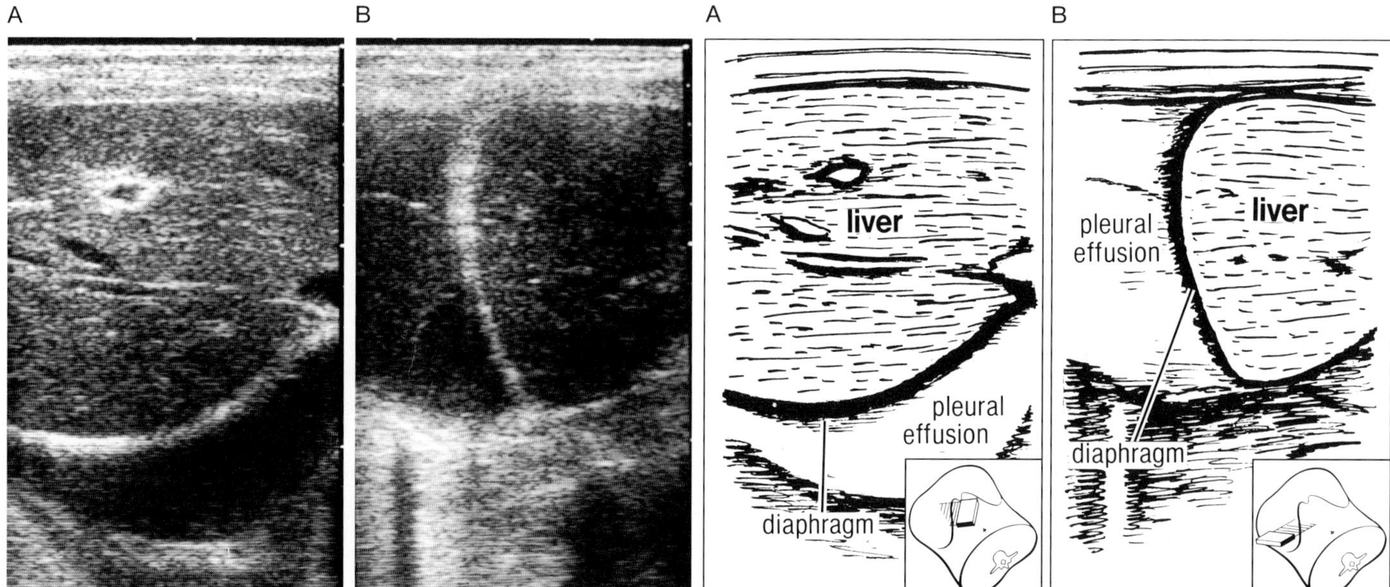

Fig. 10.21 A, B. A patient with carcinoma of the right lung. The ultrasound study was performed to rule out hepatic metastases. There is an echo-free space cephalad to the right hemidiaphragm, indicating the presence of pleural effusion. In the presence of pleural effusion, a large area of the liver immediately below the diaphragm can be clearly visualized by intercostal scanning without any blind spots

11 Glossary

Acoustic Shadowing. Absence of echoes distal to a strong reflector. Also known as shadowing.

A-Mode. A designates amplitude. Mode of operation in which the intensity of the echo is displayed as a vertical spot deflection on the distance (time) axis.

Anechoic. Refers to a structure which transmits ultrasound without reflecting sound back to its source. Synonyms include echo free, sonolucent, transonic, echolucent.

Arc scan. Refers to a method of manipulating a contact compound transducer head. The transducer head is moved over a curved surface in such a way that the ultrasound beam converges on one common point (Fig. 11.1 A). This technique is often used with a water bath for breast or thyroid imaging.

Attenuation. The process by which the intensity of an ultrasound beam is decreased as its passes through tissue by reflection, scattering, and absorption. The unit of an attenuation coefficient is dB · cm · MHz.

B-Mode. "B" designates brightness. The echo intensity is translated into degrees of brightness on the distance (time) axis of the monitor.

B-Scan. A method which displays a sectional plane of the body using B-mode. This is the principle method used for ultrasonographic imaging of the abdomen and pelvis.

Circular Scan. A method of manually moving the probe in a complete circle to obtain an image with a compound scanner, not currently in use for diagnostic ultrasonography.

C-Mode. Using B-mode data, a cross-sectional image parallel to the body surface (perpendicular to the ultrasound beam) is constructed. This mode is useful for thyroid and breast imaging.

Compound Scan. This is a method which combines linear, arc, and sector scanning techniques. The probe is moved manually, and therefore this is also referred to as contact compound scanning. Scanning is performed by manually moving an articulated transducer head over the body surface (Fig. 11.1 B). A single image is created by combining the data from several strokes of the transducer head.

Coupling Medium (Contact Medium). Olive oil, mineral oil, or gel used to eliminate the air between the probe and patient to provide a good ultrasound pathway.

Decibel (dB). Unit of power or intensity of sound. It is the ratio of the power expressed in a logarithm (to the base 10).

Doppler Method. A method of ultrasonographic diagnosis in which moving targets are interrogated with ultrasound; the frequency change of the reflected ultrasound waves is used to calculate velocity.

Dynamic Range. The range of echo intensity which is displayed. Dynamic range is expressed as the ratio (in dB) of the maximal to the minimal echo intensity.

Echo. Reflected sound. Sound is reflected from interfaces of differing acoustic impedances within the patient.

Echogenic. Refers to a substance or structure which produces echoes due to the presence of interfaces of differing acoustic impedances. Antonyms include echo free, anechoic.

Edge Enhancement. An electronic postprocessing function which makes contours of structures within the image more distinct and clear.

Enhancement. An increase in echo amplitudes from a reflector due to its location posterior to a weakly attenuating structure.

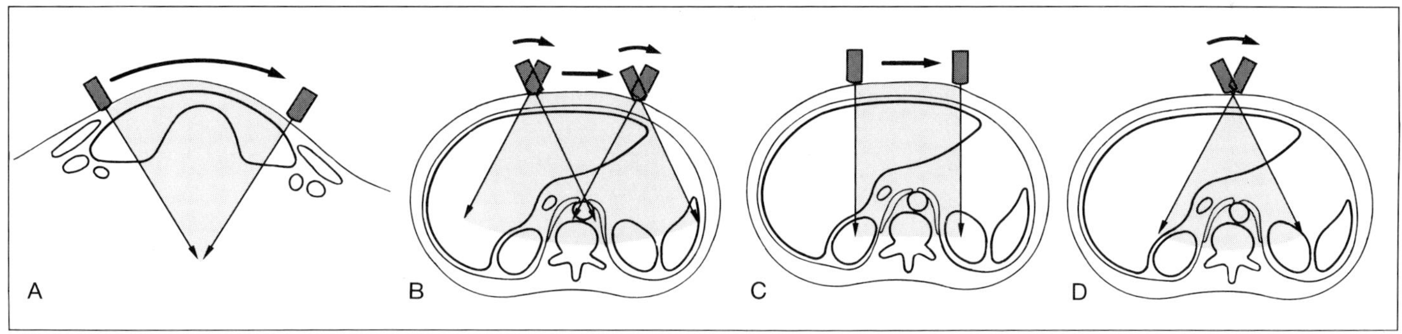

Fig. 11.1 A–D. Types of scanning. **A** Arc scan; **B** compound scan; **C** linear-scan; **D** section scan

Far Gain. Amplification of echoes returning from the far field (deep structures) in order to compensate for attenuation due to distance traveled.

Gain. Ratio of output to input power, expressed in dB, indicating the extent of amplification of the electrical signal. As gain is increased, the ultrasonographic image becomes brighter.

Gray Scale. A method of translating the electronic echo amplitude into an interpretable image. The varying amplitudes of echoes are displayed on the monitor in varying shades of gray.

Hyperechoic. Refers to a lesion or tumor which produces a stronger echo than surrounding structures or tissues.

Hypoechoic. Refers to a lesion or tumor which produces a weaker echo than surrounding structures or tissues.

Impedance. The product of the density of a substance multiplied by the sound propagation velocity within that substance. This is also referred to as the acoustic characteristic impedance, specific acoustic impedance, or simply the acoustic impedance. The fraction of ultrasound energy which is reflected is determined by the differences in the acoustic impedances at an interface.

Isoechoic. Refers to a lesion or tumor which produces an echo of the same strength as that of the surrounding structures or tissues.

Linear Scan. Multiple rectangular elements fire sequentially within the transducer head to produce a rectangular rather than a pie-shaped image (Fig. 11.1 C).

M-Mode. M designates motion. This method produces a one-dimensional time display of a moving reflector. This is primarily used in echocardiography.

Near Gain. Adjustment in the time gain control (TGC) curve to compensate for the short distance which echoes from the near field have traveled.

Noise. Random, nonuseful signal produced by the electronic circuit of the ultrasonography equipment. Differentiation from low-amplitude echoes may be difficult, and there is, therefore, interference in image interpretation.

Piezoelectric Effect. Electric current created by pressure forces. Certain types of ceramic materials can convert pressure to electricity and vice versa. Transducer elements utilize this phenomenon, which is also referred to as piezoelectricity.

Pulse Width. Time from beginning to end of a pulse. Also known as pulse duration and pulse length. Shortening the pulse width without changing the transducer frequency improves axial resolution.

Pulse Method (Pulsed Mode). Method of operation using pulsed ultrasound. Currently used for abdominal imaging.

PZT. Lead zirconate titanate. An artificial piezoelectric material that is used for most diagnostic ultrasonographic transducers.

Real Time. A system in which the time delay between the input and output of data is neglible. Moving structures can be continuously imaged.

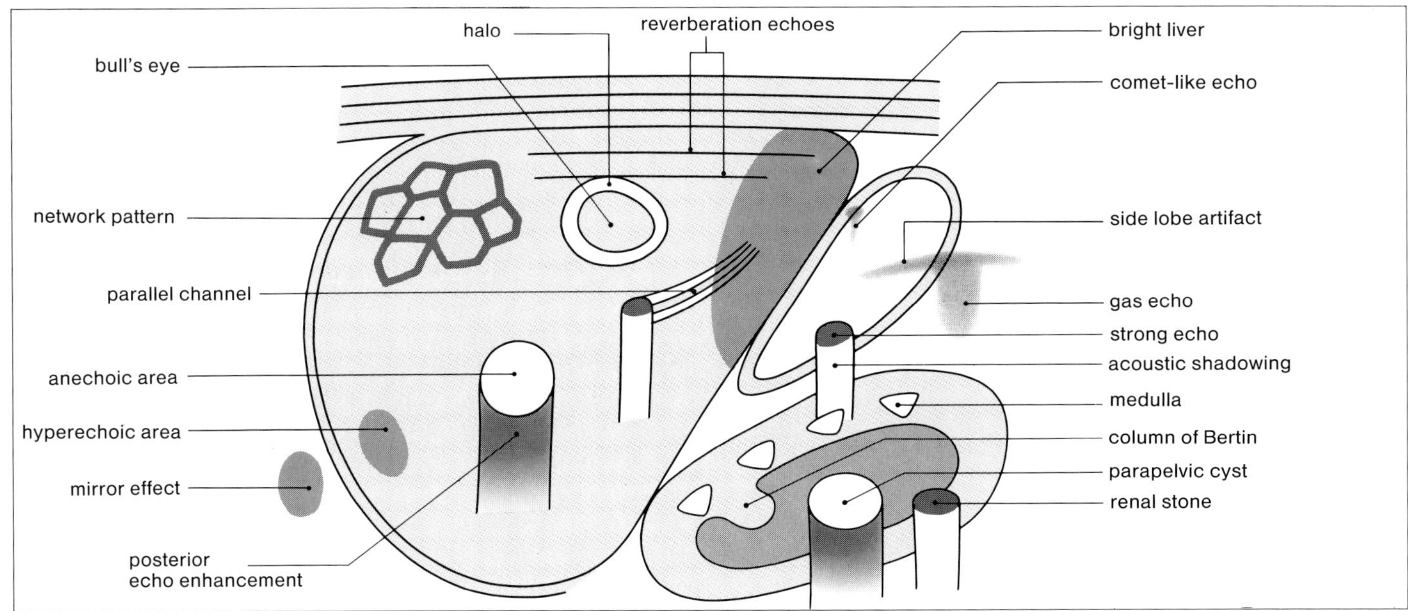

Fig. 11.2. Schematic drawing of ultrasonographic signs and findings

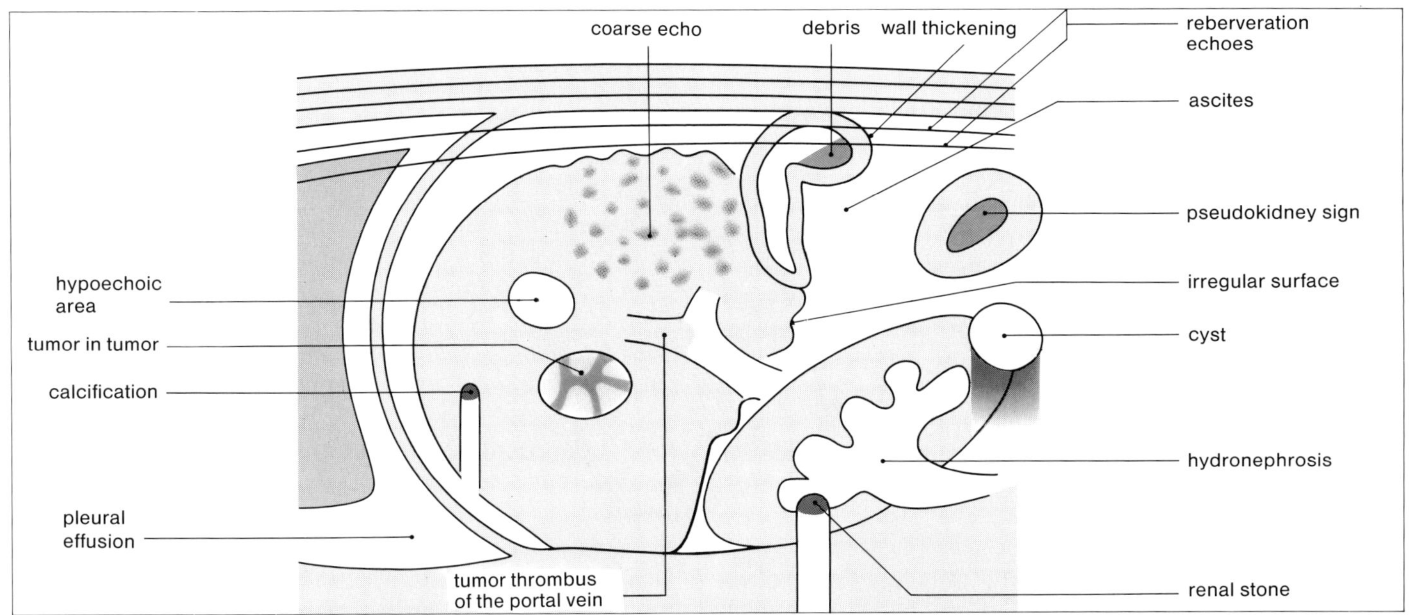

Fig. 11.3. Schematic drawing of ultrasonographic signs and findings

Reflection Method. Standard method used in diagnostic ultrasonography in which the reflected beam (echo) is used for image construction.

Refraction. Change in the direction of the ultrasound beam of passing from one substance to another. The angle of refraction is determined by Snell's law.

Rejection. Elimination of low-amplitude echoes so that they do not contribute to the image. If the rejection level is set too high, significant information can be lost.

Resolution. See "Spatial Resolution".

Reverberation. Multiple reflections of a single ultrasound pulse occurring between parallel reflecting surfaces (one of which may be the transducer) to produce an artifactual series of equally spaced parallel lines.

Scattering. Redirection of ultrasound from a reflector which is small compared to the wave length of the beam. This occurs with rough surfaces or heterogeneous substances such as a solid organ.

Sector Scanner (Mechanical Sector). A single-element transducer, or a group of single-element transducers, is moved mechanically to create a pie-shaped image. The vertical lines of the image radiate from a single point (Fig. 11.1 D).

Side Lobes. Weak ultrasound beams produced by the transducer off axis from the main beam (main lobe).

Spatial Resolution. The ability to identify two small, closely spaced reflectors as separate structures. There are two types of spatial resolution: axial (depth) and lateral.

Specular Reflection. Reflection from a wide (relative to the wave length) smooth interface, e.g., solid organ contours.

Time Gain Compensation (TGC). Correction of differences in received echo amplitudes that are due to differences in depth. Echoes returning from the far field travel a greater distance and therefore undergo greater attenuation than echoes from the near field. If the echoes from the far field are amplified more than the echoes from the near field, attenuation is compensated for. Also known as sensitivity time control (STC).

Transducer. The essential part of the ultrasonographic equipment which converts electrical energy to ultrasound energy and vice versa. The transducer both transmits and receives ultrasound.

Transducer Head. Transducer assembly containing piezoelectric crystals, and damping and matching materials within a waterproof casing. Commonly referred to as the probe or the transducer.

Transmission Method. The transmitted rather than the reflected ultrasound beam is used for diagnostic imaging. This is a method which is currently not clinically useful.

12 Exercises

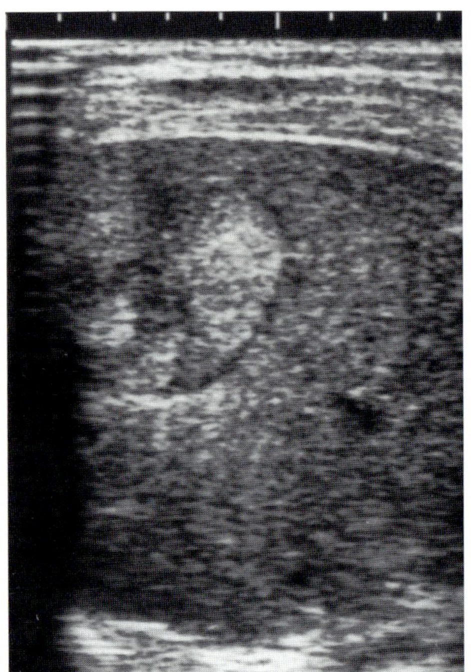

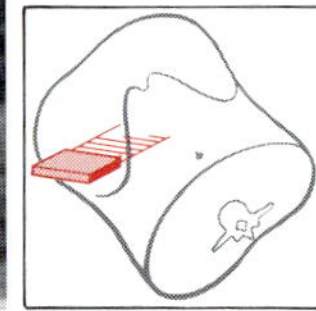

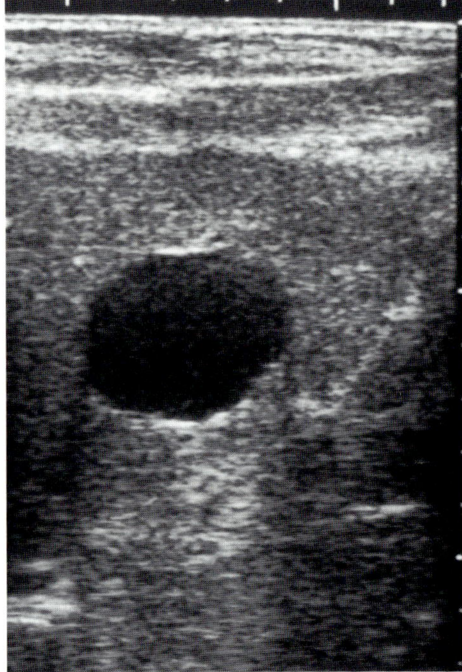

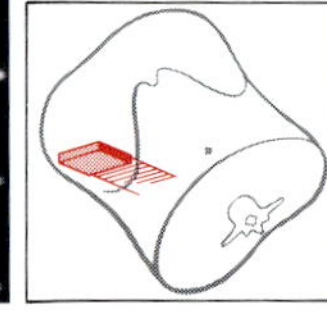

Case 1

1. What is the dark line around the hepatic tumor?
2. What is the internal echo pattern of this tumor?
3. What is your diagnosis?

Case 2

1. What is the internal echo texture of this mass?
2. The area behind the tumor appears white; what is this called?
3. What is your diagnosis?

Case 3 (See p. 54)

1. There was interval enlargement (the transverse diameter increased from 9 to 15 mm).
2. No change. It remains hypoechoic.
3. Hepatocellular carcinoma.

This is a case of slowly-growing hepatocellular carcinoma. On the initial examination, there was no definitive evidence for hepatocellular carcinoma. A regenerating nodule would have had the same appearance. On complimentary imaging examinations (CT and angiography), the tumor was not visualized. The diagnosis of hepatocellular carcinoma was made at surgery.

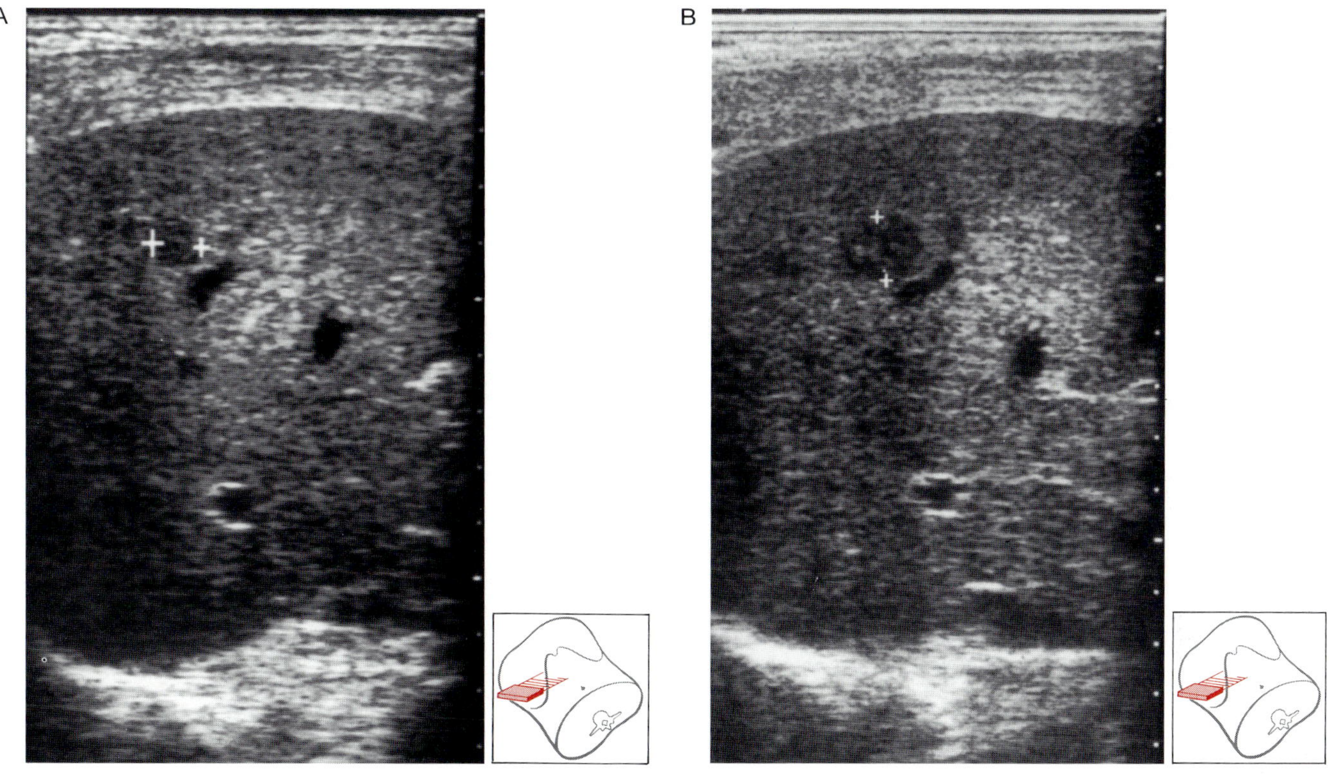

Case 3

A The initial examination; **B** 23 months after the initial examination.

1. Is there any change in the size of the tumor?
2. Is there any change in the echo pattern of the tumor?
3. What is your diagnosis?

Case 1 (See p. 50)

1. Peripheral hypoechoic band (halo).
2. Mosaic pattern or "tumor in a tumor" appearance.
3. Hepatocellular carcinoma.

This is a typical ultrasonographic image of hepatocellular carcinoma. In addition to the findings mentioned above, refractive shadows and posterior echo enhancement can be seen in hepatocellular carcinoma. However, cases with all of these characteristic findings are not very common.

Case 2 (See p. 70)

1. Complete absence of internal echo, or anechoic.
2. Posterior acoustic enhancement.
3. Hepatic cyst.

This is a typical ultrasonographic appearance of a hepatic cyst. There are fine, faint echoes within the cystic space, especially in the superficial portion, representing reverberation artifacts (see p. 22). Ignoring the reverberation echoes, the echo pattern in this case can be called anechoic.

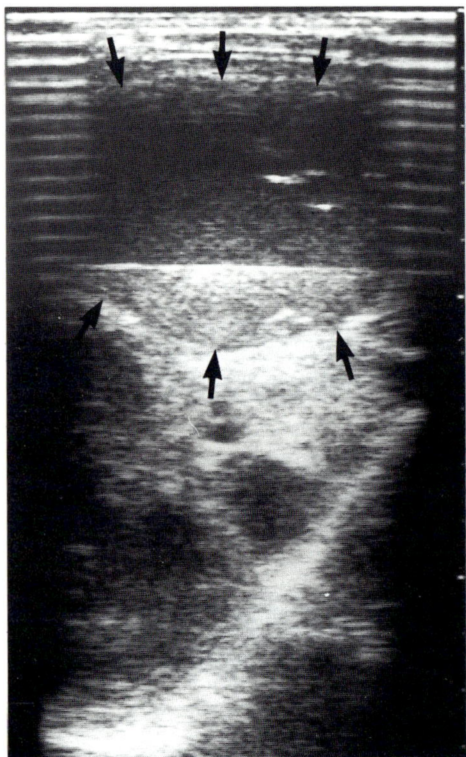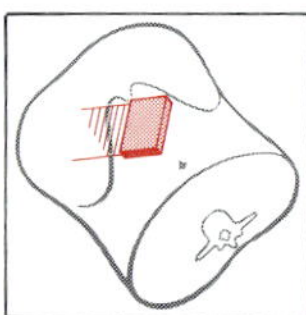

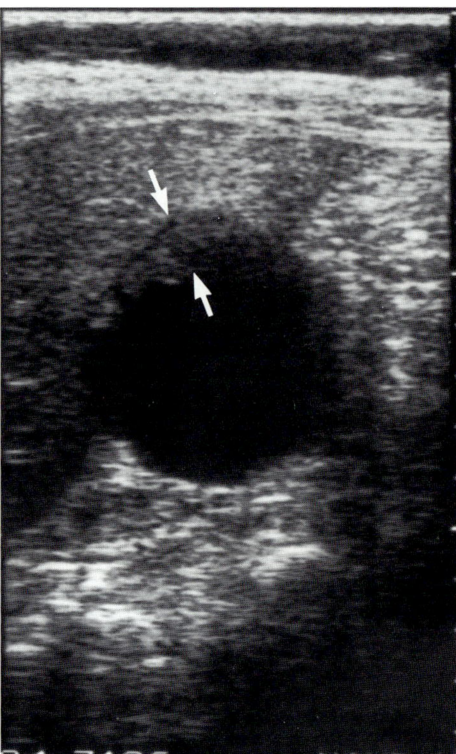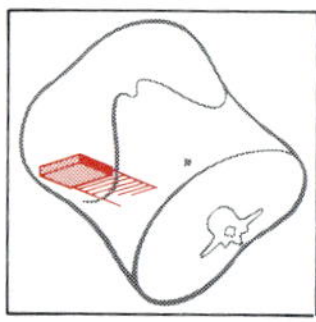

Case 4

Subcostal scan of the liver.
1. What is unusual about this mass (*arrows*)?
2. What is the internal substance of this tumor?
3. Are there any other masses?
4. What is your diagnosis?

Case 5

1. Is the tumor intra- or extrahepatic?
2. What is the internal structure of the tumor?
3. What type of tumor is this likely to be?

Case 6 (See p. 86)

1. Dilated intrahepatic bile ducts.
2. Parallel channel sign.
3. Dilated hepatic veins have a more linear course, whereas dilated intrahepatic bile ducts, as in this case, are curvilinear and tortuous. In addition, these structures have different directions.

On the static image, it is difficult to recognize that dilated structures are in continuity with one another, but during a real-time examination this is clearly evident. Hence, it is not difficult to diagnose intrahepatic biliary dilatation on real-time examination. However, when there is marked dilatation of the biliary tract, differentiation of portal veins from bile ducts becomes difficult.

Case 4 (See p. 65)

1. It is divided by a horizontal line. The superficial portion is hypoechoic, and the deep portion is hyperechoic.
2. The tumor is primarily composed of a fluid which is separated into two layers due to differences in specific gravity.
3. There are three or four hypoechoic masses, measuring 13–25 mm in size, in the deeper portion of the liver.
4. A metastatic tumor which has a tendency to degenerate and necrose. This tumor was a hepatic metastasis from ovarian carcinoma.

This is an example of a cystic tumor in which there is a fluid-fluid level. When the surface of the transducer head is not horizontal, the fluid-fluid level does not appear horizontal on the images.

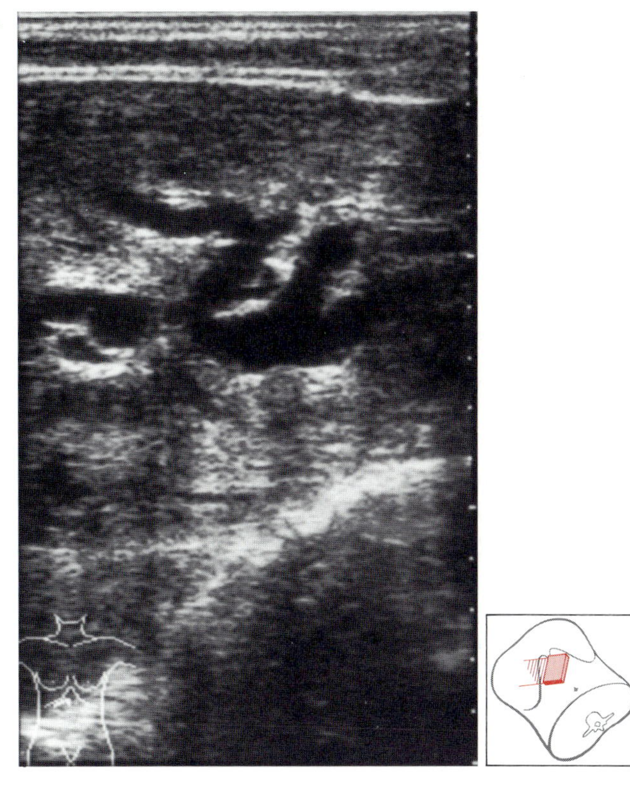

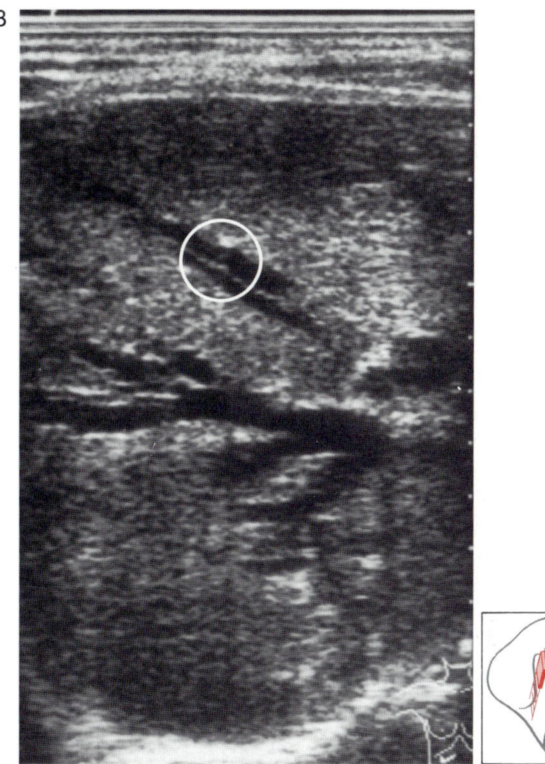

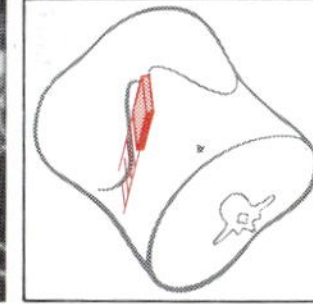

Case 6

Two images from a subcostal exam on the same patient.

1. What are the anechoic structures within the liver?
2. What is the name of the finding inside the *white circle?*
3. In general, what difference is there in the shape of dilated hepatic veins versus biliary dilatation?

Case 5 (See p. 65)

1. Approximately two-thirds of the tumor is outside the liver, but, since there is no solid organ in the region (for example, right kidney) from which it could be arising, this tumor is thought to be hepatic in origin. A mass causing compression of the liver would have clearer borders between it and the liver.
2. Most of the tumor has a cystic pattern, but a solid portion is seen near the interface with the normal liver (*arrows*).
3. A metastatic tumor characterized by a tendency toward degeneration and necrosis. This was a metastasis from ovarian carcinoma.

This tumor mimics a hepatic cyst, but a cyst should not have a solid portion within the wall. It is also unusual for a liver cyst to protrude to this extent beyond the liver contour.

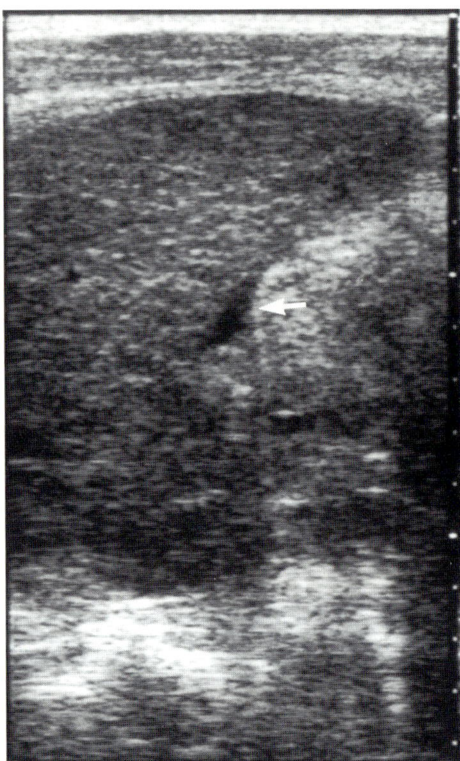
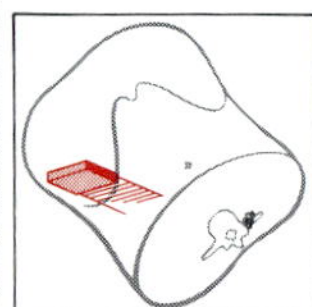

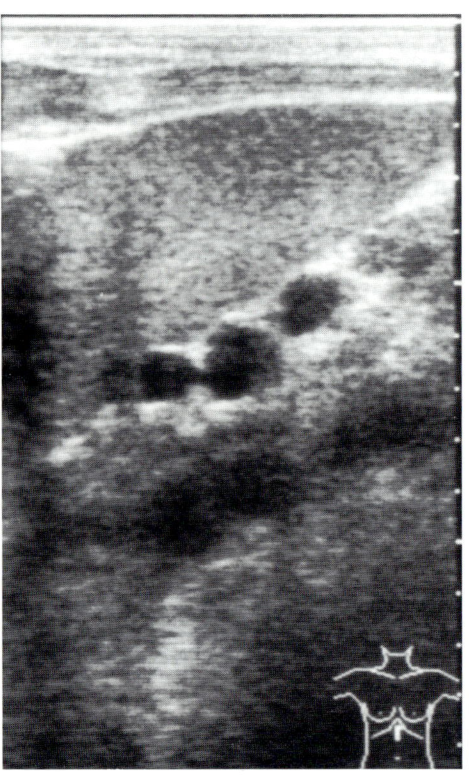
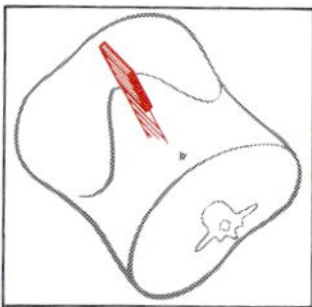

Case 7

1. How would you describe the echo texture of the liver?
2. What does the *arrow* point to?
3. What is your diagnosis?

Case 8

1. What do the three rounded masses posterior to the liver represent?
2. What is the cause of this finding?
3. A similar finding could be seen in a different site for the same reason. What would that finding be?

Case 9 (See p. 86)

1. Within the liver, there are three hyperechoic areas, each measuring 15 mm, which are surrounded by dilated tubular structures.
2. Stones in the intrahepatic biliary ducts.
3. Biliary emphysema and intrahepatic calcifications.

While stones within the gallbladder can be clearly visualized, stones within the intrahepatic biliary duct are often poorly visualized. Usually, the echoes are not very strong and are associated with weak acoustic shadowing. When there is a strong, clear echo within the liver parenchyma, it most likely represents biliary emphysema or an intrahepatic calcification.

Case 10 (See p. 88)

1. There are multiple hyperechoic areas measuring 3–10 mm within the liver.
2. Biliary emphysema.
3. Sphincterotomy of the papilla of Vater, biliary bypass surgery, or a fistula between the gallbladder and the duodenum or colon.

Compared to the stones within the intrahepatic bile ducts in case 9, the echoes are much stronger in this case. However, the acoustic shadowing is not as clear because the individual echoes are not as large since there is no biliary dilatation in this case.

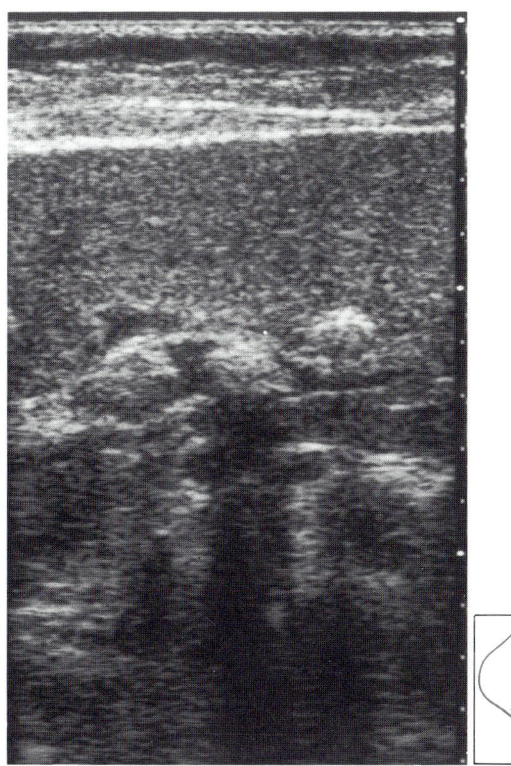
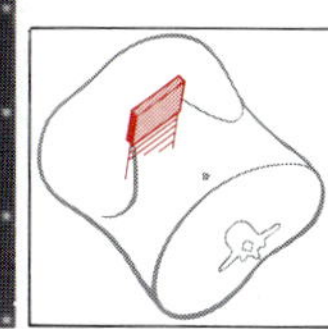

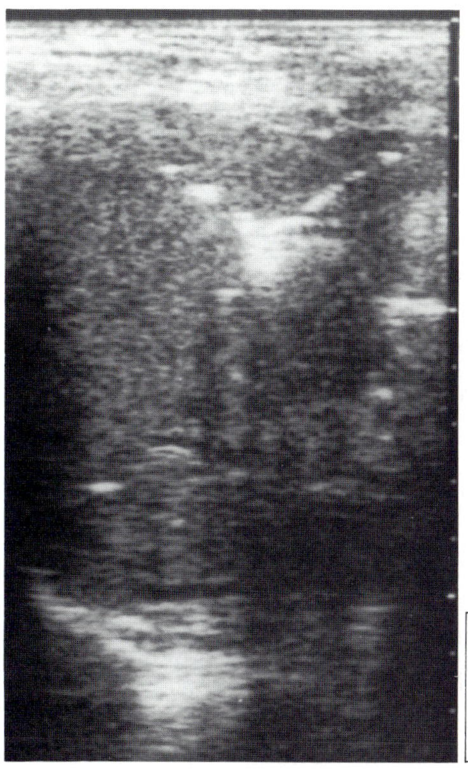
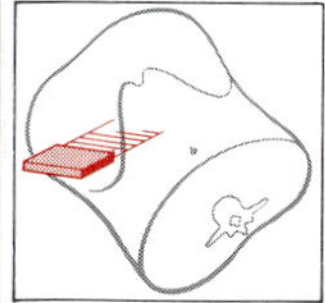

Case 9

1. What are the abnormal findings?
2. What is your diagnosis?
3. What other diseases have similar findings in the liver?

Case 10

1. What are the abnormal findings?
2. What is your diagnosis?
3. What are some causes of this entity?

Case 7 (See p. 83)

1. Coarse.
2. A-small amount of ascites.
2. Cirrhosis of the liver.

In order to recognize that the internal echo texture of the liver is coarse, comparison with the echo texture of the spleen is helpful. An obviously coarse echo pattern, as in this case, needs no comparison with the spleen.

Case 8 (See p. 80)

1. A dilated left gastric vein.
2. Portal hypertension.
3. Dilatation of the paraumbilical vein.

A dilated left gastric vein, as in this case, represents one of the routes of collateral circulation seen in portal hypertension. On the static image, this may simulate multiple enlarged lymph nodes. In a patient with portal hypertension, dilatation of the paraumbilical vein can have a similar appearance on the ultrasonographic examination.

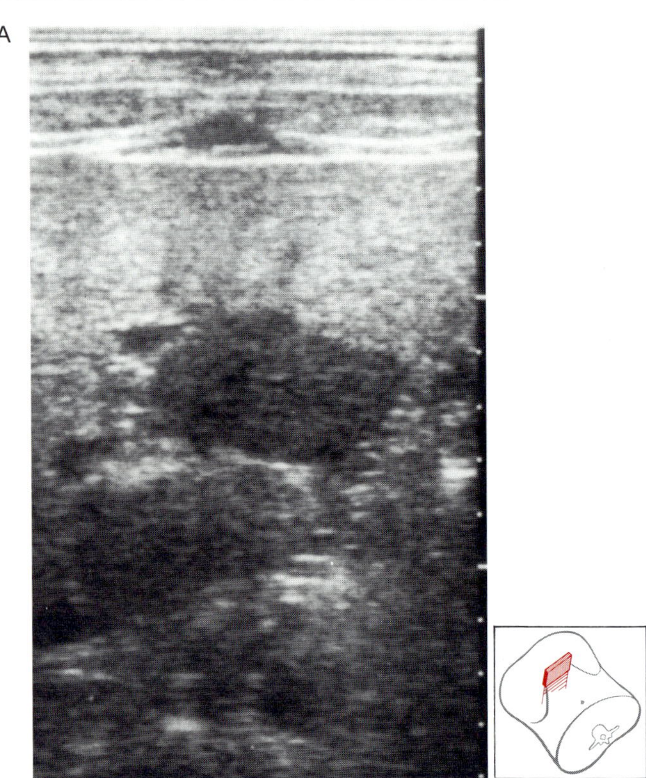

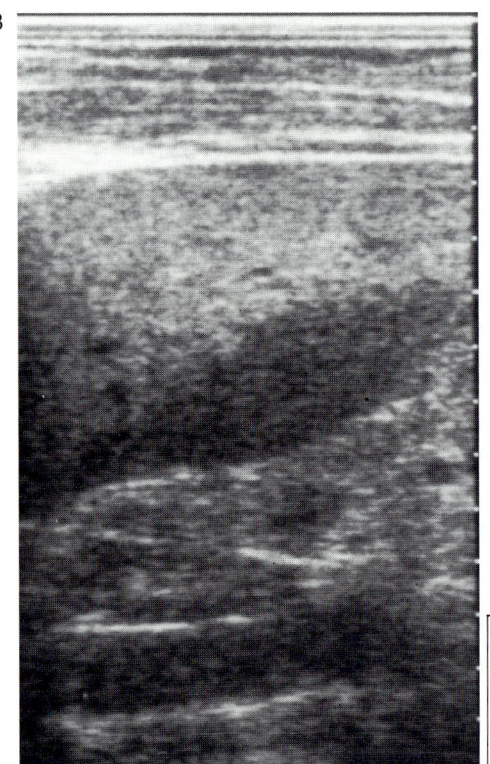

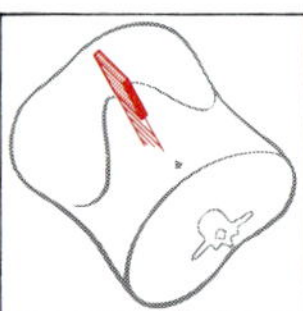

Case 11

Transverse section (**A**) and longitudinal section (**B**) of the left lobe of the liver.

1. Assuming the gain is properly set, is the overall echo-genicity of the liver normal?
2. Is there any area that has a tumor-like appearance?
3. What is your diagnosis?

Case 12 (See p. 110)

1. Yes, there is a 6-cm solid tumor on the inferior surface of the liver. The internal echo pattern is heterogeneous, and the borders of this mass are indistinct.
2. There is a hyperechoic area with associated posterior acoustic shadowing indicating a gallstone within the tumor. This is a gallbladder carcinoma containing gall-stones.

When there is a solid tumor on the undersurface of the right lobe of the liver, differentiating between hepatocellular carcinoma and gallbladder carcinoma may be difficult. When the gallbladder is not visualized, this is more likely to be gallbladder carcinoma, except in the case where the gall-bladder is shrunken secondary to gallstones. It is very rare for hepatocellular carcinoma or metastatic tumor to the liver to invade the gallbladder and causing nonvisualization of the gallbladder on the ultrasonographic images.

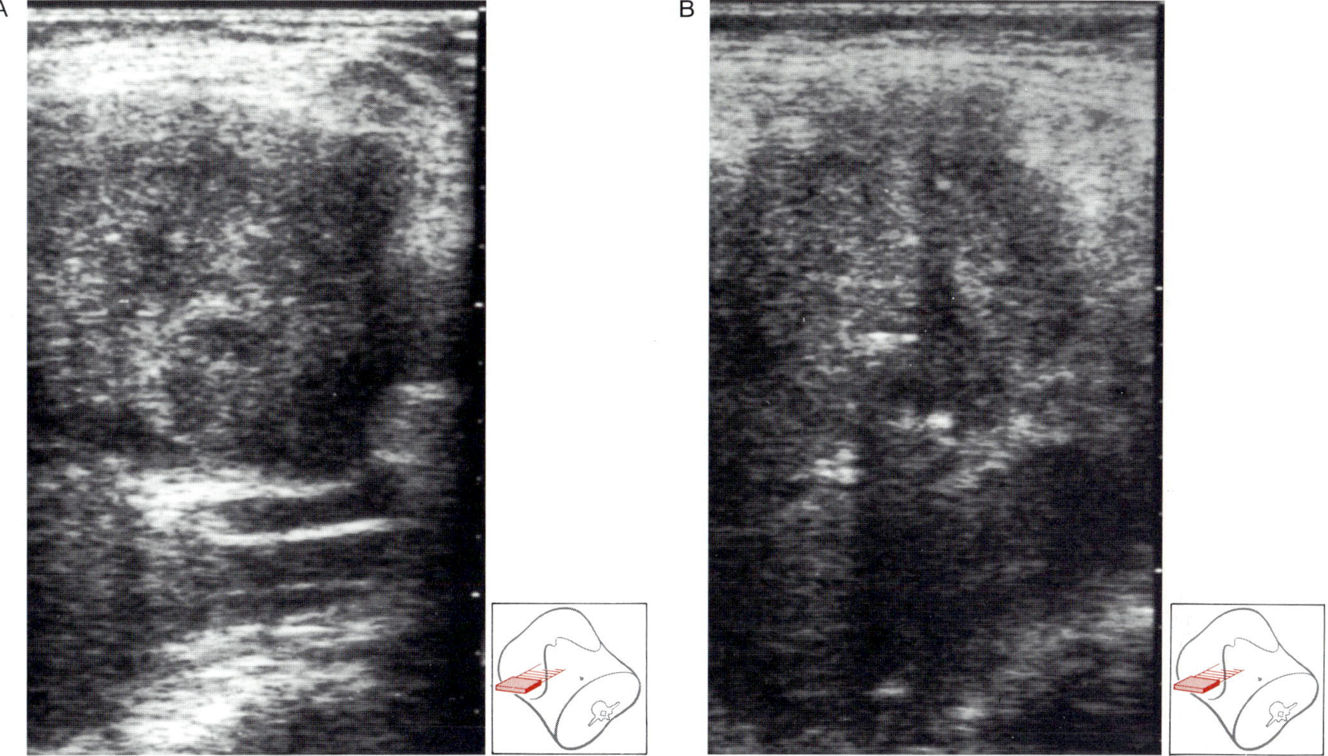

Case 12

Two intercostal images on the same patient. These were obtained in order to visualize the gallbladder.

1. Is there any tumor-like abnormality on these images?
2. There are findings suggesting the origin of the tumor in **B**. What are these?

Case 11 (See p. 84)

1. No, it is increased.
2. There is a hypoechoic, tumor-like area in the posterior portion of the lateral segment of the left lobe of the liver.
3. The tumor-like area represents residual normal liver parenchyma in a fatty liver simulating a hypoechoic mass. This is referred to as a fat-spared area. This pattern of involvement is referred to as focal fatty infiltration of the liver.

It is not rare to find focal fatty infiltration of the liver, as in this case. The fat-spared area is often seen around the gallbladder or anterior to the transverse portion of the left branch of the portal vein. A mildly fatty liver may be recognized on the basis of nonuniform fatty deposition.

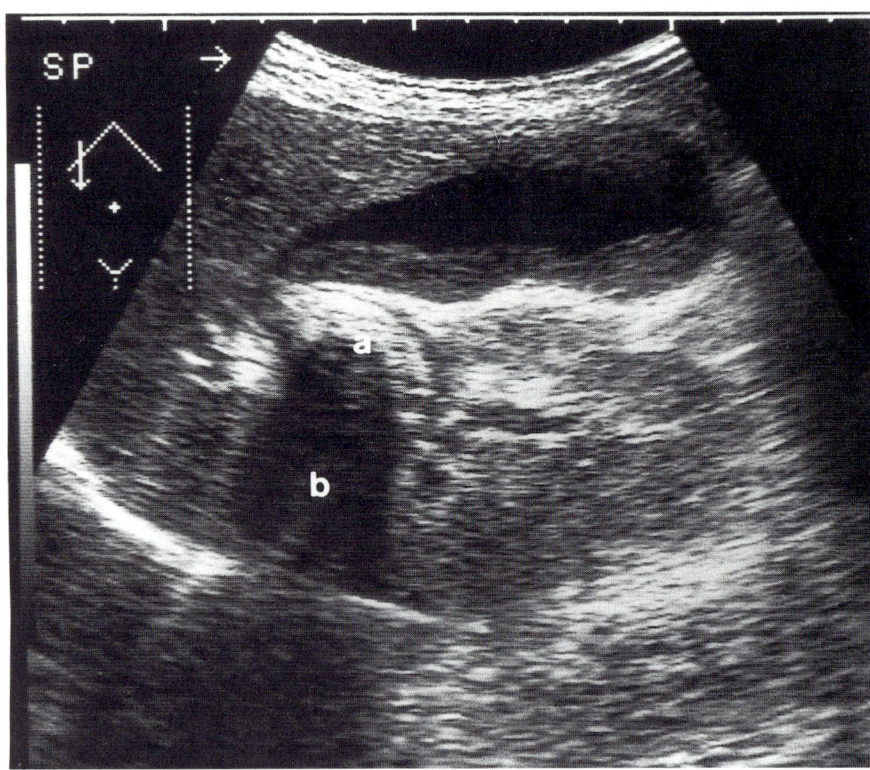

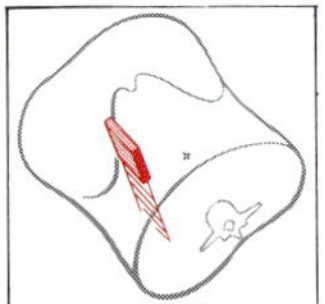

Case 13

1. What is in the lumen of the gallbladder?
2. Is the gallbladder wall thickened?
3. Are there any gallstones?

Case 14 (See p. 108)

1. No, there is thickening of the wall, and the central layer appears anechoic (the wall has a three-layer appearance). These findings indicate severe inflammation.
2. There is a 12-mm crescent-shaped hyperechoic area at the neck of the gallbladder. There is also evidence of weak echoes, suggesting bile sludge.

This is a typical appearance of acute cholecystitis secondary to gallstones. Other lesions which cause thickening of the gallbladder wall include cirrhosis of the liver, adenomyomatosis of the gallbladder, acute hepatitis, and carcinoma of the gallbladder. Among these, only acute cholecystitis and some cases of cirrhosis of the liver cause a three-layer pattern in the gallbladder wall.

Case 15

1. The wall is slightly thickened.
2. The lumen is small.
3. The stomach, filled with food (*a*), is visualized adjacent to the gallbladder.

Usually, ultrasonographic examination of the gallbladder is performed in a fasting patient. In a patient who has not been fasting, the gallbladder will be contracted with a slightly thickened wall. The thickened wall will appear homogeneous. Food within the stomach is often identified, confirming that the patient has not been fasting.

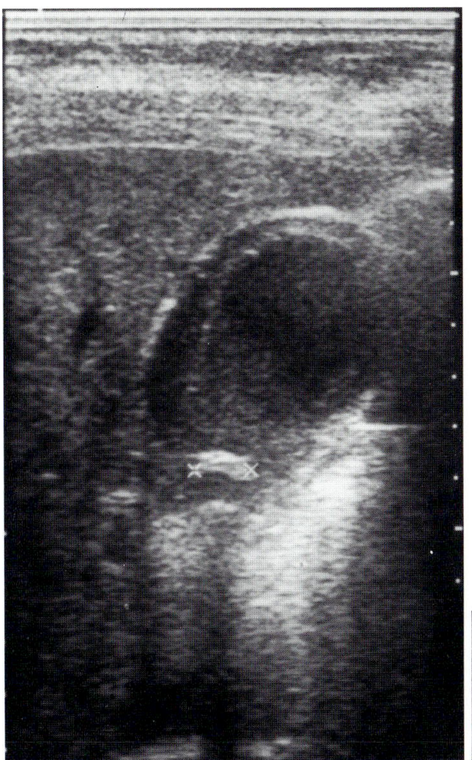

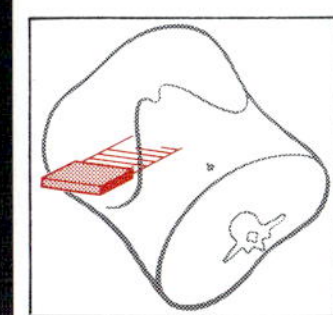

Case 14

1. Is the wall of the gallbladder normal?
2. Are there any abnormalities within the gallbladder?

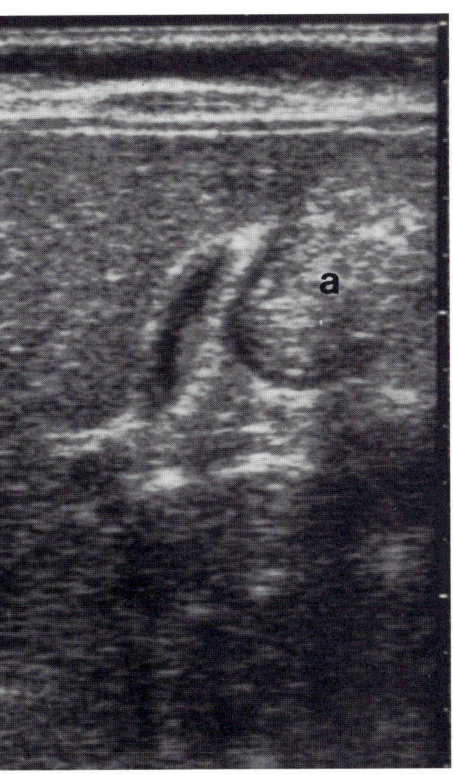

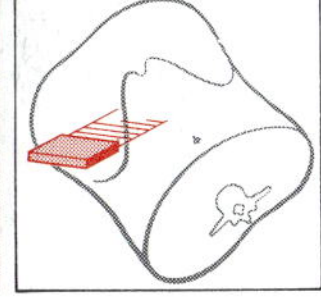

Case 15

1. Is the wall of the gallbladder thickened?
2. What is the size of the lumen of the gallbladder?
3. What is the cause of these findings?

Case 13 (See p. 105)

1. There is a collection of finely echogenic material with a fluid-fluid level suggesting bile sludge.
2. There is no wall thickening.
3. There is gallstone. There is a large incacerated gallstone at the neck (*a*). However, this is difficult to identify because of the normal curving course of the gallbladder neck. This abnormal echo appears to be outside the gallbladder. This is associated with distinct acoustic shadowing (*b*).

When the gallbladder is folded on itself and is separated into several segments or chambers, it can be difficult to identify gallstones. This is especially true when one of these gallbladder segments is filled with multiple stones. Gallstones within a separate segment in the region of the gallbladder fundus may be overlooked because of overlapping intestinal gas or because of reverberation artifacts from the abdominal wall.

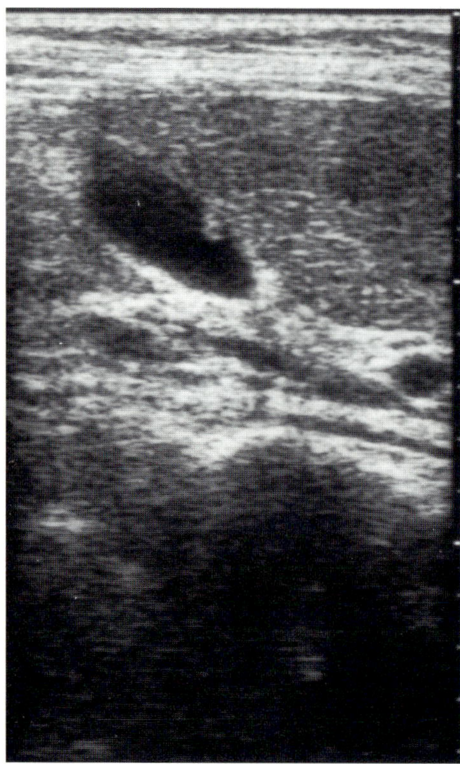
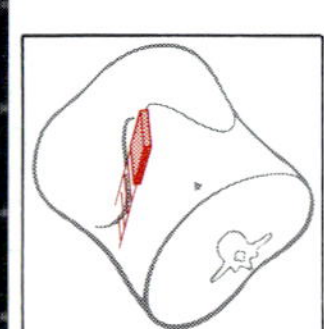
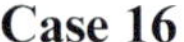

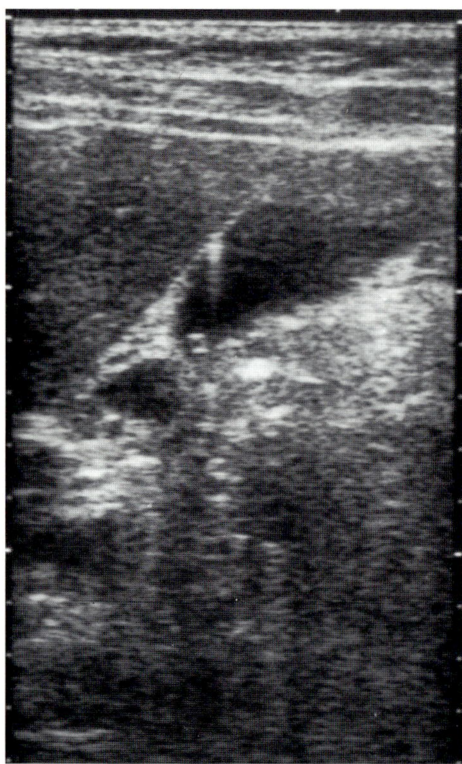
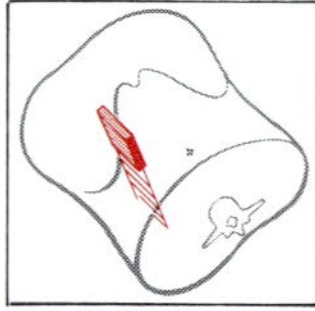

Case 16

1. What is the abnormal finding?
2. What is your differential diagnosis?
3. What is the most likely diagnosis in this case?

Case 17

1. What is the abnormal finding?
2. What is this called?
3. What entities can cause this finding?

Case 18 (See p. 102)

1. No, intestinal gas is compressed against the gallbladder.
2. The shadow, in this case, is a dirty shadow caused by intestinal gas. A gallstone of this size would have much cleaner acoustic shadowing.

Without careful observation, this patient would have been diagnosed as having cholelithiasis. During the examination, gallstones can be easily excluded because of absence of movement with changes in the patient's position. On this static image alone, there is enough evidence to exclude gallstones; that is, the width of the apparent gallstone is different from that of the acoustic shadowing. Acoustic shadowing from an actual gallstone should be the same width as the stone.

Case 19 (See p. 113)

1. Gallbladder carcinoma, bile sludge.
2. It should be observed whether the abnormal echo collection moves when the patient's position is changed. In this case, it did move, showing that what appears to be tumor is actually inspissated bile sludge.

This patient had a previous erroneous diagnosis of tumor of the gallbladder. Apparently, the previously detected abnormality was somewhat rounded and resembled a solid tumor. This is not a very common type of sludge, but statistically these findings more likely represent bile sludge than cancer of the gallbladder.

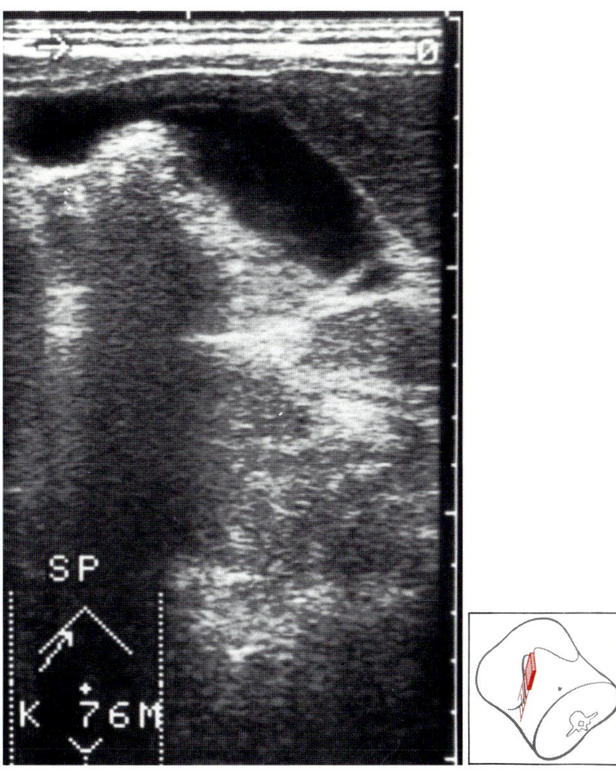

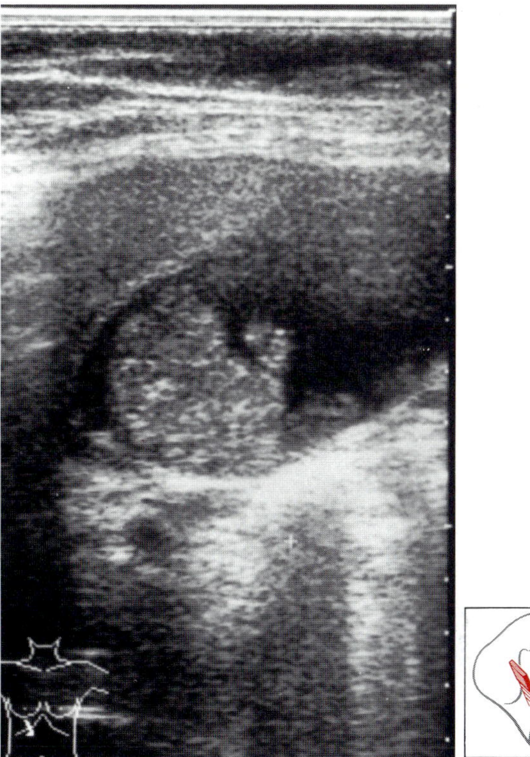

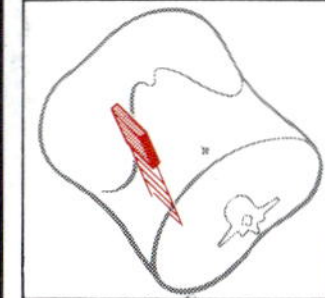

Case 18

Subcostal scan of the gallbladder.
1. Is there a gallstone?
2. What finding is crucial to the answer to question 1?

Case 19

There is an abnormal collection of echoes near the neck of the gallbladder.
1. What is in your differential diagnosis?
2. What maneuver should be performed in this case?

Case 16 (See p. 112)

1. There is an abnormal echogenic focus, measuring 5 mm, on the anterior wall of the gallbladder.
2. Cholesterol polyp, adenoma of the gallbladder, papilloma, or cancer of the gallbladder.
3. Cholesterol polyp.

A small echogenic focus projecting from the wall of the gallbladder, which does not move when the patient's position is changed, is often encountered. It is difficult to differentiate the four different entities described above. It is a general consensus that surgery is recommended when the polypoid area is more than 10 mm in size because of a higher chance of the polyp representing a carcinoma.

Case 17 (See p. 98)

1. There is a hyperechoic area on the anterior wall of the gallbladder associated with a tail which projects into the lumen.
2. Comet-like echo.
3. Intramural stones, small cholesterol polyps.

This comet-like echo represents a reverberation artifact caused by the anterior and posterior wall of a small structure resulting in an interesting pattern on the ultrasonographic image. This phenomenon can also be seen along the posterior wall of the gallbladder, but, because of prominent through-transmission beyond the posterior wall, this finding cannot be easily recognized.

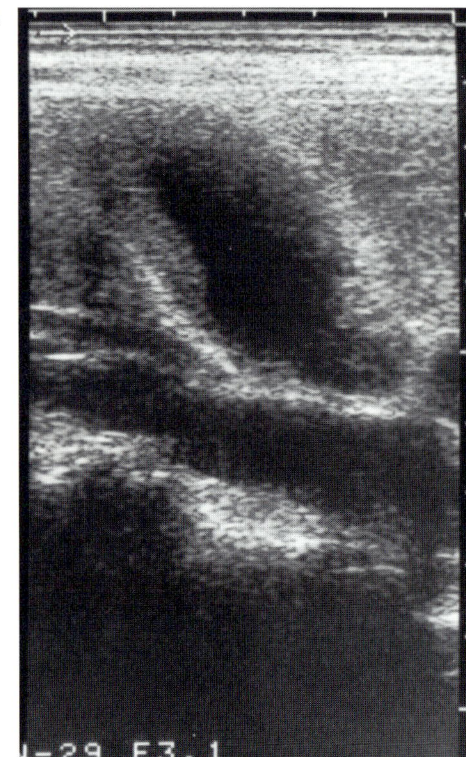
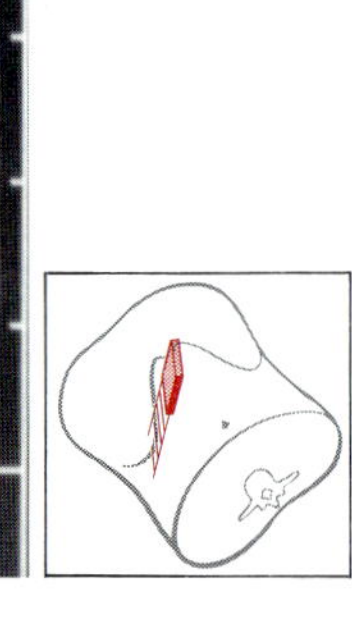
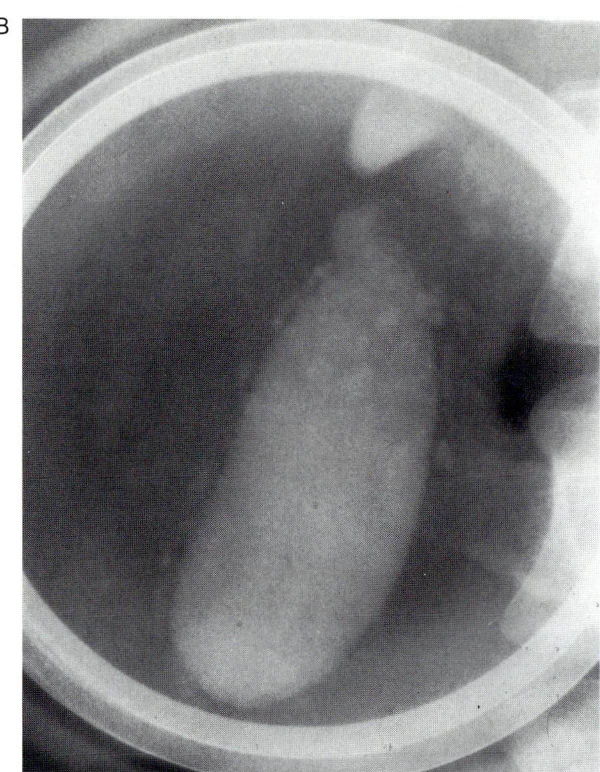

Case 20

A subcostal scan of the gallbladder (**A**) and a film of an oral cholecystogram with compression (**B**).
1. What is the state of the gallbladder wall?
2. Are there any abnormal echoes within the lumen of the gallbladder?
3. What is the differential diagnosis based only on the ultrasonographic image?
4. What is your diagnosis?

Case 21

1. On the anterior wall of the gallbladder.
2. Hyperechoic areas with associated acoustic shadowing. This is a dirty shadow instead of a clean shadow, which is seen in association with cholelithiasis.
3. Emphysematous cholecystitis versus air within the lumen of the gallbladder.
4. Air within the lumen of the gallbladder. This air entered the gallbladder at the time of endoscopic retrograde cholangiopancreatographic examination. This air is thought to be within the lumen of the gallbladder because it is located only anteriorly. This moved when the patient's position was changed.

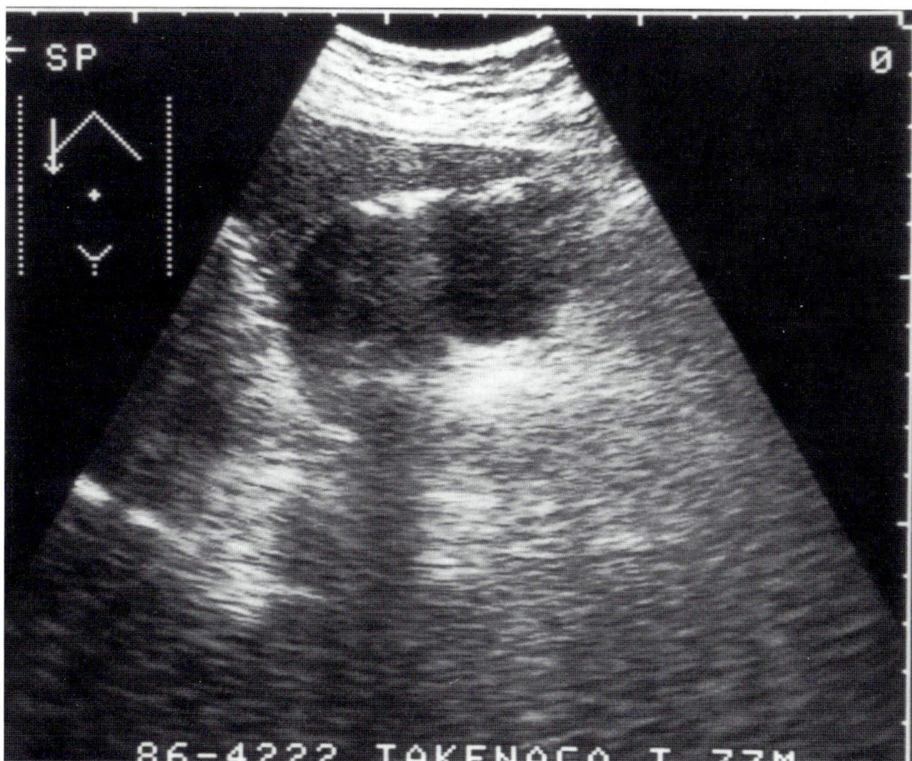
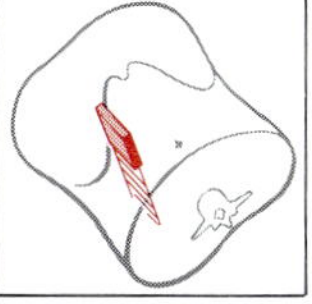

Case 21

1. Where is the abnormal finding?
2. What is the abnormality?
3. What is your differential diagnosis?
4. What is your diagnosis?

Case 20 (See p. 114)

1. The wall of the gallbladder is thickened.
2. There are no abnormal echoes within the lumen of the gallbladder.
3. Cholecystitis, cancer of the gallbladder, cirrhosis of the liver, acute hepatitis, and adenomyomatosis of the gallbladder.
4. This is a generalized type of adenomyomatosis of the gallbladder. On the cholecystogram, contrast is seen in the Rokitansky-Aschoff sinuses within the thickened gallbladder wall.

Note that the fundal type is the most common form of adenomyomatosis. The fundal type has a characteristic shape and it can be diagnosed on the ultrasonographic examination alone. However, differentiation of the generalized type from other disease entities causing thickening of the gallbladder wall is difficult. The Rokitansky-Aschoff sinus is only rarely visualized on the ultrasonographic examination.

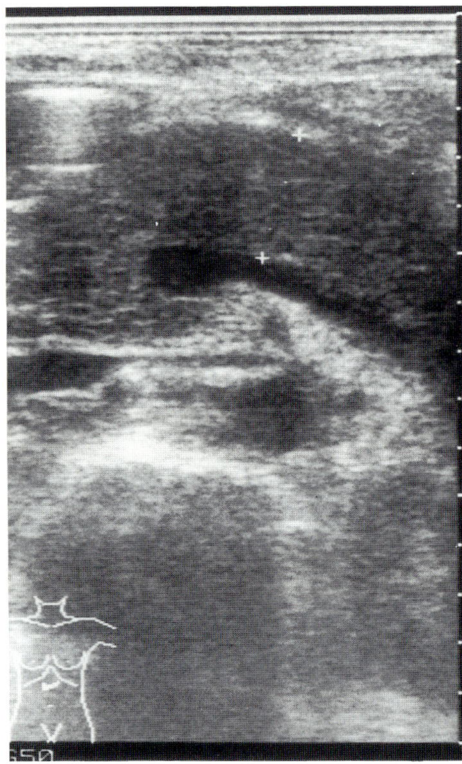

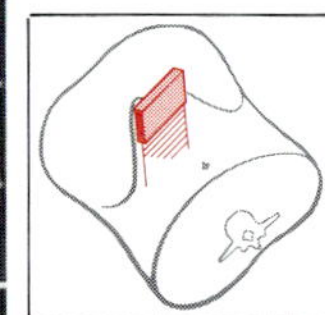

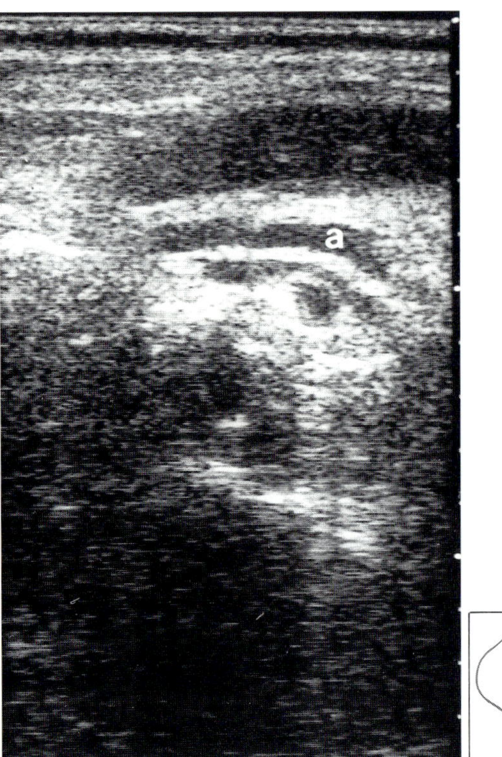

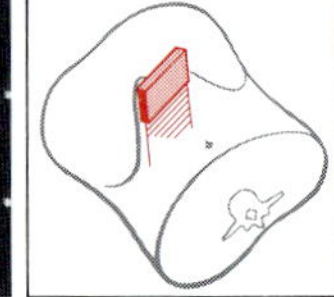

Case 22

1. What is the thickness of the body of the pancreas?
2. What is your diagnosis?

Case 23

1. What is the abnormal finding in the pancreas?
2. What are the differential diagnostic considerations?

Case 24 (See p. 136, 138, 139)

1. The main pancreatic duct (*a*) is dilated, measuring 5 mm.
2. The pancreatic calcifications are visualized as hyperechoic areas in image **B**.
3. Image **B** demonstrates a 16 × 16-mm pseudocyst (*b*) in the pancreatic head.
4. Chronic pancreatitis.

Pancreatic calcifications are the only findings on the ultrasonographic examination which are specific for chronic pancreatitis. Pancreatic pseudocysts can be secondary to trauma. Dilatation of the main pancreatic duct can also be secondary to obstruction of the duct due to a mass in the head of the pancreas (for example, cancer of the pancreatic head).

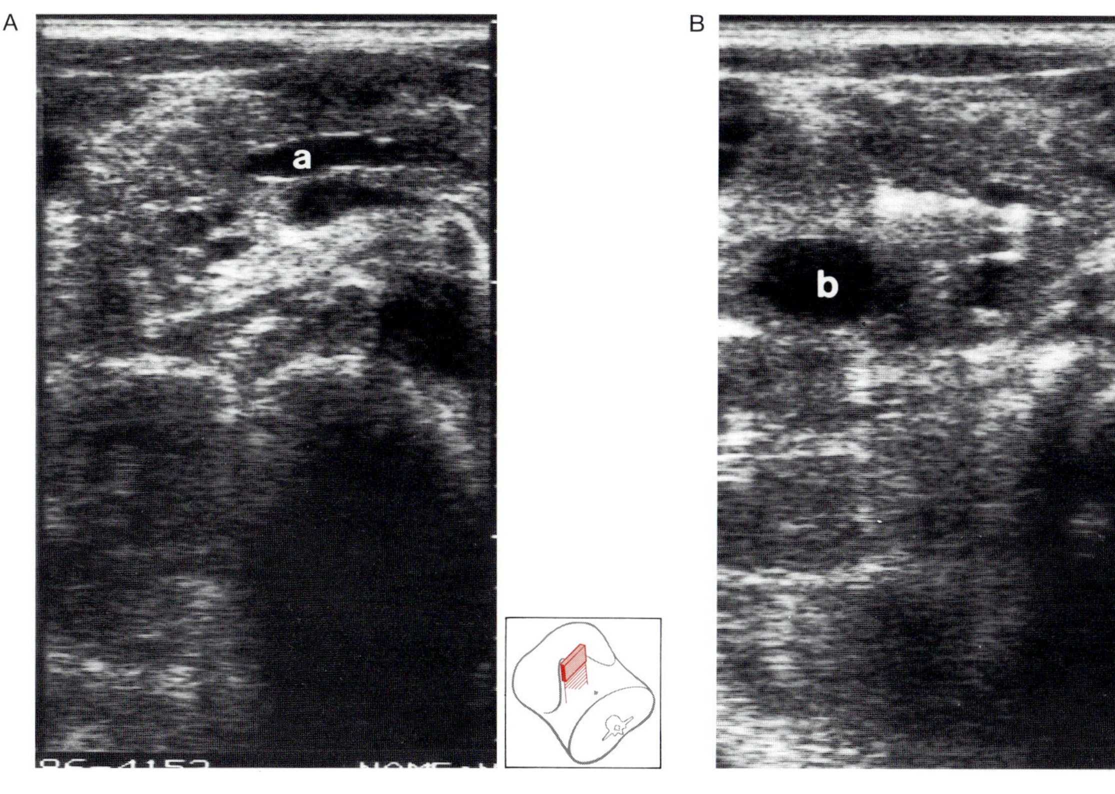

Case 24

Two transverse sections of the pancreas on the same patient.

1. In what way is the main pancreatic duct abnormal?
2. Are there pancreatic calcifications?
3. Are there any other abnormalities?
4. What is your diagnosis?

Case 22 (See p. 134)

1. It is thickened and measures 27 mm.
2. Acute pancreatitis. The differential diagnosis of increased thickness of the pancreas also includes chronic pancreatitis and pancreatic carcinoma.

Acute pancreatitis with significant enlargement of the pancreas (football size) has been described in the literature; however, from my experience with cases in Japan, acute pancreatitis is often associated with mild enlargement, as in this case. On CT, the inflammatory changes in the surrounding tissues secondary to leakage of pancreatic fluid can be clearly visualized. CT is superior to ultrasonography in evaluating cases of acute pancreatitis.

Case 23 (See p. 136)

1. The main pancreatic duct (*a*) is dilated. The pancreatic parenchyma appears hyperechoic relative to normal, but this is of no clinical significance.
2. Chronic pancreatitis, cancer of the head of the pancreas, and cancer of the duodenal papilla.

An increased echo level of the pancreatic parenchyma is relatively frequent in older or obese patients. In both instances, this increased echo level is secondary to fatty deposition in the pancreatic tissue. This finding has no clinical significance. In this case, the dilatation of the main pancreatic duct is smooth, a nonspecific finding.

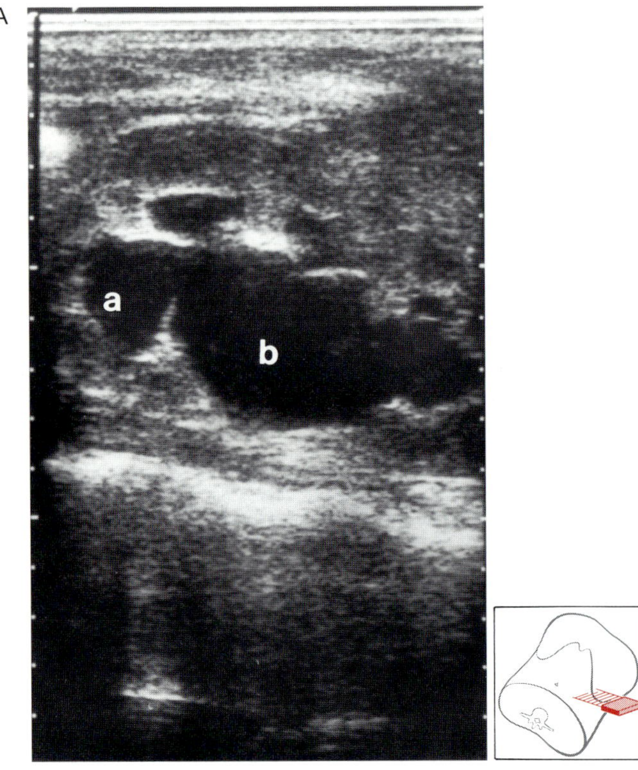

Case 25

Two ultrasonographic images of the left kidney in different patients.

1. Is the central echo complex normal?
2. What are the possible diagnoses for the case shown in **B**?
3. What single diagnosis applies to both images?

Case 26 (See p. 162)

1. Upper pole of the right kidney.
2. Diffusely increased.
3. There is no acoustic shadowing.
4. Renal hamartoma or angiomyolipoma.

Renal hamartoma (angiomyolipoma) is frequently found incidentally. Most are approximately 3 cm in size. On CT examination, fatty tissue in these tumors has a CT number below zero, and they are therefore easily recognized.

Case 27 (See p. 157)

1. In the central portion of the left renal sinus.
2. There is a hyperechoic area measuring 8 mm in dimension, accompanied by clear acoustic shadowing.
3. Nephrolithiasis.

Small gallstones measuring 2–3 mm can easily be detected, whereas a renal stone must be as large as 1 cm in dimension to be accurately diagnosed on ultrasonography. This is because the renal central echo complex is filled with strong echoes, and small stones cannot be differentiated from these. Acoustic shadowing must be present to definitely diagnose renal stones.

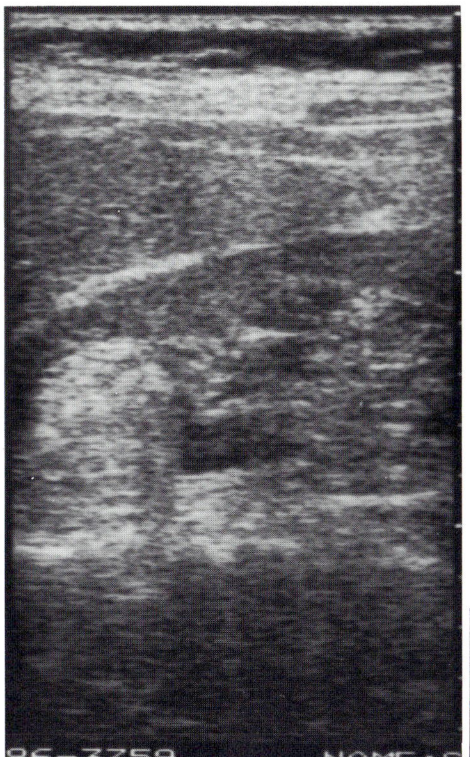

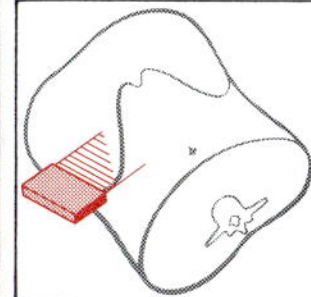

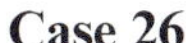

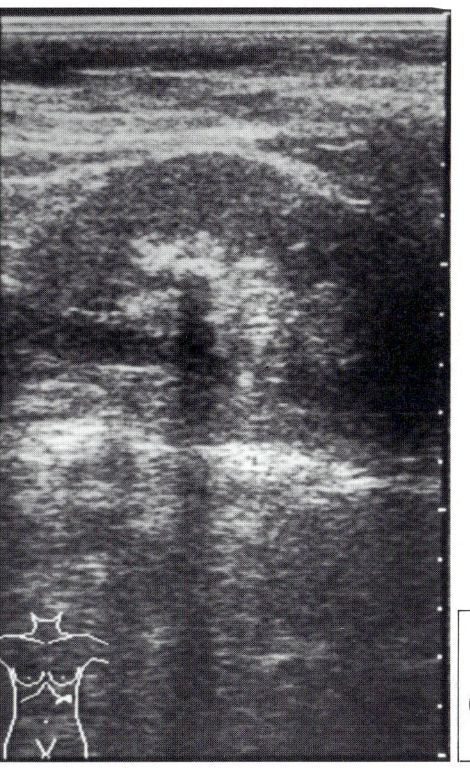

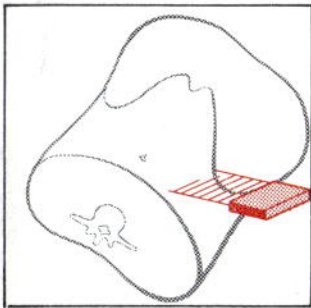

Case 26

1. What is the location of the renal tumor?
2. What is the echo level of the renal tumor?
3. Is there any acoustic shadowing?
4. What is your diagnosis?

Case 27

1. Where is the abnormality?
2. What is the abnormality?
3. What is your diagnosis?

Case 25 (See p. 156)

1. No, there is no central echo complex (see p. 151).
2. Multiple renal cysts, hydronephrosis.
3. Hydronephrosis. In image **A**, the anechoic structures communicate. Images of multiple renal cysts are not as complicated as this. The *a* marks dilated renal calyces, and *b* indicates the dilated renal pelvis.

These two cases demonstrate typical ultrasonographic findings of hydronephrosis. As hydronephrosis advances, the parenchymal echoes are lost, and ultrasonographically the kidney has the appearance of a multicystic tumor. A more specific diagnosis cannot be made. On the other hand, differentiation between very mild hydronephrosis and physiologic dilatation of the renal collecting system (due to a filled urinary bladder or overhydration) or a prominent vein can be quite difficult.

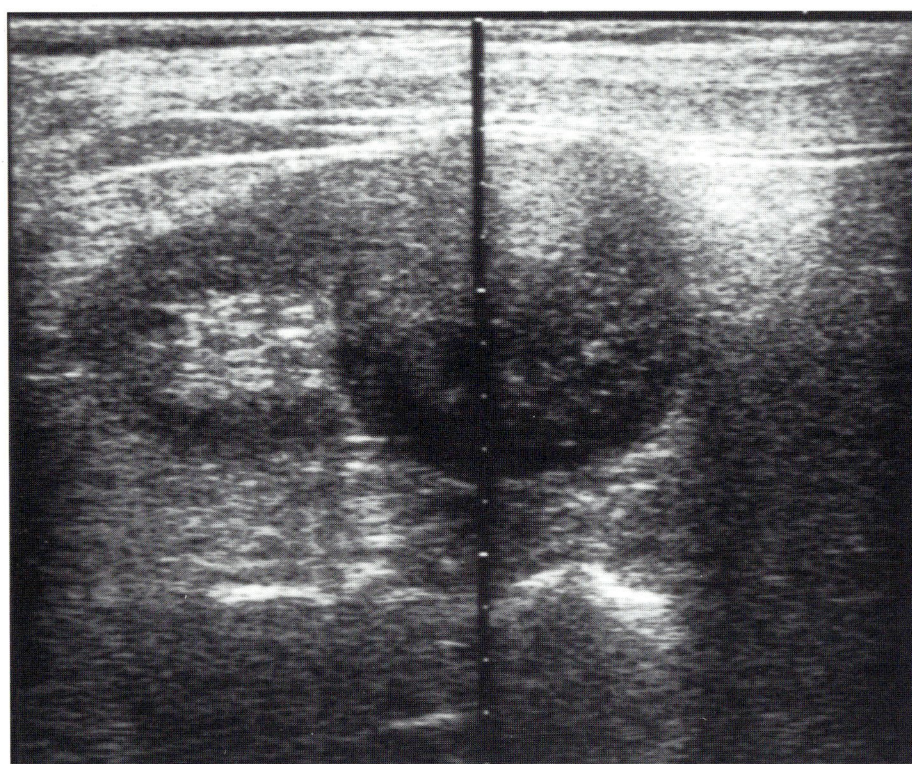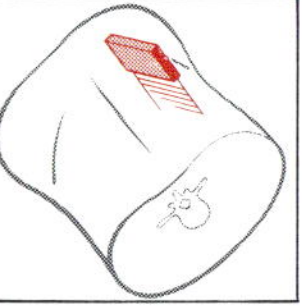

Case 28

1. What is the location of this tumor?
2. What is the size of this tumor?
3. What is the internal echo pattern of this tumor?
4. What is your diagnosis?

Case 29 (See p. 186)

1. There is no mass in the liver.
2. The abnormality is in the stomach.
3. The wall of the stomach is markedly thickened in a diffuse manner with a linear strong echo in the central portion. This is referred to as a pseudokidney sign.
4. Advanced gastric carcinoma.

Ultrasonography cannot be used as a screening examination to rule out disease of the gastrointestinal tract as it is not sensitive for these lesions. However, advanced disease, especially mass-forming lesions, can be visualized on an ultrasonographic examination. It is not unusual for a cancer of the gastrointestinal tract to be discovered on an ultrasonographic examination.

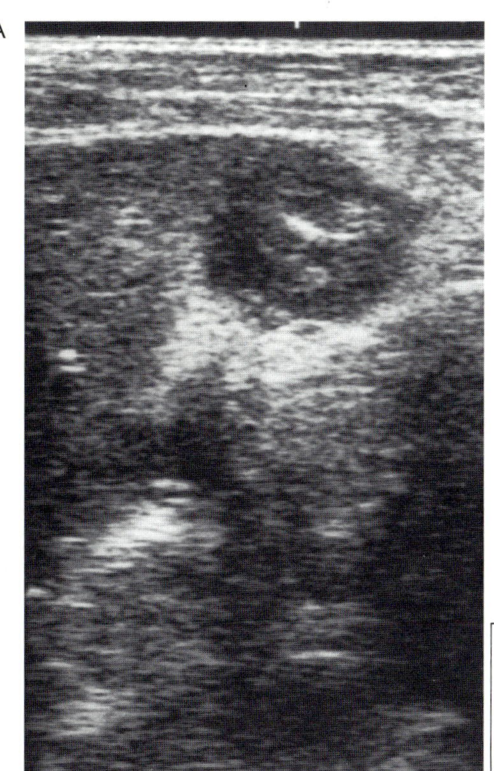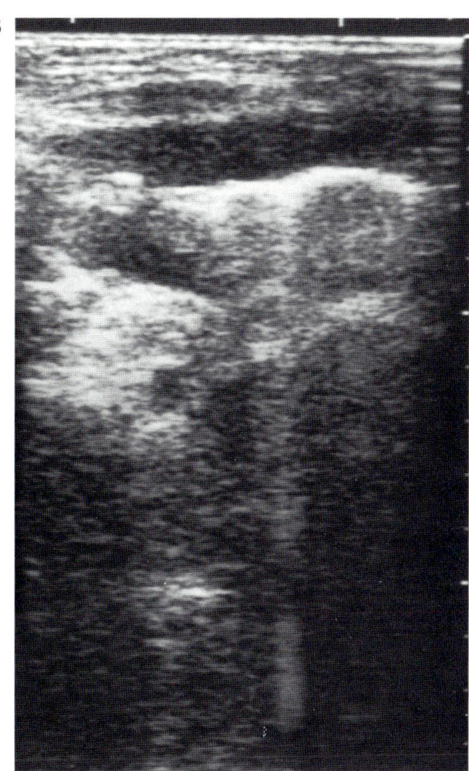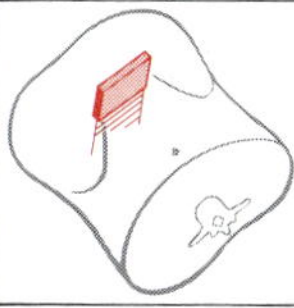

Case 29

1. Is there a tumor in the liver on the image in **A**?
2. Where is the lesion?
3. What are the findings?
4. What is your diagnosis?

Case 28 (See p. 158)

1. Lower pole of the right kidney.
2. Maximal dimension of 65 mm.
3. The overall echo level is similar to that of the renal parenchyma, although there are hypoechoic areas within it.
4. Renal cell carcinoma.

In Japan, renal cell carcinoma is much less frequent than hepatocellular carcinoma. The postoperative prognosis is much better for renal cell carcinoma compared to hepatocellular carcinoma. If a renal cell carcinoma is detected before it become symptomatic, there is a high likelihood of surgical cure. During examination of the upper abdomen, it is important to visualize not only the liver and the gallbladder, but also the kidneys.